Neonatal Brain Injury

Gerda Meijler • Khorshid Mohammad
Editors

Neonatal Brain Injury

An Illustrated Guide for Clinicians Counselling Parents and Caregivers

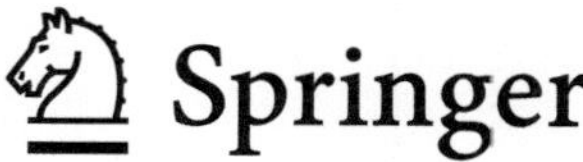

Editors
Gerda Meijler
Department of Neonatology
Isala Women and Children's Hospital
Zwolle, The Netherlands

Khorshid Mohammad
Section of Newborn Critical Care
Department of Pediatrics
Alberta Children's Hospital
and University of Calgary
Calgary, AB, Canada

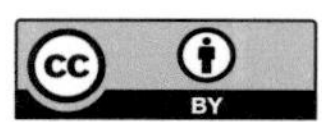

ISBN 978-3-031-55974-7   ISBN 978-3-031-55972-3   (eBook)
https://doi.org/10.1007/978-3-031-55972-3

This Springer imprint is published by the registered company Springer Nature Switzerland AG
The registered company address is: Gewerbestrasse 11, 6330 Cham, Switzerland

If disposing of this product, please recycle the paper.

Foreword

As Henrik Ibsen said in 1906 *A picture is worth a thousand words,* and this has been taken literally by the skilled illustrations and representations presented in this highly valuable illustrated guide to neonatal brain injury. The experienced editors Drs. Meijler and Mohammad have been assisted by many other leaders in the field of neonatal neurology, including Drs. Cowan, de Vries, Steggerda, Leijser, Martinez-Biarge, and El-Dib. Beautiful illustrations have been created under their guidance by Amanda Gautier. An understanding of the neonatal brain can be challenging for many—from neonatologists and caregivers in the neonatal intensive care unit, community pediatric providers and therapists, and most importantly, the families of the infants who are affected. This illustrated guide is a powerful companion to any clinician and caregiver to provide insights pictorially. It provides images that can be easily translated to the common representation of brain imaging, such as the images acquired with a cranial ultrasound. This allows valuable insights to apply imaging for an individual infant, providing additional confidence and assistance in counseling a family related to findings such as intraventricular hemorrhage. This atlas provides representation of the patterns of the common forms of brain injury in the newborn, clearly depicting where and what is influenced in the newborn brain. The guide also portrays common diagnostic and management approaches, such as lumbar puncture studies and drainage of cerebrospinal fluid by temporizing devices. At a stressful time for many families with a small or sick infant, the capability to have greater insights and understanding that this atlas provides is invaluable. As a clinician guiding colleagues and counseling families, I cannot count the thousands of times that I have drawn illustrations on paper and whiteboards. This atlas will now take the place of my amateur illustrations with skilled accurate artistic renderings that will be used again and again. This is a must-have book in the armamentarium of any clinician caring for the high-risk newborn infant, and its pictures are truly worth thousands of words.

Center for Neonatal Research,   Terrie Eleanor Inder
Children's Hospital of Orange
County, Orange, CA, USA

University of California Irvine,
Irvine, CA, USA

Acknowledgements

The publication of this open-access book was made possible through financial resources generated from cranial ultrasound courses conducted at the Hammersmith Hospital, Imperial College, London, UK, under the auspices of the Genesis Research Trust. The authors are the main contributors to these courses.

The authors are grateful to CardioNova Foundation, Amsterdam, the Netherlands, for funding the illustrations in this book. These were drawn by Amanda Gautier-Ronopawiro, Drachten, the Netherlands (gautierillustration.com).

Contents

Contributors

Frances M. Cowan Department of Paediatrics, Imperial College London, London, UK

Mohamed El-Dib Neonatal Neurocritical Care, Department of Pediatrics, Division of Newborn Medicine, Brigham and Women's Hospital, Boston, MA, USA

Department of Pediatrics, Harvard Medical School, Boston, MA, USA

Lara M. Leijser Section of Newborn Critical Care, Department of Pediatrics, Cumming School of Medicine, University of Calgary, Calgary, AB, Canada

Miriam Martinez-Biarge Department of Paediatrics, Imperial College Healthcare NHS Trust, London, UK

Gerda Meijler Department of Neonatology, Isala Women and Children's Hospital, Zwolle, The Netherlands

Khorshid Mohammad Section of Newborn Critical Care, Department of Pediatrics, Alberta Children's Hospital and University of Calgary, Calgary, AB, Canada

Sylke J. Steggerda Department of Pediatrics, Division of Neonatology, Willem-Alexander Children's Hospital, Leiden University Medical Center (LUMC), Leiden, The Netherlands

Linda S. de Vries Department of Neonatology, University Medical Center Utrecht (UMCU), Utrecht, The Netherlands

Department Pediatrics, Division Neonatology, Willem Alexander's Children Hospital, Leiden University Medical Center (LUMC), Leiden, The Netherlands

Introduction on Development, Maturation, and Vulnerability of the Neonatal Brain and Factors Contributing to Injury

Gerda Meijler and Khorshid Mohammad

Abbreviations

PLIC	Posterior limb of the internal capsule
pre-Ols	Pre-myelinating oligodendrocytes
WMI	White matter injury

G. Meijler (✉)
Department of Neonatology, Isala Women and Children's Hospital, Zwolle, The Netherlands
e-mail: gmeijler@gmail.com

K. Mohammad
Section of Newborn Critical Care, Department of Pediatrics, Alberta Children's Hospital and University of Calgary, Calgary, AB, Canada
e-mail: mkhorshi@ucalgary.ca; khorshid.mohammad@albertahealthservices.ca

© The Author(s) 2024
G. Meijler, K. Mohammad (eds.), *Neonatal Brain Injury*,
https://doi.org/10.1007/978-3-031-55972-3_1

1.1 For Parents

The brain of the newborn baby is still immature and undergoes essential and rapid growth and development. Important maturational processes include the folding of the brain surface, which enables enlargement of the brain surface without needing too much space; the "wiring" of the nerve cell extensions with insulating material, enabling fast conduction of electrical impulses between nerve cells; the formation of synapses that connect different nerve cells with each other; and the programmed elimination of abundant nerve cells and synapses.

The immaturity of the newborn's brain combined with its rapid development renders the brain of the newborn infant vulnerable to injury and abnormal growth and development. This is especially true for the brains of preterm-born infants. Therefore, problems around and after birth, such as traumatic delivery or oxygen shortage during delivery, or illness during the first weeks after birth may lead to brain injury or abnormal brain development. On the other hand, the abundance of nerve cells and synapses gives the brain "plasticity," meaning that injury does not necessarily result in significant impairment. In addition, the young nervous system is capable of learning and adapting, again meaning that injury does not always lead to functional problems. Thus, early intervention in infants with brain injury may help the infant to develop as normally as possible and to cope with possible impairments. Besides the prevention of brain injury, early detection and diagnosis are therefore of utmost importance.

1.2   For Professionals

Human brain development is a very protracted and highly orchestrated process that starts in the early embryonic phase and proceeds until adulthood (Fig. 1.1) [1].

During the fetal period, brain development is rapid and critical. It comprises neuronal and glial cell proliferation and migration, a massive increase in volume and weight, layering of the cerebral wall, cortical folding, establishment of connectivity, apoptosis and programmed elimination of synapses, and beginning of myelination.

In the case of preterm birth, essential brain growth and maturation need to take place outside of the protective in utero-environment, while the infant is cared for in an incubator in a neonatal (intensive care) unit and undergoes many (sometimes painful and/or stressful) medical and nursing procedures.

The critical brain development during this period explains the vulnerability of the preterm brain. The preterm brain is susceptible to injury from ischemic, hemorrhagic, inflammatory, and infective insults [2].

In this chapter, we provide an overview of the most important developmental processes that take place during the preterm and neonatal period and that largely determine preterm brain injury. We also explain brain maturation disturbance (dysmaturation). Cerebellar development will be described in the chapter on cerebellar injury (See Chap. 4).

1. Neuronal and glial cell proliferation and migration.
2. Increase in volume and weight.
3. Gyration and sulcation.

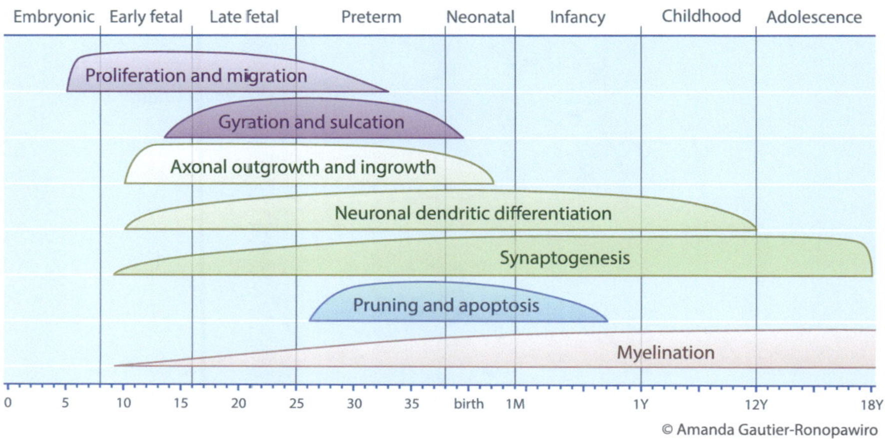

Fig. 1.1 Timeline of important human brain developmental processes from the embryonic phase until adolescence. (© Amanda Gautier-Ronopawiro)

4. Development of connectivity.
5. Apoptosis and programmed elimination of synapses.
6. Myelination.
7. Dysmaturation.

1.2.1 Neuronal and Glial Cell Proliferation and Migration

The bulk of cell proliferation takes place in the germinal matrix (Fig. 1.2): a transient, highly cellular and vascular embryological and fetal structure located in the lateral ventricular wall that gives origin to neural and glial precursor cells.

In the germinal matrix, neuronal precursor cells divide into two identical clones. One of these clones will migrate along a radial glial cell toward the cortex or deep gray matter, and the other clone will further divide and then start its journey along the glial cell.

The cortex is built up by different layers of cells: the "oldest" (first arriving) cells will end up in the most inner layer of the cortex, while newer cells will form a layer on top of this. This process goes on until the cortex consists of six separate cell layers, each containing differentiated neurons, in an inside-out orientation: the first arriving cells forming the most inner layer and the latest arriving cells forming the most outer layer (Fig. 1.3).

Because of its high cellularity and vascularity, combined with poor vascular support, the germinal matrix is one of the most vulnerable brain structures in the very preterm infant. It is abundantly present between 14 and 26 weeks gestation.

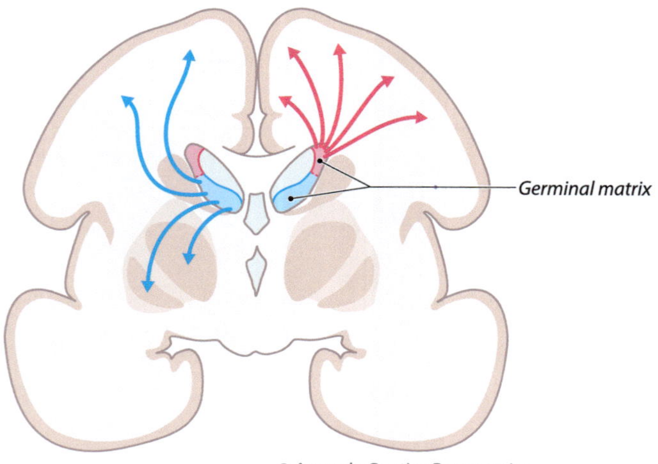

Fig. 1.2 The germinal matrix is a transient highly cellular and vascular structure beneath the ventricular ependyma and is most prominent on the head of the caudate nucleus. In the germinal matrix, neuronal and glial precursor cells proliferate and subsequently migrate toward their final destinations (© Amanda Gautier-Ronopawiro)

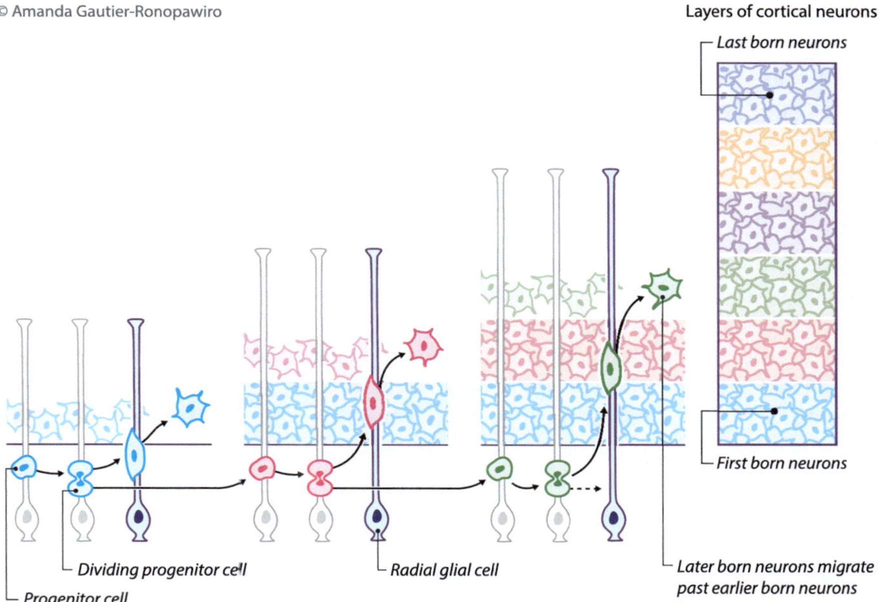

Fig. 1.3 The process of proliferation in and migration from the germinal matrix. The cortical layers are shown: the oldest neurons end in the most inner layer of the cortex, while the newest neurons end in the most superficial cortical layer. (© Amanda Gautier-Ronopawiro)

Afterward, it undergoes regression, and after 34 weeks gestation, only some remnants remain [3, 4].

In preterm neonates the vast majority of intracranial hemorrhages thus arise in the germinal matrix (see Chap. 3).

1.2.2 Increase in Volume and Weight

Due to massive cell proliferation, impressive brain growth takes place during the fetal period: between 26 and 40 weeks gestation, brain weight increases more than twofold and brain volume almost fivefold [5–8]. There is a linear growth pattern of brain structures between 25 and 37 weeks gestation [7], and between 20 and 40 weeks gestation, there is a 90% increase in brain weight [6].

1.2.3 Gyration and Sulcation

In the early fetal period, the brain surface is smooth. The development of the cerebral gyri and sulci is a sequential and orderly process that starts around the 14th week of gestation with the formation of the lateral fissure (or Sylvian fissure). The process of gyration and sulcation is probably driven by several mechanisms, including exponential brain growth within the confinement of the hard skull, and complex mechanical forces in the cortex and the underlying white matter [9, 10]. Gyration enables maximizing the number of cortical neurons and minimizing the total fiber length within the skull [11].

The sulci can be classified into primary sulci (the pericallosal, cingulate, parieto-occipital, hippocampal sulci) and secondary sulci (including the central, precentral and postcentral, intraparietal, frontal, temporal, calcarine, and occipital sulci). The primary and secondary sulci develop in a predictable, fixed sequence and are symmetric in location [12–14].

The primary sulci appear shortly after mid-gestation, followed by the secondary sulci between 25 and 30 weeks gestation. Tertiary sulci are branches of the primary and secondary sulci and are variable in appearance and development [15].

In general, the development of gyri and sulci is most rapid in the area of the central sulcus and the medial occipital area, while the development is slowest in the frontobasal and frontopolar areas and the anterior part of the temporal lobe [16]. There is a lag between the development of the cortical surface at postmortem and detection of gyri and sulci with ultrasound and MRI.

For the normal sequence of gyral and sulcal development, we refer to the previous literature [17, 18].

Several factors such as antenatal brain injury, antenatal infection, and genetic and metabolic disorders may directly affect the processes of proliferation and migration and of gyration and sulcation, resulting in variable neurodevelopmental delay, epilepsy, and motor problems [9, 15, 17, 19].

1.2.4 Development of Connectivity

Before midgestation, there is no direct connection between the cortex and the rest of the central nervous system. With developing connectivity, axons are formed and axonal branches multiply. During the second half of gestation, axons extend branches to numerous cortical and subcortical targets, until each neuron connects with thousands of other neurons [19].

The newborn brain undergoes rapid and massive connectivity modeling and remodeling through two simultaneous, interactive, and complex processes: progressive and regressive. Both are guided by predetermined genetic factors and modifiable epigenetic and environmental factors which allow for brain plasticity and adaptive mechanisms.

The progressive process is mainly due to the generation of new synapses, dendrites, and axons [20, 21], while the regressive process is due to pruning of unused or unnecessary connections [22]. The balance between both processes, and complex interactive relationship makes our neuronal circuits and functional networks: "neurons that fire together wire together" (Donald Hebb, cited from [23].

1.2.5 Apoptosis and Programmed Elimination of Synapses

Neurons and glial cells that fail to participate in a functioning network die through a process called programmed cell death or apoptosis; the cell shrinks, the nucleus condenses and fragments, and there is a lack of inflammatory reaction by the dying cell. Eventually the dead cells get removed by macrophages [24]. This type of programmed cell death is an essential part of brain development during proliferation and migration and should be differentiated from cell death due to injury or aging. Synaptic pruning on the other hand seems to be triggered by signals from the neuronal cell itself, inviting microglia to prune the unused synapses flagged by complements [25, 26].

1.2.6 Myelination

Myelination of the central nervous system starts relatively late, in the third trimester of pregnancy, and proceeds slowly until birth. It accelerates after birth and progresses rapidly during infancy, slower thereafter, and continues into adulthood [27, 28]. Myelination follows a fixed, predictable, and orderly pattern and sequence. The most basic "rules" of myelination are as follows: anatomic brain regions responsible for primitive functions myelinate earlier than anatomic regions responsible for phylogenetically advanced functions; myelination parallels function; tracts myelinate in the direction of impulse conduction; and myelination proceeds from caudal to rostral, posterior to anterior, and central to peripheral. Thus, myelination in the central nervous system starts in the brainstem and then moves to the cerebellum and pons, followed by the deep gray matter and finally the central and peripheral white matter [17, 28–34].

In the central nervous system, myelin is produced by a certain type of glial cells, the oligodendrocyte. Oligodendrocytes wrap a myelin sheath in tight spirals around the axons (Fig. 1.4).

The axons carry electrical signals from one nerve cell to another. Myelinated axons enable rapid action potential transmission and thereby support brain

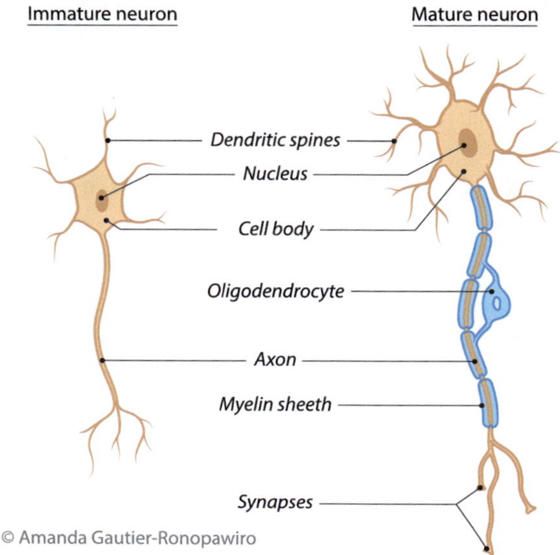

Fig. 1.4 Immature and mature neurons in the central nervous system: the immature neuron is unmyelinated and not yet connected to other neurons. The axon of the mature neuron is covered with myelin (produced by mature oligodendrocytes). The mature neuron connects with thousands of other neurons through its axon that sends impulses to other neurons, and extensive dendritic spines that receive impulses from other neurons. (© Amanda Gautier-Ronopawiro)

connectivity. The insulating myelin sheaths are discontinuous, resulting in so-called saltatory conduction, whereby the action potential "jumps" from one so-called node of Ranvier over a long myelinated stretch of the axon to the next node of Ranvier and so on until it reaches the axon terminal. The nodes of Ranvier are very short unmyelinated parts of the axon interspersed between the adjacent long myelinated internodes.

As myelination is extremely important for the speed of impulse conduction and myelin provides axonal protection, it is essential for normal nervous system functioning.

Myelin is white, due to its high fat content. In the mature brain, it is abundantly present in the white matter (thus the name "white matter") which contains the connecting fibers and is mainly populated by axons.

Abnormal and/or delayed myelination plays a major role in neonatal brain injury. Oligodendrocytes undergo critical maturation during the third trimester of gestation. During the fetal period and in the case of preterm birth, the preterm period, the immature white matter is abundantly populated by pre-myelinating oligodendrocytes (pre-Ols). These immature oligodendrocytes are not yet capable of myelination and are highly susceptible to hypoxic-ischemic and inflammatory injury. Especially in the very preterm infant, injury to the white matter may therefore lead to widespread myelination disturbances. Diffuse white matter injury (WMI) is associated with abnormalities in gray matter structures, including the cerebral and cerebellar cortex, thalamus, basal ganglia, and hippocampus [35].

Diffuse WMI and its associated gray matter injury are probably at least partly responsible for the cognitive disabilities that are frequently encountered in children born very prematurely (see Chap. 5) [2, 36–38].

In the full-term neonate, active myelination takes place in, among others, the internal capsule and the deep gray matter. Due to their high metabolic demands, these brain regions are highly susceptible to hypoxic-ischemic injury. In the full-term infant, severe hypoxic-ischemic events (e.g., perinatal asphyxia) may therefore lead to deep gray matter injury and abnormal myelination of the posterior limb of the internal capsule (PLIC) (see Chap. 8) [39–42].

1.2.7 Brain Maturation Disturbance (Dysmaturation)

With the advances in technology and care, the more severe types of preterm brain injury are declining [43–45]. However, milder forms of brain injury are increasingly recognized [46, 47]. Nowadays there is also increasing attention for so-called neuronal dysmaturation: arrested neuronal development rather than necrosis and apoptosis [48]. In cases with dysmaturation, no overt injury is present, and there is no obvious delay in myelination. However, around term equivalent age (TEA) volumes of the white matter and deep gray matter are reduced, and the extracerebral spaces are wide. It is thought that independent of WMI and myelination delay, neuronal maturation is impaired [49]. This impaired neuronal maturation may be related to undernutrition, pain, and stress. Besides WMI, primary neuronal dysmaturation may be responsible for the cognitive problems that are so often encountered in children born very prematurely.

This new concept of dysmaturation opens possibilities for new neuroprotective strategies and a wider window of opportunity to improve neurodevelopmental outcomes through positive parenting and an interactive nurturing environment [50, 51].

References

1. Kostovic I, Sedmak G, Judas M. Neural histology and neurogenesis of the human fetal and infant brain. Neuroimage. 2019;188:743–73.
2. Volpe JJ. Brain injury in premature infants: a complex amalgam of destructive and developmental disturbances. Lancet Neurol. 2009a;8(1):110–2.
3. Del Bigio MR. Cell proliferation in human ganglionic eminence and suppression after prematurity-associated haemorrhage. Brain. 2011;134(Pt 5):1344–61.
4. Ballabh P. Pathogenesis and prevention of intraventricular hemorrhage. Clin Perinatol. 2014;41(1):47–67.
5. Guihard-Costa AM, Larroche JC. Growth velocity of some fetal parameters. I. Brain weight and brain dimensions. Biol Neonate. 1992;62(5):309–16.
6. Kinney HC. The near-term (late preterm) human brain and risk for periventricular leukomalacia: a review. Semin Perinatol. 2006;30(2):81–8.
7. Clouchoux C, Guizard N, Evans AC, du Plessis AJ, Limperopoulos C. Normative fetal brain growth by quantitative in vivo magnetic resonance imaging. Am J Obstet Gynecol. 2012;206(2):173e171–8.
8. Jarvis D, Akram R, Mandefield L, Paddock M, Armitage P, Griffiths PD. Quantification of total fetal brain volume using 3D MR imaging data acquired in utero. Prenat Diagn. 2016;36(13):1225–32.
9. Budday S, Steinmann P, Kuhl E. Physical biology of human brain development. Front Cell Neurosci. 2015;9:257.
10. Striedter GF, Srinivasan S, Monuki ES. Cortical folding: when, where, how, and why? Annu Rev Neurosci. 2015;38:291–307.
11. Zilles K, Palomero-Gallagher N, Amunts K. Development of cortical folding during evolution and ontogeny. Trends Neurosci. 2013;36(5):275–84.
12. Chi JG, Dooling EC, Gilles FH. Gyral development of the human brain. Ann Neurol. 1977;1(1):86–93.
13. Feess-Higgins A, Larroche JC. Development of the human foetal brain. An anatomical atlas. Paris: Masson; 1987.
14. Nishikuni K, Ribas GC. Study of fetal and postnatal morphological development of the brain sulci. J Neurosurg Pediatr. 2013;11(1):1–11.
15. Raybaud C, Widjaja E. Development and dysgenesis of the cerebral cortex: malformations of cortical development. Neuroimaging Clin N Am. 2011;21(3):483–543. vii
16. van der Knaap MS, Wezel-Meijler G, Barth PG, Barkhof F, Ader HJ, Valk J. Normal gyration and sulcation in preterm and term neonates: appearance on MR images. Radiology. 1996;200(2):389–96.
17. Barkovich AJ, Mukherjee P. Normal development of the neonatal and infant brain, skull and spine. In: Barkovich AJ, Raybaud C, editors. Pediatric neuroimaging. Philadelphia: Lippincott Williams & Wilkins; 2012. p. 20–81.
18. Govaert P, Triulzi F, Dudink J. The developing brain by trimester. Handb Clin Neurol. 2020;171:245–89.
19. Raybaud C, Ahmad T, Rastegar N, Shroff M, Al Nassar M. The premature brain: developmental and lesional anatomy. Neuroradiology. 2013;55(Suppl 2):23–40.

20. Knickmeyer RC, Gouttard S, Kang C, Evans D, Wilber K, Smith JK, Hamer RM, Lin W, Gerig G, Gilmore JH. A structural MRI study of human brain development from birth to 2 years. J Neurosci. 2008;28(47):12176–82.
21. Tau GZ, Peterson BS. Normal development of brain circuits. Neuropsychopharmacology. 2010;35(1):147–68.
22. Levitt P. Structural and functional maturation of the developing primate brain. J Pediatr. 2003;143(4 Suppl):S35–45.
23. Lowel S, Singer W. Selection of intrinsic horizontal connections in the visual cortex by correlated neuronal activity. Science. 1992;255(5041):209–12.
24. Rakic S, Zecevic N. Programmed cell death in the developing human telencephalon. Eur J Neurosci. 2000;12(8):2721–34.
25. Paolicelli RC, Bolasco G, Pagani F, Maggi L, Scianni M, Panzanelli P, Giustetto M, Ferreira TA, Guiducci E, Dumas L, Ragozzino D, Gross CT. Synaptic pruning by microglia is necessary for normal brain development. Science. 2011;333(6048):1456–8.
26. Stevens B, Allen NJ, Vazquez LE, Howell GR, Christopherson KS, Nouri N, Micheva KD, Mehalow AK, Huberman AD, Stafford B, Sher A, Litke AM, Lambris JD, Smith SJ, John SW, Barres BA. The classical complement cascade mediates CNS synapse elimination. Cell. 2007;131(6):1164–78.
27. Yakovlev P, Lecours A. The myelogenetic cycles of regional maturation of the brain in early life. In: Minkowski A, editor. Regional development of the brain in early life. Oxford: Blackwell; 1967. p. 3–17.
28. Brody BA, Kinney HC, Kloman AS, Gilles FH. Sequence of central nervous system myelination in human infancy. I. An autopsy study of myelination. J Neuropathol Exp Neurol. 1987;46(3):283–301.
29. Gilles FH, Dooling E, Fulchiero A. Sequence of myelination in the human fetus. Trans Am Neurol Assoc. 1976;101:244–6.
30. Kinney HC, Brody BA, Kloman AS, Gilles FH. Sequence of central nervous system myelination in human infancy. II. Patterns of myelination in autopsied infants. J Neuropathol Exp Neurol. 1988;47(3):217–34.
31. Barkovich AJ. Concepts of myelin and myelination in neuroradiology. AJNR Am J Neuroradiol. 2000;21(6):1099–109.
32. Counsell SJ, Maalouf EF, Fletcher AM, Duggan P, Battin M, Lewis HJ, Herlihy AH, Edwards AD, Bydder GM, Rutherford MA. MR imaging assessment of myelination in the very preterm brain. AJNR Am J Neuroradiol. 2002;23(5):872–81.
33. van der Knaap MS, Valk J. Myelin and white matter. In: van der Knaap MS, Valk J, editors. Magnetic resonance of myelination and myelin disorders. Berlin, Heidelberg: Springer; 2005. p. 1–20.
34. Welker KM, Patton A. Assessment of normal myelination with magnetic resonance imaging. Semin Neurol. 2012;32(1):15–28.
35. Back Stephen A, Volpe Jospeh J. Encephalopathy of Prematurity: Pathophysiology. Chapter 19 In: Volpe's Neurology of the Newborn, Elsevier 7th edition. 2025.
36. Volpe JJ. The encephalopathy of prematurity—brain injury and impaired brain development inextricably intertwined. Semin Pediatr Neurol. 2009b;16(4):167–78.
37. Keunen K, Kersbergen KJ, Groenendaal F, Isgum I, de Vries LS, Benders MJ. Brain tissue volumes in preterm infants: prematurity, perinatal risk factors and neurodevelopmental outcome: a systematic review. J Matern Fetal Neonatal Med. 2012;25(Suppl 1):89–100.
38. Ophelders D, Gussenhoven R, Klein L, Jellema RK, Westerlaken RJJ, Hutten MC, Vermeulen J, Wassink G, Gunn AJ, Wolfs T. Preterm brain injury, antenatal triggers, and therapeutics: timing is key. Cells. 2020;9(8):1871.
39. Barkovich AJ, Westmark K, Partridge C, Sola A, Ferriero DM. Perinatal asphyxia: MR findings in the first 10 days. AJNR Am J Neuroradiol. 1995;16(3):427–38.
40. Martin E, Barkovich AJ. Magnetic resonance imaging in perinatal asphyxia. Arch Dis Child Fetal Neonatal Ed. 1995;72(1):F62–70.

41. Cowan FM, de Vries LS. The internal capsule in neonatal imaging. Semin Fetal Neonatal Med. 2005;10(5):461–74.
42. Mrelashvili A, Ferriero Donna M, Inder Terrie E, Volpe Jospeh J. Hypoxic-ischemic injury in the term infant: clinical-neurological features, diagnosis, imaging, management and prognosis. In: Volpe J, editor. Volpe's neurology of the newborn. Philadelphia: Elsevier; 2025. p. 643–96.
43. Hamrick SE, Miller SP, Leonard C, Glidden DV, Goldstein R, Ramaswamy V, Piecuch R, Ferriero DM. Trends in severe brain injury and neurodevelopmental outcome in premature newborn infants: the role of cystic periventricular leukomalacia. J Pediatr. 2004;145(5):593–9.
44. Groenendaal F, Termote JU, van der Heide-Jalving M, van Haastert IC, de Vries LS. Complications affecting preterm neonates from 1991 to 2006: what have we gained? Acta Paediatr. 2010;99(3):354–8.
45. van Haastert IC, Groenendaal F, Cuno SPM, et al. Decreasing incidence and severity of cerebral palsy in prematurely born children. J Pediatr. 2011;159:86–91.
46. Volpe JJ. Neurobiology of periventricular leukomalacia in the premature infant. Pediatr Res. 2001;50(5):553–62.
47. Rezaie P, Dean A. Periventricular leukomalacia, inflammation and white matter lesions within the developing nervous system. Neuropathology. 2002;22(3):106–32.
48. Back SA, Miller SP. Brain injury in premature neonates: a primary cerebral dysmaturation disorder? Ann Neurol. 2014;75(4):469–86.
49. Volpe JJ. Primary neuronal dysmaturation in preterm brain: important and likely modifiable. J Neonatal Perinatal Med. 2020;14:1–6.
50. Kolb B, Gibb R. Searching for the principles of brain plasticity and behavior. Cortex. 2014;58:251–60.
51. Kolb B, Harker A, Gibb R. Principles of plasticity in the developing brain. Dev Med Child Neurol. 2017;59(12):1218–23.

Normal Anatomy

2

Gerda Meijler

2.1 For Parents and Professionals

This chapter includes important, clearly illustrated brain structures that may be affected in neonatal brain injury. It also shows the territories of the main arteries of the brain that play a role in perinatal stroke (see Chaps. 6 and 9).

These illustrations enable professionals to explain the location and meaning of lesions to parents (Figs. 2.1, 2.2, 2.3, 2.4, 2.5, 2.6, 2.7, 2.8, 2.9, 2.10, 2.11, and 2.12).

G. Meijler (✉)
Department of Neonatology, Isala Women and Children's Hospital, Zwolle, The Netherlands
e-mail: gmeijler@gmail.com

© The Author(s) 2024
G. Meijler, K. Mohammad (eds.), *Neonatal Brain Injury*,
https://doi.org/10.1007/978-3-031-55972-3_2

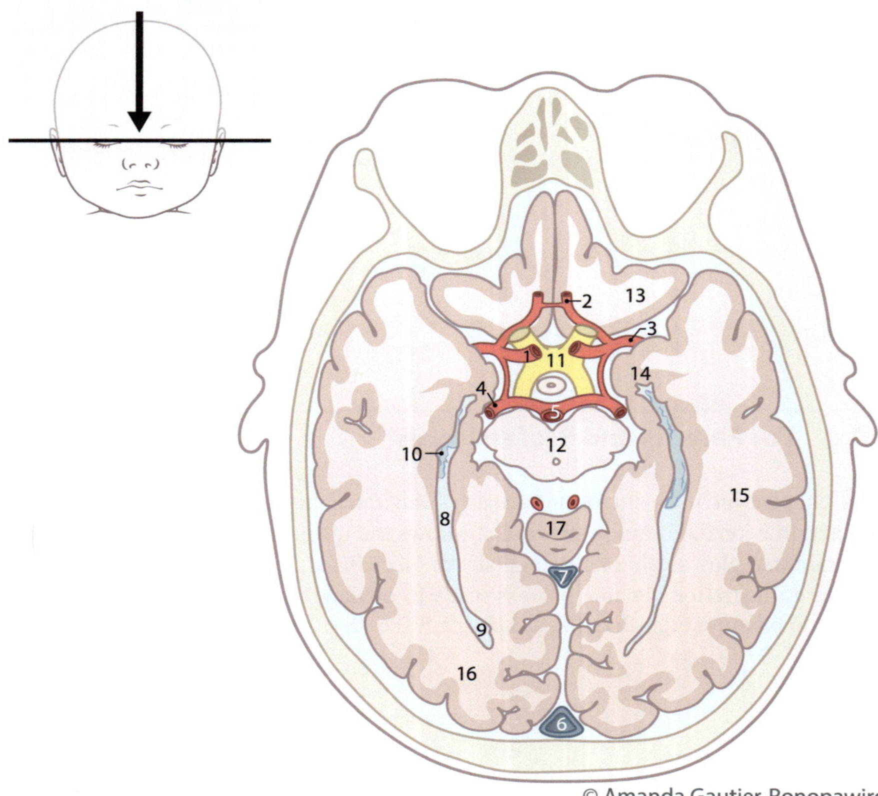

Fig. 2.1 Low axial plane. (1) Internal carotid artery. (2) Anterior cerebral artery. (3) Middle cerebral artery. (4) Posterior cerebral artery. (5) Basilar artery. (6) Superior sagittal sinus. (7) Straight sinus. (8) Lateral ventricle (temporal horn). (9) Lateral ventricle (occipital horn). (10) Choroid plexus. (11) Optic chiasm. (12) Midbrain (mesencephalon). (13) Frontal lobe. (14) Hippocampal gyrus (of temporal lobe). (15) Temporal lobe. (16) Occipital lobe. (17) Cerebellar vermis (upper part). (© Amanda Gautier-Ronopawiro)

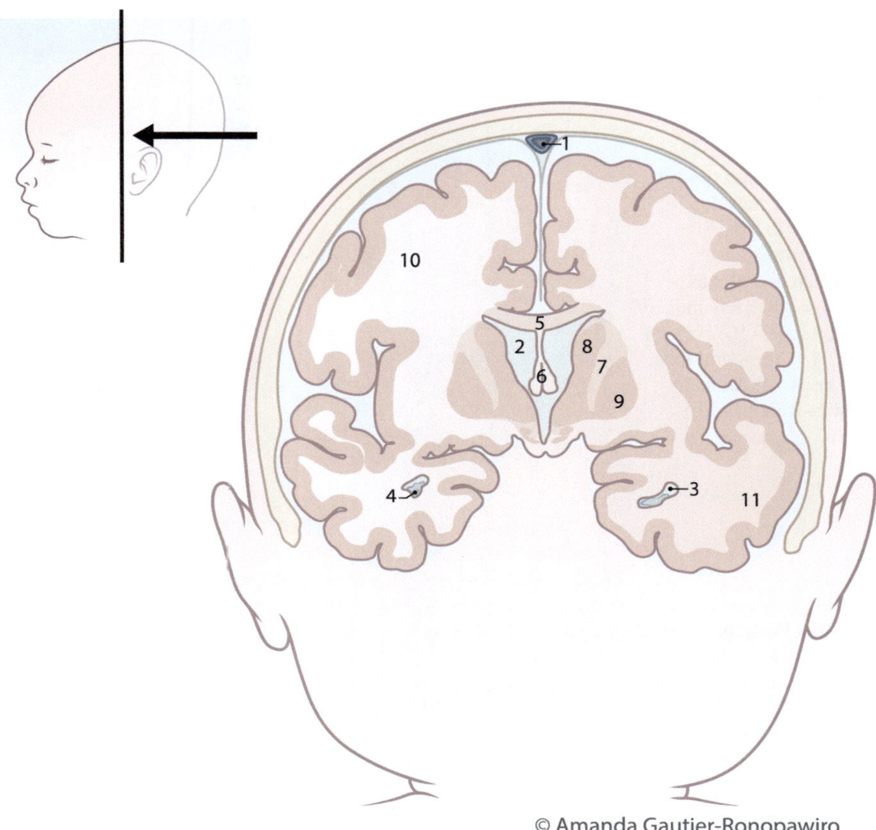

Fig. 2.2 Anterior coronal plane. (1) Superior sagittal sinus. (2) Lateral ventricle (frontal horn). (3) Lateral ventricle (temporal horn). (4) Choroid plexus (in temporal horn). (5) Corpus callosum (genu). (6) Septum pellucidum. (7) Internal capsule (anterior limb). (8) Caudate nucleus (head). (9) Putamen. (10) Frontal lobe. (11) Temporal lobe. (© Amanda Gautier-Ronopawiro)

Fig. 2.3 Mid-coronal plane. (1) Superior sagittal sinus. (2) Middle cerebral artery (branches of). (3) Lateral ventricle (body). (4) Third ventricle. (5) Corpus callosum (body). (6) Internal capsule (posterior limb). (7) Lentiform nucleus (putamen and globus pallidus). (8) Thalamus. (9) Frontal lobe. (10) Parietal lobe. (11) Temporal lobe. (12) Pons. (© Amanda Gautier-Ronopawiro)

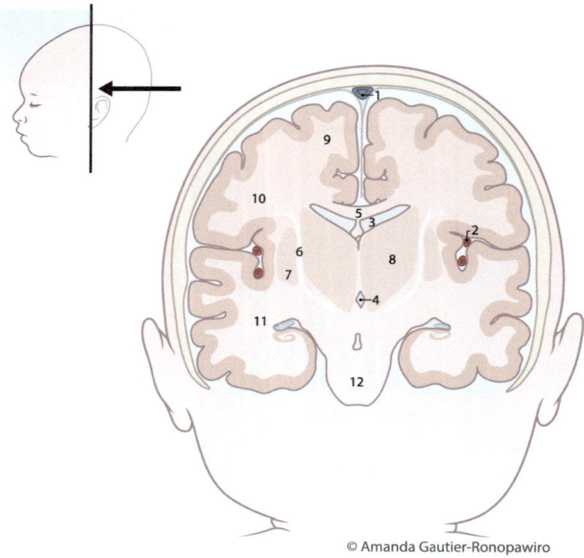

Fig. 2.4 Posterior coronal plane. (1) Superior sagittal sinus. (2) Internal cerebral vein. (3) Middle cerebral artery (branch of). (4) Insular artery (branch of middle cerebral artery). (5) Body of lateral ventricle containing choroid plexus. (6) Corpus callosum (body). (7) Thalamus. (8) Mesencephalon (Midbrain). (9) Frontal lobe. (10) Parietal lobe. (11) Temporal lobe. (© Amanda Gautier-Ronopawiro)

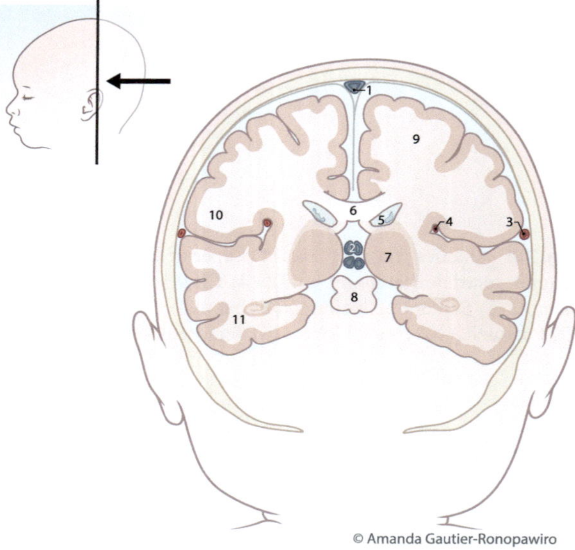

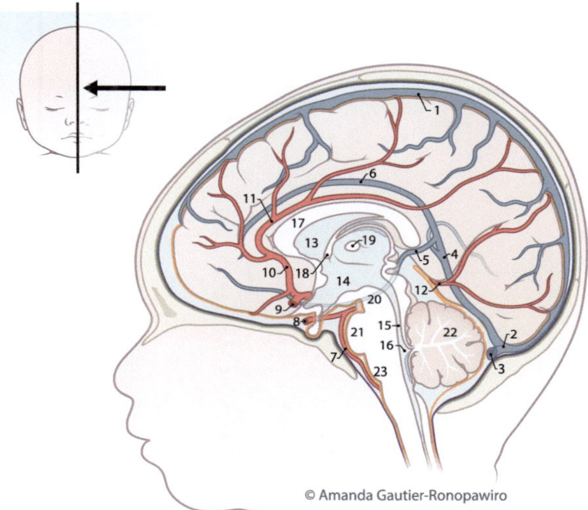

Fig. 2.5 Mid-sagittal plane. (1) Superior sagittal sinus. (2) Confluence of sinuses (Torcular Herophili). (3) Transverse sinus (beginning of). (4) Straight sinus. (5) Vein of Galen. (6) Inferior sagittal sinus. (7) Basilar artery. (8) Internal carotid artery. (9) Anterior communicating artery. (10) Anterior cerebral artery. (11) Pericallosal artery. (12) Posterior cerebral artery. (13) Cavum septum pellucidum. (14) Third ventricle. (15) Aqueduct of Sylvius. (16) Fourth ventricle. (17) Corpus callosum. (18) Fornix. (19) Interthalamic adhesion. (20) Midbrain (mesencephalon). (21) Pons. (22) Cerebellum (vermis). (23) Medulla oblongata. (© Amanda Gautier-Ronopawiro)

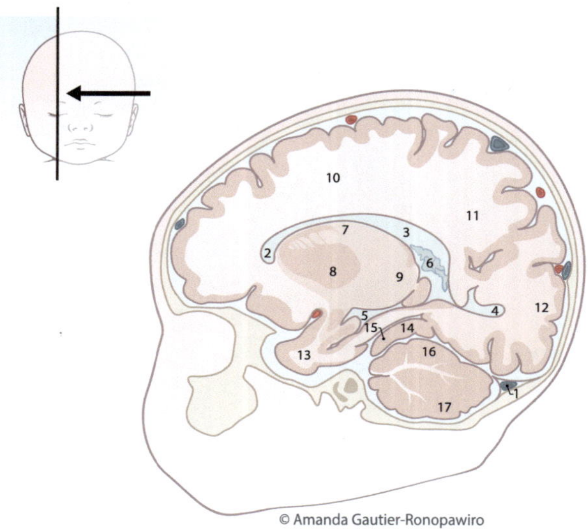

Fig. 2.6 Para-sagittal plane. (1) Transverse sinus. (2) Lateral ventricle (frontal horn). (3) Lateral ventricle (body). (4) Lateral ventricle (occipital horn). (5) Lateral ventricle (temporal horn). (6) Choroid plexus. (7) Caudate nucleus. (8) Lentiform nucleus (putamen and globus pallidus). (9) Thalamus. (10) Frontal lobe. (11) Parietal lobe. (12) Occipital lobe. (13) Temporal lobe. (14) Parahippocampal gyrus (temporal lobe). (15) Hippocampus (temporal lobe). (16) Cerebellar hemisphere (superior cerebellar lobe). (17) Cerebellar hemisphere (inferior cerebellar lobe). (© Amanda Gautier-Ronopawiro)

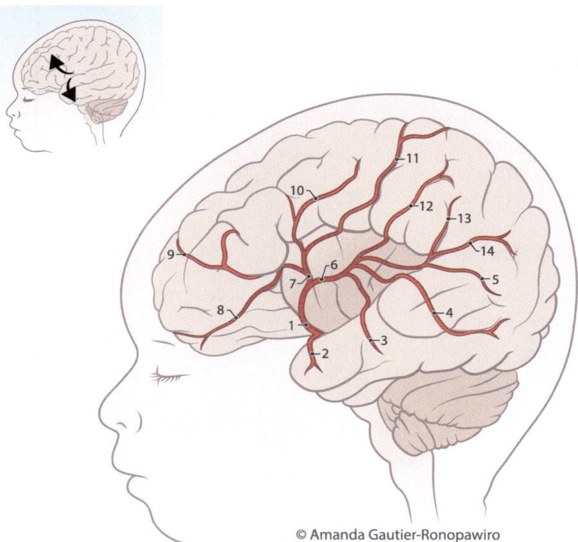

Fig. 2.7 Arterial blood supply lateral brain surface, territory of the middle cerebral artery. (1) Middle cerebral artery (MCA). (2) Frontal temporal branch. (3) Middle temporal branch. (4) Posterior temporal branch. (5) Branch to angular gyrus. (6) Inferior terminal branch. (7) Superior terminal branch. (8) Lateral frontobasal artery. (9) Prefontal artery. (10) Artery of precentral sulcus. (11) Artery of central sulcus. (12) Artery of postcentral sulcus. (13) Anterior parietal artery. (14) Posterior parietal artery. (© Amanda Gautier-Ronopawiro)

Fig. 2.8 Ventricular system. (1) Lateral ventricle (frontal horn). (2) Lateral ventricle (body). (3) Lateral ventricle (occipital horn). (4) Lateral ventricle (temporal horn). (5) Foramen of Monro. (6) Third ventricle. (7) Aqueduct of Sylvius. (8) Fourth ventricle. (9) Foramina of Luschka (lateral apertures). (10) Foramen of Magendie (median aperture). (© Amanda Gautier-Ronopawiro)

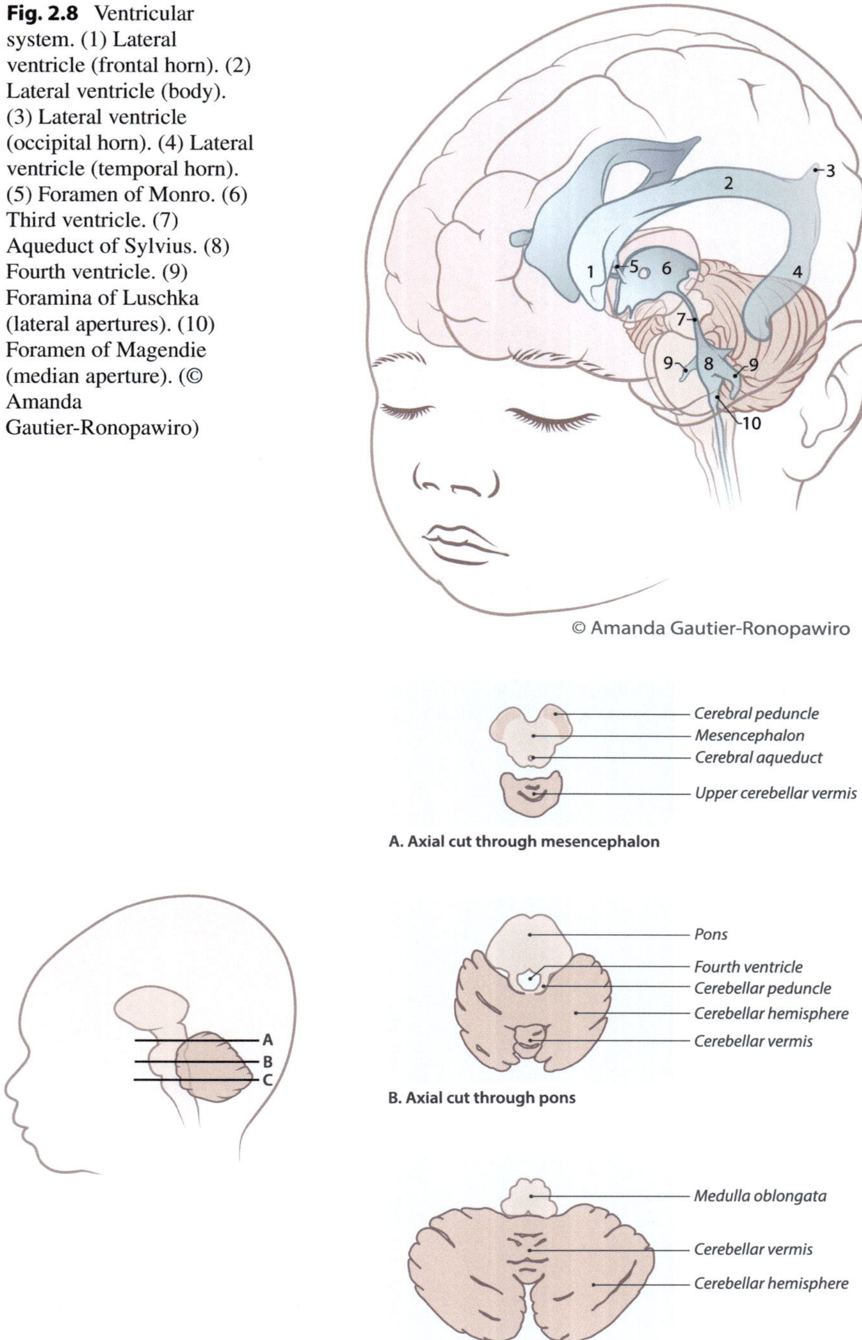

Fig. 2.9 Axial views of the brain stem and cerebellum. (© Amanda Gautier-Ronopawiro)

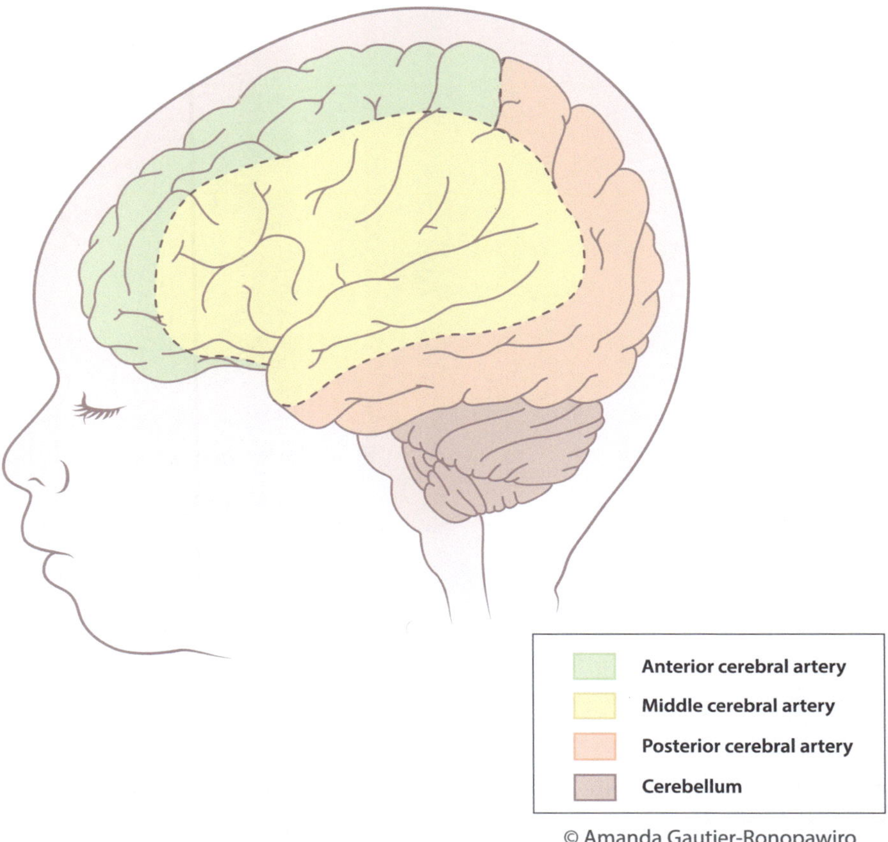

Fig. 2.10 Territories of the major cerebral arteries, lateral surface. (© Amanda Gautier-Ronopawiro)

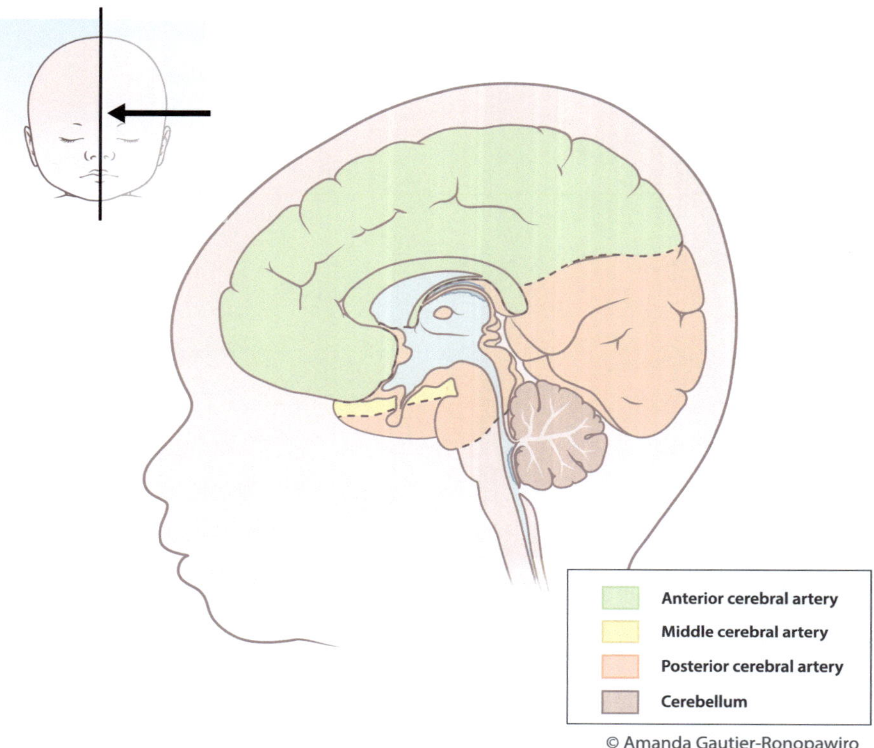

Fig. 2.11 Territories of the major cerebral arteries, medial surface. (© Amanda Gautier-Ronopawiro)

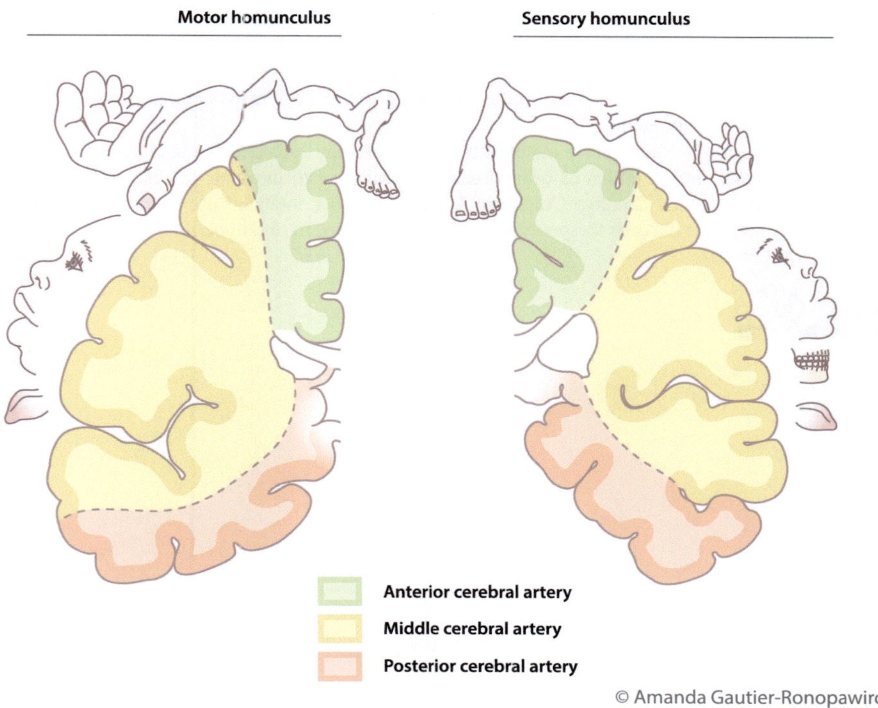

Fig. 2.12 Motor and sensory homunculus in relation to arterial territories. (© Amanda Gautier-Ronopawiro)

Further Reading

1. Feess-Higgins A, Larroche JC. Development of the human foetal brain. An anatomical atlas. Paris: Masson; 1987.
2. Griffiths PD, Morris J, Larroche J-C, Reeves M. Atlas of fetal and postnatal brain MR. Philadelphia, PA: Mosby Elsevier; 2010.
3. Meijler G, Steggerda SJ. Neonatal Cranial Ultrasonography. 3rd ed. Cham: Springer; 2019.
4. Sobotta Atlas of Anatomy. Head, Neck and Neuroanatomy. 16th Edition, 2018. Elsevier Health, Europe.

Part II

Preterm Brain Injury

Intraventricular Hemorrhage and Post-Hemorrhagic Ventricular Dilatation

3

Lara M. Leijser and Linda S. de Vries

Abbreviations

AHW	Anterior horn width
CSF	Cerebrospinal fluid
c-PVL	Cystic periventricular leukomalacia
cUS	Cranial ultrasound
FOHR	Fronto-occipital horn ratio
FTHR	Fronto-temporal horn ratio
GA	Gestational age
GMH	Germinal matrix hemorrhage
IVH	Intraventricular hemorrhage
LP	Lumbar puncture
NEL	Neuro-endoscopic lavage
PHVD	Post-hemorrhagic ventricular dilatation
PLIC	Posterior limb of the internal capsule
PVHI	Periventricular hemorrhagic infarction
SWI	Susceptibility weighted imaging
TEA	Term-equivalent age
TOD	Thalamo-occipital distance
VI	Ventricular index

L. M. Leijser (✉)
Section of Newborn Critical Care, Department of Pediatrics, Cumming School of Medicine, University of Calgary, Calgary, AB, Canada
e-mail: lara.leijser@ucalgary.ca

L. S. de Vries
Department of Neonatology, University Medical Center Utrecht (UMCU), Utrecht, The Netherlands

Department of Pediatrics, Division of Neonatology, Willem-Alexander Children's Hospital, Leiden University Medical Center (LUMC), Leiden, The Netherlands
e-mail: l.s.de_vries@lumc.nl

© The Author(s) 2024
G. Meijler, K. Mohammad (eds.), *Neonatal Brain Injury*,
https://doi.org/10.1007/978-3-031-55972-3_3

3.1   For Parents

A bleed (or hemorrhage) is commonly seen in the brain of infants that are born too early (preterm, prematurely). Bleeds mostly occur in the lining of the two normal fluid-filled spaces in the brain (one on either side) called the lateral ventricles. This lining is called the germinal matrix. During the early stages of brain development, the germinal matrix is important because it contains many immature cells that develop into nerve cells and supportive (so-called glial) cells. During pregnancy, these immature cells travel from the germinal matrix to the cortex of the brain. The cortex is the outermost layer of the brain that contains billions of nerve cells that send signals to each other. Most nerve cells have reached the cortex by 24 weeks into the pregnancy. From that time onward, the germinal matrix starts to shrink, and almost all of it will have disappeared by the expected delivery date.

3.1.1   Why Did My Baby Develop a Hemorrhage?

The germinal matrix also contains many small and fragile blood vessels. In a sick preterm infant, the amount of blood that flows through these small vessels can vary considerably. The variations in blood flow and pressure may rupture the fragile vessels of the germinal matrix, resulting in a bleed.

A bleed in the brain of a preterm infant nearly always starts in the germinal matrix and is therefore called a germinal matrix hemorrhage or GMH (Fig. 3.1a). Due to the location of the germinal matrix in the wall of the lateral ventricles, the hemorrhage may break through the wall and extend into the fluid-filled lateral ventricle. In that case, the hemorrhage is called an intraventricular hemorrhage or IVH (Fig. 3.1b). Germinal matrix or intraventricular hemorrhages mostly develop in the first 3 days after birth. A hemorrhage can be seen in the lateral ventricle on one side (unilateral) or on both sides (bilateral) of the brain. The size of the hemorrhage in the ventricle can vary from small to large. In most cases, the hemorrhage is small. However, in some cases, there is so much blood in the lateral ventricle that it causes a sudden enlargement of the ventricle (Fig. 3.1c). In rare cases, blood is also seen in the brain tissue surrounding the lateral ventricle, called parenchymal hemorrhage (Fig. 3.1d, e). Germinal matrix and intraventricular hemorrhages are usually detected with an ultrasound examination of the brain.

About 20% of preterm infants that are born before 30 weeks of pregnancy develop a germinal matrix and/or intraventricular hemorrhage (GMH-IVH). Fortunately, most of the hemorrhages are small, so-called grade I and II hemorrhages (Fig. 3.1a, b). These small hemorrhages do not have a serious effect on the short-term development of the infant, but it is still unclear whether they have some effect in the long term. In the case of a large hemorrhage in the ventricle (grade III; Fig. 3.1c) or blood in the brain tissue (Fig. 3.1d, e), there is a risk of enlargement of the ventricles and problems with the development of the infant later in life.

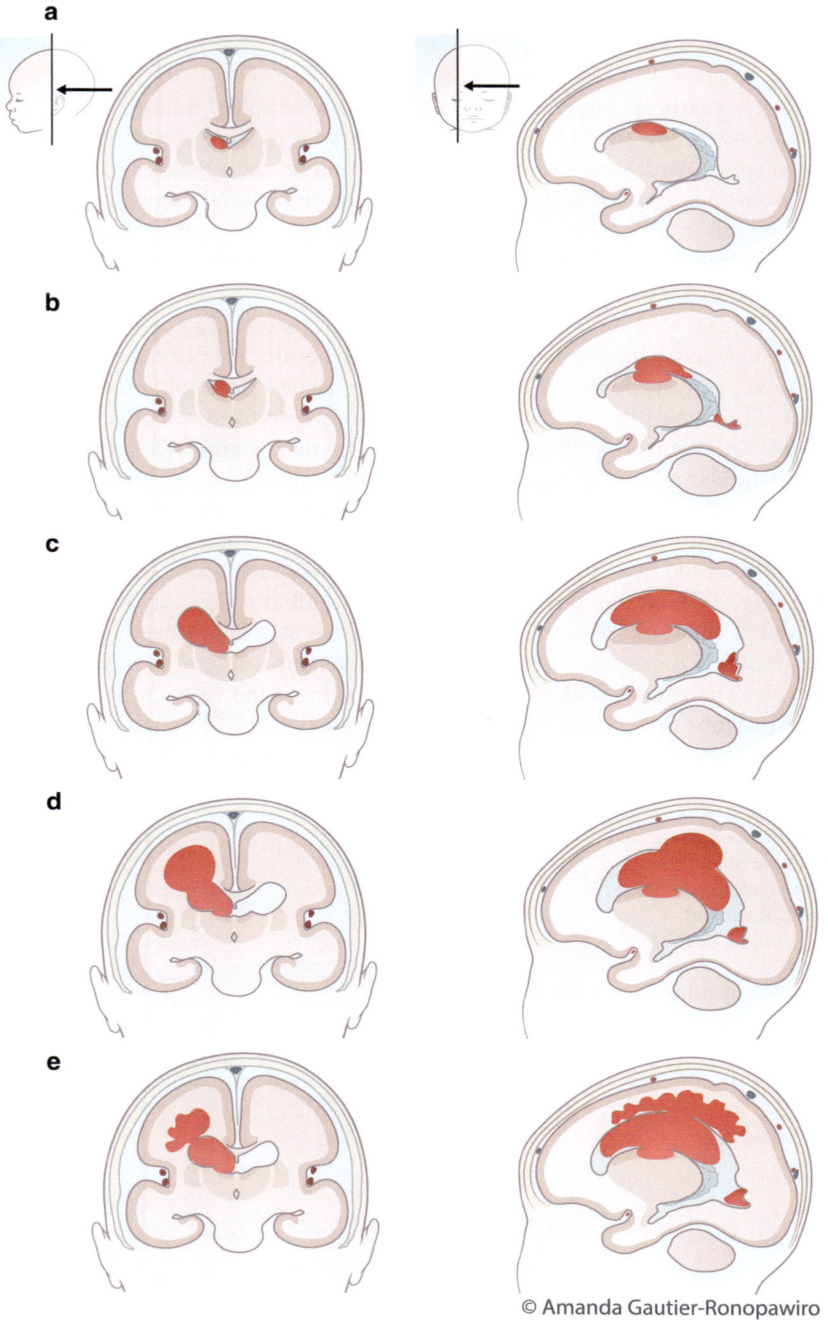

Fig. 3.1 Schematic drawings of coronal and sagittal views of the brain showing: (**a**) unilateral germinal matrix hemorrhage; (**b**) unilateral grade II intraventricular hemorrhage; (**c**) unilateral grade III intraventricular hemorrhage; (**d, e**) unilateral intraventricular hemorrhage with parenchymal hemorrhage (called periventricular hemorrhagic infarction). (© Amanda Gautier-Ronopawiro)

3.1.2   What Is the Treatment If My Baby Is Diagnosed with a Hemorrhage?

The lateral ventricles contain fluid, called the cerebrospinal fluid (CSF). The CSF normally flows downward from the lateral ventricles to the spaces around the brain and the spinal cord, where it is absorbed by blood vessels (Fig. 3.2). If the flow of CSF is obstructed by a blood clot in the ventricles or the CSF is not absorbed by the blood vessels, CSF may accumulate in the ventricles. Accumulation of CSF may lead to enlargement of the ventricles, called post-hemorrhagic ventricular dilatation (PHVD) (Fig. 3.3).

PHVD may develop 7–14 days after the development of a hemorrhage and can also be detected using ultrasound imaging of the brain. PHVD can become worse over time and can cause pressure on the brain tissue surrounding the lateral ventricles. The size of the ventricles should therefore be followed closely. This can be done with measurements of the ventricles on ultrasound. When the ventricles become too large for the age of the infant, treatment may be needed as too much pressure on the surrounding brain tissue may cause injury to the brain. The size of the ventricles can be reduced by draining CSF from the lateral ventricles. The first method used to do this is a puncture from the lumbar space (lumbar puncture [LP]) (Fig. 3.4). Draining some CSF from the lumbar space may be sufficient to resolve PHVD. If the effect of the LP is not sufficient or if LPs need to be repeated more than 3–5 times, the next step is to ask the neurosurgeon to implant a small reservoir. The reservoir is placed under the skin of the infant's head and connected to a tube that ends in one of the lateral ventricles. CSF can then be removed

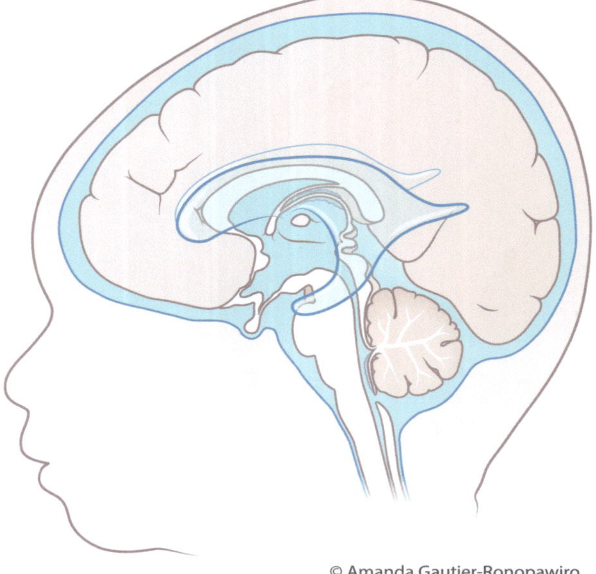

Fig. 3.2 Schematic drawing of the mid-sagittal view of the brain showing the ventricular system and cerebrospinal fluid (CSF) outflow tract. (© Amanda Gautier-Ronopawiro)

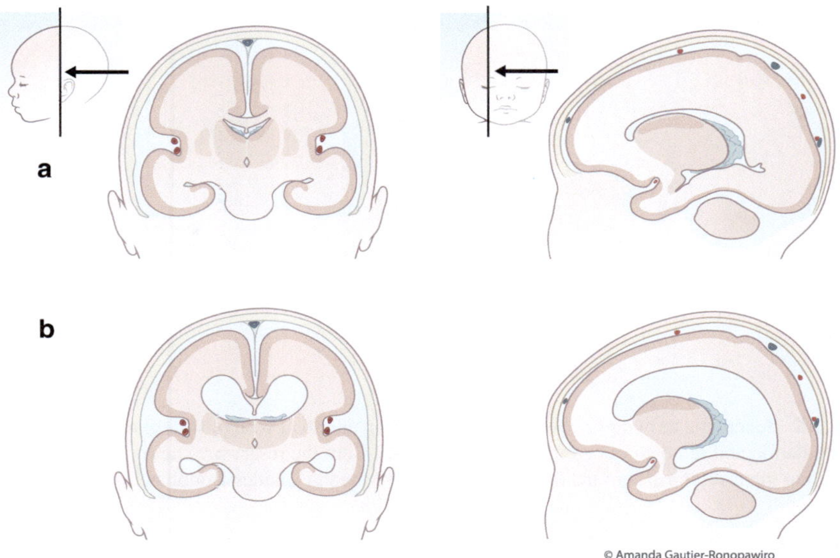

Fig. 3.3 Schematic drawings of coronal and sagittal views of the brain showing post-hemorrhagic ventricular dilatation. (© Amanda Gautier-Ronopawiro)

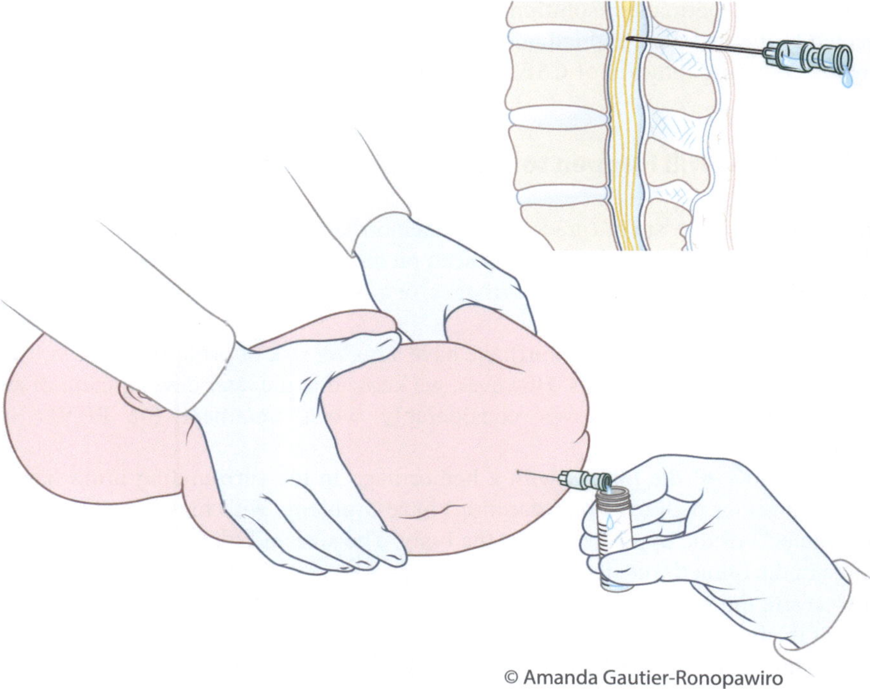

Fig. 3.4 Schematic drawing of lumbar puncture procedure in newborn infant; also showing the spinal cord, vertebrae, and lumbar space. (© Amanda Gautier-Ronopawiro)

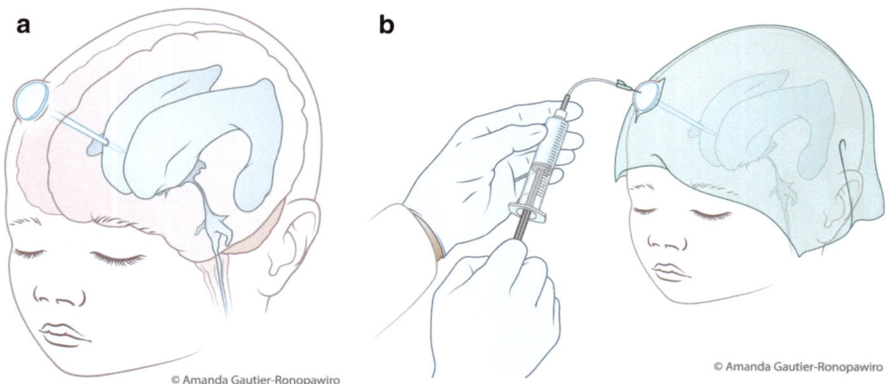

Fig. 3.5 Schematic drawings of ventricular reservoir in an infant with post-hemorrhagic ventricular dilatation and removal of cerebrospinal fluid (CSF) from the reservoir. The tip of the tube connected to the reservoir lies in the lateral ventricle. (© Amanda Gautier-Ronopawiro)

from the reservoir 1–2 times per day to reduce the size of the ventricles (Fig. 3.5). In most cases, removal of CSF from the ventricles is enough to resolve PHVD in 1–2 weeks. However, in about 40% of infants who need a reservoir, the CSF removal through the reservoir is not sufficient to keep the ventricles small enough so that they do not cause too much pressure on the surrounding brain tissue. In those cases, a permanent solution, called a shunt, is needed. A tube is then connected to the reservoir and led under the infant's skin to the abdomen. The shunt enables ongoing removal of CSF from the lateral ventricles into the abdomen.

3.1.3   What Will Happen to My Baby (Prognosis)?

Infants who have a small (grade I or II) hemorrhage mostly do well later in life. However, if additional brain injury is seen on an ultrasound and/or MRI examination, such as small cerebellar hemorrhages or white matter injury, the development of the infant may be affected.

Infants with a grade III hemorrhage have a higher risk of problems later in life, especially if PHVD develops. However, we know that the later development of an infant with PHVD improves considerably when treatment for PHVD is started early.

About 50% of the infants with a hemorrhage in the surrounding brain tissue (periventricular hemorrhagic infarction) have problems with motor development (movement) of the opposite side of the body. The size and location of the hemorrhage in the brain tissue determine whether problems with movement develop and how severe the problems will be. Ultrasound imaging, or better an MRI examination of the brain, around the expected delivery date can help with the prediction of motor development. MRI can show the connections between nerve cells (called nerve fibers) in the brain that are involved in controlling movement. When these connection are not visible on MRI on the side of the hemorrhage, an infant likely develops a one-sided problem with movement (on the other side of the body). The majority of the children with a one-sided movement problem will be able to walk without support by the age of 24–30 months. When the infant has other risk factors for problems with later development (such as extremely low gestational age at birth), the child may develop additional problems (e.g., learning and/or behavioral problems).

Over the past decades, we have learned a lot about factors that both reduce and increase the risk for preterm infants to develop a germinal matrix or intraventricular hemorrhage. Corticosteroids, given to the pregnant mother to boost lung maturation in the fetus when she is at risk of a preterm delivery, protect against the development of hemorrhages. We have also learned that gentle handling of a preterm infant, keeping the head in the midline during the first 3 days after birth and an individualized approach to intensive care treatments the infant may need are all important measures to reduce the risk of hemorrhages. The search for other risk factors is ongoing, so we can further reduce the occurrence of hemorrhages.

3.2 For Professionals

3.2.1 Pathogenesis

Germinal matrix hemorrhage (GMH) and intraventricular hemorrhage (IVH) typically originate from the germinal matrix (Fig. 3.1a–d). The germinal matrix, also called the ganglionic eminence, is a highly cellular and vascularized structure that is transient, related to its role in brain development. It is the initial site for neuronal and glial cell proliferation and differentiation before the cells migrate to other parts of the brain including the cortex and the deep gray matter [1] (see Chap. 1). The germinal matrix area is most abundant over the head and body of the caudate nucleus, at the level of the foramen of Monro. It is also present in the roof of the temporal horns and occipital horns of the lateral ventricles. When cell migration is complete around 24 weeks gestation, the germinal matrix area gradually regresses, and it has fully involuted by term-equivalent age (TEA) (Fig. 1.2, Chap. 1).

The germinal matrix is described as an "immature vascular rete" as its vessels are primitive and cannot be classified as arterioles, venules, or capillaries. The vessels in the germinal matrix occupy border zones between cerebral arteries and the venous outflow collection zone from the deep white matter. The vessels are thin-walled, lack structural support, and are metabolically active. As a result, the walls have increased permeability, rendering them vulnerable to injury and hemorrhage, particularly when exposed to hypoxia and/or fluctuations in cerebral blood flow [2]. The hemorrhage can be confined to the germinal matrix (i.e., GMH). It can also disrupt the ependymal lining, at the interface of the lateral ventricles filled with cerebrospinal fluid (CSF), and extend into the lateral ventricle to become an IVH [3]. IVHs vary in extent of the hemorrhage filling the lateral ventricles and presence of ventricular dilatation (see below).

In addition, there can be parenchymal involvement. The parenchymal venous outflow occurs through a fan-shaped collection of short and long medullary veins. These veins drain blood into the germinal matrix and subsequently into the terminal vein, lying below the germinal matrix [4] (Fig. 3.6). A GMH-IVH can result in impaired venous drainage of the medullary veins and subsequent congestion and stasis of blood and therewith infarction of the periventricular white matter. Cells in the infarcted area can become necrotic, eventually resulting in a cystic evolution of the periventricular white matter. The cystic evolution can be a single cyst communicating with the ipsilateral lateral ventricle, a so-called porencephalic cyst, or multiple cysts not or partly communicating with the lateral ventricle [5–8].

Regardless of the gestational age (GA) at birth, most GMH-IVHs develop within the first few days of birth. This is related to accelerated maturation of the germinal matrix after birth [2]. It is not uncommon to detect a hemorrhage soon after admission; in 16%, a hemorrhage is diagnosed within 1 h of birth, and in up to 50% within 6 h of birth [9].

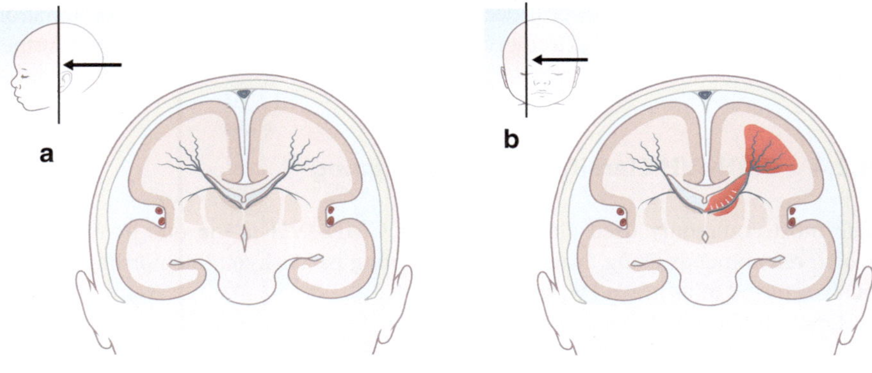

Fig. 3.6 Location and trajectory of medullary and terminal veins in coronal view. (**a**) Normal unobstructed trajectory; (**b**) triangular-shaped hemorrhage following rupture of distended veins in the white matter due to impaired venous drainage. (© Amanda Gautier-Ronopawiro)

3.2.2 Risk Factors

GMH-IVHs have a multifactorial origin. In line with the etiology and impaired cerebral autoregulation in preterm infants, an important risk factor for GMH-IVH is fluctuations in cerebral blood flow related to changes in systemic blood pressure [10, 11]. Other factors that have been described to cause fluctuations in cerebral blood flow include anemia, hypercarbia, acidemia, hypoglycemia, hypoxia, and abrupt elevations in systemic blood pressure (due to use of inotropes, rapid volume expansion with fluid boluses, and seizures) [12].

3.2.3 Incidence

The incidence of GMH-IVH is usually reported for all grades combined and depends on the GA and birthweight range described. Related to the evolution of the germinal matrix during fetal and preterm brain development, the incidence of GMH-IVH decreases with increasing GA. The incidence of GMH-IVH was as high as 45% in a study looking at infants born <1000 g [13] and 38% in a recent study looking at infants with a GA between 24 and 28 weeks [14]. Others have specifically studied infants with a severe hemorrhage (see below). In a large study by Yeo and colleagues, a slight decrease in incidence of GMH-IVH (all grades) was seen over time in infants <32 weeks gestation, from 23.6% in 1995–2000 to 21.4% in 2007–2012 [15]. The authors also looked at the subgroup of infants with severe hemorrhage and reported a decrease from 6.6% to 5%. For infants born ≤27 weeks gestation, the incidences were higher: 34.9% for all grades and 11.6% for the severe hemorrhages during the most recent study period. While the incidence of GMH-IVH has gradually declined over the past decades, its multifactorial origin, in combination with increased survival of extremely preterm infants, has so far challenged further incidence reduction.

3.2.4 GMH-IVH Classification and Imaging

The most commonly used classification for GMH-IVH is the one by Volpe [2], which recommends using three grades and noting parenchymal hemorrhage (previously referred to as grade IV) separately.

- Grade I: Germinal matrix hemorrhage (Fig. 3.1a).
- Grade II: Intraventricular hemorrhage without ventricular dilatation (Fig. 3.1b).
- Grade III: Intraventricular hemorrhage with acute ventricular dilatation (clot fills >50% of the ventricle) (Fig. 3.1c).
- Periventricular hemorrhagic infarction (PVHI), including description of size and location (Fig. 3.1d, e).

Cranial ultrasound (cUS) remains the preferred tool to screen the preterm infant's brain for GMH-IVH development and progress. However, a low-grade IVH (grade I and II) can be missed with cUS, especially when it develops in unusual locations such as the temporal or occipital horn of the lateral ventricle. When comparing with MRI, including a sequence called susceptibility-weighted imaging (SWI), the sensitivity of cUS for low-grade IVH was found to be as low as 60% [16]. To better distinguish a grade I from a grade II hemorrhage, performing cUS through the posterior fontanel can be helpful as this allows for better visualization of presence of blood in the occipital horn [17, 18].

Severe hemorrhages (grade III and PVHI) and larger grade II hemorrhages are well visualized with cUS. The diagnosis of a grade III hemorrhage should be made in the acute phase when the clot is filling the ventricle for >50%, causing acute distention of the lateral ventricle (which should not be confused with post-hemorrhagic ventricular dilatation [PHVD; see below]).

A PVHI can vary in shape, size, and location and all these characteristics should be reported. The shape can be globular with the parenchymal lesion communicating with the lateral ventricle (Fig. 3.7c). Such PVHI may evolve into a porencephalic cyst that communicates with the lateral ventricle. A PVHI can also be triangular in shape, with the tip of the triangle pointing toward the lateral ventricle and be partly or completely separate from the lateral ventricle (Fig. 3.7a, b). In the latter case, the PVHI may (initially) evolve into multiple small cysts instead of one large cystic lesion. When these cysts are not communicating with the lateral ventricle, they are sometimes incorrectly diagnosed as cystic periventricular leukomalacia (c-PVL). Multiple cystic lesions due to PVHI are mostly unilateral (ipsilateral to the side of the IVH), while c-PVL is mostly bilateral and preceded by a period of bilateral inhomogeneous echogenicity in the periventricular white matter (see Chap. 5). The size and location of a PVHI and number of lobes involved can be best assessed from a sagittal cUS plane. A coronal plane can be used to assess the presence of a midline shift, which is sometimes present [19, 20].

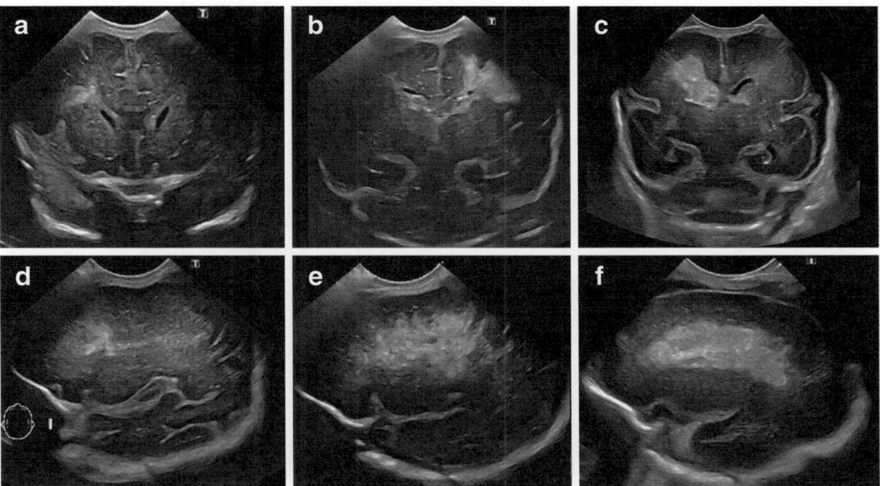

Fig. 3.7 cUS images of three preterm infants with PVHI. Top row showing coronal images and lower row showing parasagittal images. (**a** and **d**) Small PVHI, triangular in shape, involving the frontal lobe; (**b** and **e**) larger PVHI, also triangular in shape, involving the fronto-parietal lobes; (**c** and **f**) large globular shaped PVHI clearly communicating with the lateral ventricle. See Figs. 3.9 and 3.10 for MRI correlate at term-equivalent age

Infants with a large IVH have a considerable (30–50%) risk to develop PHVD [21]. PHVD usually develops between 7 and 14 days after the onset of the hemorrhage, when CSF accumulates in the ventricular system due to an imbalance between the production and the outflow and reabsorption of CSF. PHVD can be transient or slowly or rapidly progressive. The onset and progress of PHVD can be followed with cUS measurements of ventricular size, for which thresholds in relation to infant postmenstrual and postnatal age have been described. The measurements that are most often performed are the ventricular index (VI, width of midline of the brain to the lateral border of the ventricle in third coronal plane), the anterior horn width (AHW, diagonal width between the walls of the anterior horn at its widest point in third coronal plane), the thalamo-occipital distance (TOD, distance between the outermost point of the thalamus at its junction with the choroid plexus and the outermost part of the occipital horn in the parasagittal plane), and fronto-temporal or fronto-occipital horn ratio (FTHR/FOHR, widest distance of the frontal horns plus temporal or occipital horns, respectively, divided by twice the largest bi-parietal distance) (Fig. 3.8). A recent study showed that the intra-observer and inter-observer reliability are best for the VI and AHW [22]. To avoid a delay in intervention for PHVD (see below), cUS including ventricular measurements should be repeated, and measurements plotted in a graph several times per week when a GMH-IVH has been diagnosed [23, 24].

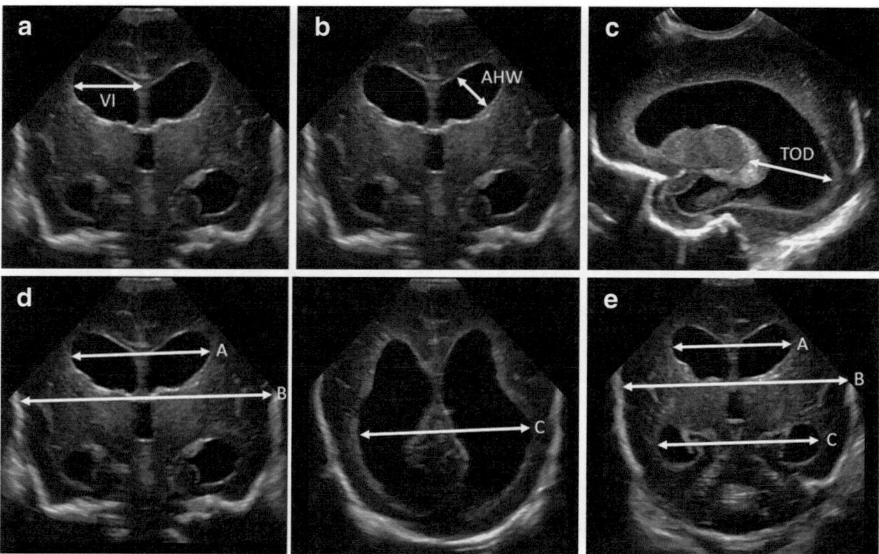

Fig. 3.8 Coronal and parasagittal cUS images showing measurements of the lateral ventricles. (**a**) Ventricular index (VI); (**b**) anterior horn width (AHW); (**c**) thalamo-occipital distance (TOD); (**d**) fronto-occipital horn ratio (FOHR; A + C/2 × B); (**e**) fronto-temporal horn ratio (FTHR; A + C/2 × B)

3.2.5 Prognosis (See Also Table 3.1)

The initial studies on neurodevelopmental outcomes related to low-grade GMH-IVH were based on cUS assessment [28]. One could therefore not be certain about additional subtle brain lesions, such as subtle white matter injury or small cerebellar hemorrhages, that may influence prognosis. A recent study reported on outcomes at 8 years in preterm infants born at <28 weeks gestation and found children with a grade I or II GMH-IVH to be at higher risk for cerebral palsy than those without GMH-IVH (OR 2.24, 95% CI 1.21–4.16). However, the authors did not exclude infants with c-PVL, as they suggested this to be along the causal pathway of an IVH [25]. Other recent studies, using MRI with advanced imaging techniques around TEA, suggest that neurodevelopmental outcome is less favorable in infants with low-grade IVH compared with those without IVH [29–31].

The neurodevelopmental outcome following IVH grade III depends on the evolution of the IVH and the presence of associated white matter injury and/or PHVD. The prognosis is more favorable without the development of PHVD; if PHVD does develop, the outcome depends on the severity and the timing of intervention. Therefore, once the diagnosis of a severe IVH is made, it is important to perform cUS frequently to diagnose and follow the progress of PHVD so intervention can be initiated timely, based on cUS findings rather than waiting for clinical symptoms of increased intracranial pressure to develop [23, 32].

Table 3.1 Prognosis for neurodevelopmental outcome [14, 25–27]

cUS finding (maximum extent)	Conjunctive MRI findings at TEA (Carefully assess site and extent of lesions and PLIC myelination)	Prognosis (See [a] below table for important note)
2-year outcome		
No GMH-IVH	No GMH, IVH, CBH, or WM injury	Favorable (no CP and Bayley composite scores >85)
Low-grade IVH	No WM injury or CBH	Low risk of CP and/or mild motor delay
Low-grade IVH	Non-cystic WM abnormalities and/or punctate CBH	Mild risk of mostly ambulant CP and/or mild motor delay (adverse motor outcome more likely if PLIC myelination delayed/absent at TEA and/or lesions adjacent to the CST)[b]
5-year outcome		
Low-grade IVH	*Not specified*	15–20% risk of moderate to severe NDI, similar to infants without IVH (Epipage-2 study)
2-year outcome		
Grade III IVH without progressive PHVD	*Not specified*	Mild risk of (mostly mild, ambulant) CP when isolated Moderate risk of (mostly mild, ambulant) CP when associated with WM lesions (in particular if PLIC myelination is delayed/absent)[b] *and* 30–40% risk of (mild-moderate) cognitive impairment
Grade III IVH with progressive PHVD	*Not specified*	Mild risk of CP when isolated and PHVD treated early based on US measurements of ventricular size Moderate risk of CP when isolated but PHVD treated after onset of clinical symptoms of increased ICP *and* At risk for cognitive impairment especially when associated with WMI and/or treated after onset of clinical symptoms
5-year outcome		
Grade III IVH	*Not specified*	35–40% risk of moderate-severe NDI, including up to 20% risk of CP (Epipage-2 study)
2-year outcome		

(continued)

Table 3.1 (continued)

cUS finding (maximum extent)	Conjunctive MRI findings at TEA (Carefully assess site and extent of lesions and PLIC myelination)	Prognosis (See [a] below table for important note)
PVHI without and with progressive PHVD	*Not specified*	Higher risk of CP when parietal lobe is involved as compared to other lobes (~ 50% risk of USCP), in particular if PLIC myelination delayed/absent[b] *and* At risk for cognitive, behavioral, and/or visual impairment, the latter in particular with temporal lobe involvement
5-year outcome		
PVHI	*Not specified*	35–65% risk of moderate-severe NDI (Epipage-2 study)

CBH cerebellar hemorrhage, *CP* cerebral palsy, *CST* corticospinal tract, *GMH-IVH* germinal matrix-intraventricular hemorrhage, *ICP* intracranial pressure, *NDI* neurodevelopmental impairment, *PHVD* post-hemorrhagic ventricular dilatation, *PLIC* posterior limb of internal capsule, *PVHI* periventricular hemorrhagic infarction, *PWML* punctate white matter lesion, *TEA* term-equivalent age, *USCP* unilateral spastic cerebral palsy, *WM* white matter

[a]Described risks are based on the average reported occurrence of neurodevelopmental deficits across the very preterm population with GMH-IVH. However, risks are influenced by multiple factors, such as lower gestational age and weight at birth, prematurity-related morbidity, and required interventions. The severity of deficits can span the spectrum from mild to severe. The table thus provides an indication, but risk needs to be assessed on an individual basis in view of other risk factors for NDI

[b]If cysts do not involve the corticospinal tract and the extent of myelination of the PLIC is normal for age, motor outcome in the normal range without cerebral palsy is expected

Performing an MRI at TEA is recommended to assess possible additional injury to the periventricular white matter and cerebellum. MRI at this age also contributes to the assessment of maturational features of the brain, such as myelination, which may help with prognostication. Neurosurgical intervention for PHVD may also result in additional brain injury, such as piercing of the corpus callosum during reservoir insertion or periventricular or subcortical bleeds following a fast reduction in ventricular volume, which can also be diagnosed with MRI [33, 34].

The prognosis related to a PVHI depends on the size and location of the lesion. Motor sequelae are most common in preterm infants with a lesion in the parietal white matter and rare for lesions in the frontal or temporal white matter. Behavioral, visual, and cognitive problems are especially common in infants with a PVHI in the temporal lobe [35]. The location of the PVHI can be best assessed on a cUS in the parasagittal plane (see Fig. 3.7). In this plane, one can assess the number of lobes involved and whether the trigonal area is affected [36]. In the coronal view, one can best assess whether the PVHI is unilateral or bilateral and whether there is a midline shift. A score can be used to assess PVHI severity [19, 37].

Performing an MRI at TEA is highly recommended in case of (suspected) PVHI as MRI allows assessment of myelination of the posterior limb of the internal capsule (PLIC). An asymmetry in myelination between both sides of the brain is a strong predictor of subsequent development of unilateral spastic cerebral palsy (Fig. 3.9). When the MRI is performed at discharge, the infant is often <37 weeks gestation, and myelination is still absent or insufficient to assess asymmetry. Performing an MRI during the first week after the development of PVHI can contribute to the prediction of motor outcome, when combining assessment of the site and size of the lesion from conventional images with assessment of the PLIC using diffusion weighted imaging (Fig. 3.10) [38]. This is especially useful in the case of bilateral injury, as redirection of care may be considered with bilateral PLIC involvement.

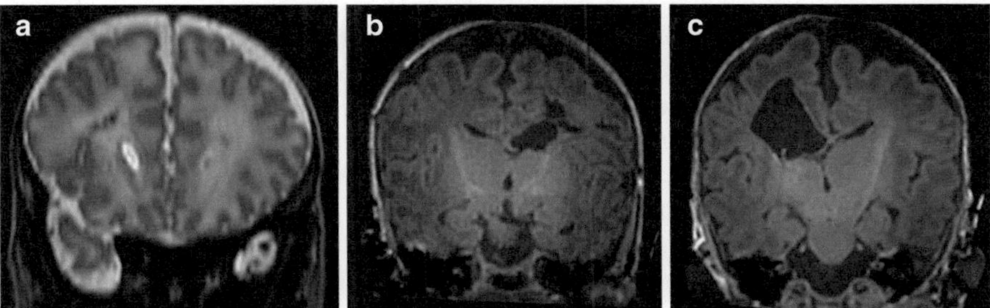

Fig. 3.9 MRIs at TEA of the three preterm infants shown in Fig. 3.7. (**a**) T2-weighted sequence, coronal view reconstructed from 3D image, still showing remnants of blood seen as low signal intensity in the right frontal lobe; (**b**) T1-weighted sequence, coronal view, showing cysts in the white matter, separate from the lateral ventricle as well as asymmetry of myelination of the PLIC; (**c**) T1-weighted sequence, coronal view, showing a large porencephalic cyst and absence of myelination of the PLIC on the affected side

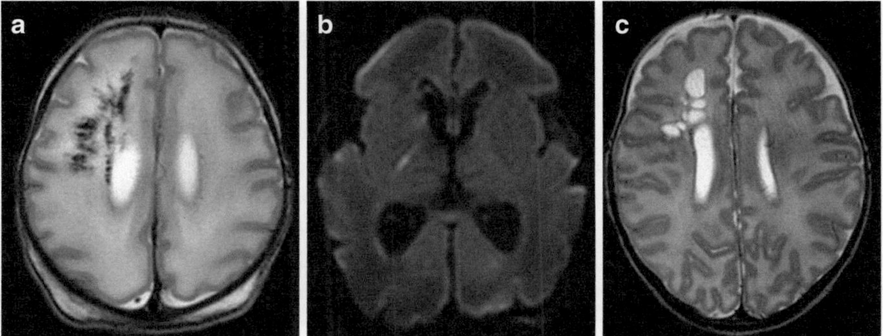

Fig. 3.10 Brain MRI of a preterm infant (31 weeks gestation) performed in the first week after birth. (**a**) Showing a PVHI on the T2-weighted sequence and (**b**) showing diffusion restriction of the middle part of the PLIC. (**c**) MRI at TEA in the same infant shows multi-cystic evolution on the T2-weighted sequence. The child developed unilateral spastic cerebral palsy, level I on the GMFCS

In a recent study, mortality was reported to be as high as 40% with increased PVHI severity score, being associated with a higher likelihood of death. Less than half (42%) of the survivors assessed at 2 years corrected age developed cerebral palsy. Involvement of the trigonal area was strongly associated with the development of cerebral palsy. In infants with a grade III IVH, associated PHVD (in 36% of the infants) was an independent risk factor for poorer cognitive and motor outcomes ($P < 0.001$ for both) [37].

3.2.6 Prevention and Treatment

Proven effective preventive measures for GMH-IVH consist of antenatal administration of corticosteroids to promote lung maturation and postnatal maintenance of circulatory and respiratory stability to avoid rapid fluctuations in cerebral blood flow. The introduction and use of neonatal care bundles, aimed at the prevention of GMH-IVH by targeting multiple risk factors simultaneously, have been associated with a reduction in the incidence of IVH [12, 39]. Also, it has been reported to reduce the progression in size of the IVH following its diagnosis [39]. The neonatal care bundles include maintaining the head in the midline position, tilting the head end of the incubator and avoidance of flushing/rapid withdrawal of blood, sudden elevation of the legs, and reduction in use of inotropes and fluid boluses.

At present, no treatment is available for GMH-IVH and management is conservative. Once a hemorrhage has been diagnosed, serial cUS is needed to follow the progression of the hemorrhage and the development of PHVD. Close cUS monitoring of PHVD development, including frequent ventricular measurements, allows for timely intervention. Growing evidence suggests that intervention started once ventricular size is increasing, resulting in better neurodevelopmental outcome compared to waiting for clinical symptoms of increased intracranial pressure (sunsetting, apneic spells, rapid increase in head circumference) [20, 32, 40, 41].

Initiation of intervention should be considered when the VI has crossed the 97th percentile and is approaching the p97 + 4 mm line, combined with an AHW >6 mm [23]. LPs can be the first intervention method and be performed a total of 3–5 times, with maximum frequency of once per day and depending on cUS measurements. However, when LPs are unsuccessful, not well tolerated by the infant or do not lead to a reduction in ventricular size, it is better to consult the neurosurgical team and discuss the insertion of a ventricular access device (e.g., reservoir) or subgaleal shunt. Punctures from a reservoir, starting with 10 mL/kg of CSF per day divided over two punctures, will help to reduce ventricular size and remove blood-stained fluid. Care should be taken to perform the punctures under sterile conditions (gown, mask gloves, and surgical scrubbing) and to remove the CSF slowly (1 mL/min). cUS with ventricular measurements should be performed every (other) day, and a decision is made to increase or decrease the amount of CSF removed based on the measurements. If punctures are still needed after 4–6 weeks, a challenge is performed (stop or halve the amount punctured) to assess whether the infant is indeed dependent on the punctures. If this is the case, a decision will be made to insert a ventriculo-peritoneal shunt when the infant has gained enough weight (mostly 2–2.5 kg), the protein level in the CSF has come down to 1–1.5 mg/dL, and the red cell count in the CSF is less than 100/mm^3.

At present, CSF drainage through LPs, reservoir tapping, or permanent shunting has proven effective for the treatment of PHVD. Other techniques have been introduced for treatment of PHVD, such as neuro-endoscopic lavage (NEL) and a combination of ventriculo-external drainage with urokinase insertion during a 2-week period [42, 43]. Also, a phase I study in nine preterm infants, all with PVHI, showed intraventricular administration of mesenchymal stem cells to be safe, feasible, and promising to reduce the inflammatory response related to severe IVH [44]. A phase II study is currently underway to assess the potential beneficial effects of stem cells on IVH evolution and PHVD development. These studies show promise toward optimized prevention and treatment of IVH and PHVD.

3.3 Conclusion

GMH-IVH remains common in preterm infants, with the incidence increasing with decreasing GA. Most GMH-IVHs are detected with cUS, which is an easy bedside tool to screen for GMH-IVH and the development of clinically significant complications, including PVHI and PHVD which may require timely intervention. Brain MRI around TEA is of additional value in the case of IVH as it is more sensitive to detect associated white matter injury and cerebellar hemorrhage and enables assessment of myelination. Low-grade IVHs without associated brain injury or complications are generally associated with a low risk of long-term sequelae, while the risk of abnormal neurodevelopmental outcomes increases with presence of severe IVHs, associated brain injury, and PHVD (in particular when treated late in its development).

References

1. Del Bigio MR. Cell proliferation in human ganglionic eminence and suppression after prematurity-associated haemorrhage. Brain. 2011;134(Pt 5):1344–61. https://doi.org/10.1093/brain/awr052.
2. Inder TE, Perlman JM, Volpe JJ. Preterm intraventricular hemorrhage/posthemorrhagic hydrocephalus. In: Volpe JJ, editor. Volpe's neurology of the newborn, 7th. Philadelphia: Elsevier; 2024. p. 777.
3. Dawes W. Secondary brain injury following neonatal intraventricular hemorrhage: the role of the ciliated ependyma. Front Pediatr. 2022;10:887606. https://doi.org/10.3389/fped.2022.887606.
4. Takashima S, Mito T, Ando Y. Pathogenesis of periventricular white matter hemorrhages in preterm infants. Brain Dev. 1986;8(1):25–30. https://doi.org/10.1016/s0387-7604(86)80116-4.
5. Robinson S. Neonatal posthemorrhagic hydrocephalus from prematurity: pathophysiology and current treatment concepts. J Neurosurg Pediatr. 2012;9:242–58. https://doi.org/10.3171/2011.12.PEDS11136.
6. Volpe JJ. Neurologic outcome of prematurity. Arch Neurol. 1998;55:297. https://doi.org/10.1001/archneur.55.3.297.
7. Bassan H. Intracranial hemorrhage in the preterm infant: understanding it, preventing it. Clin Perinatol. 2009;36:737–62. https://doi.org/10.1016/j.clp.2009.07.014.

8. de Vries LS, Roelants-van Rijn AM, Rademaker KJ, van Haastert IC, Beek FJ, Groenendaal F. Unilateral parenchymal haemorrhagic infarction in the preterm infant. Eur J Paediatr Neurol. 2001;5(4):139–49. https://doi.org/10.1053/ejpn.2001.0494.

9. Al-Abdi SY, Al-Aamri MA. A systematic review and meta-analysis of the timing of early intraventricular hemorrhage in preterm neonates: clinical and research implications. J Clin Neonatol. 2014;3:76–88. https://doi.org/10.4103/2249-4847.134674.

10. Soul JS, Hammer PE, Tsuji M, Saul JP, Bassan H, Limperopoulos C, Disalvo DN, Moore M, Akins P, Ringer S, Volpe JJ, Trachtenberg F, du Plessis AJ. Fluctuating pressure-passivity is common in the cerebral circulation of sick premature infants. Pediatr Res. 2007;61:467. https://doi.org/10.1203/pdr.0b013e31803237f6.

11. Noori S, Seri I. Hemodynamic antecedents of peri/intraventricular hemorrhage in very preterm neonates. Semin Fetal Neonatal Med. 2015;20:232. https://doi.org/10.1016/j.siny.2015.02.004.

12. Murthy P, Zein H, Thomas S, Scott JN, Abou Mehrem A, Esser MJ, Lodha A, Metcalfe C, Kowal D, Irvine L, Scotland J, Leijser L, Mohammad K. Neuroprotection care bundle implementation to decrease acute brain injury in preterm infants. Pediatr Neurol. 2020;110:42–8. https://doi.org/10.1016/j.pediatrneurol.2020.04.016.

13. Stoll BJ, Hansen NI, Bell EF, Walsh MC, Carlo WA, Shankaran S, Laptook AR, Sánchez PJ, Van Meurs KP, Wyckoff M, Das A, Hale EC, Ball MB, Newman NS, Schibler K, Poindexter BB, Kennedy KA, Cotten CM, Watterberg KL, D'Angio CT, DeMauro SB, Truog WE, Devaskar U, Higgins RD, Eunice Kennedy Shriver National Institute of Child Health and Human Development Neonatal Research Network. Trends in care practices, morbidity, and mortality of extremely preterm neonates, 1993-2012. JAMA. 2015;314(10):1039–51. https://doi.org/10.1001/jama.2015.10244.

14. Law JB, Wood TR, Gogcu S, Comstock BA, Dighe M, Perez K, Puia-Dumitrescu M, Mayock DE, Heagerty PJ, Juul SE. Intracranial hemorrhage and 2-year neurodevelopmental outcomes in extremely preterm infants. J Pediatr. 2021;238(21):124–134.e10. https://doi.org/10.1016/j.jpeds.2021.06.071.

15. Yeo KT, Thomas R, Chow SS, Bolisetty S, Haslam R, Tarnow-Mordi W, Lui K, Australian and New Zealand Neonatal Network. Improving incidence trends of severe intraventricular haemorrhages in preterm infants <32 weeks gestation: a cohort study. Arch Dis Child Fetal Neonatal Ed. 2020;105(2):145–50. https://doi.org/10.1136/archdischild-2018-316664.

16. Parodi A, Morana G, Severino MS, Malova M, Natalizia AR, Sannia A, Rossi A, Ramenghi LA. Low-grade intraventricular hemorrhage: is ultrasound good enough? J Matern Fetal Neonatal Med. 2015;28(S1):2261–4. https://doi.org/10.3109/14767058.2013.796162.

17. Correa F, Enríquez G, Rosselló J, Lucaya J, Piqueras J, Aso C, Vázquez E, Ortega A, Gallart A. Posterior Fontanelle sonography: an acoustic window into the neonatal brain. AJNR Am J Neuroradiol. 2004;25(7):1274–82.

18. Meijler G, Steggerda SJ. Neonatal cranial ultrasonography. 3rd ed. Cham: Springer; 2019.

19. Bassan H, Benson CB, Limperopoulos C, Feldman HA, Ringer SA, Veracruz E, Stewart JE, Soul JS, Disalvo DN, Volpe JJ, du Plessis AJ. Ultrasonographic features and severity scoring of periventricular hemorrhagic infarction in relation to risk factors and outcome. Pediatrics. 2006;117(6):2111–8.

20. Cizmeci MN, de Vries LS, Ly LG, van Haastert IC, Groenendaal F, Kelly EN, Traubici J, Whyte HE, Leijser LM. Periventricular hemorrhagic infarction in very preterm infants: characteristic sonographic findings and association with neurodevelopmental outcome at age 2 years. J Pediatr. 2020a;217:79–85.e1. https://doi.org/10.1016/j.jpeds.2019.09.081.

21. Groulx-Boivin E, Paquette M, Khairy M, Beltempo M, Dudley R, Ferrand A, Guillot M, Bizgu V, Garfinkle J. Spontaneous resolution of post-hemorrhagic ventricular dilatation in preterm newborns and neurodevelopment. Pediatr Res. 2023;94:1428. https://doi.org/10.1038/s41390-023-02647-6. Online ahead of print.

22. Leijser LM, Scott JN, Roychoudhury S, Zein H, Murthy P, Thomas SP, Mohammad K. Calgary Neonatal neuro-critical care program. Post-hemorrhagic ventricular dilatation: inter-observer reliability of ventricular size measurements in extremely preterm infants. Pediatr Res. 2020;90(2):403–10. https://doi.org/10.1038/s41390-020-01245-0.

23. El-Dib M, Limbrick DD, Inder T, Whitelaw A, Kulkarni AV, Warf B, Volpe JJ, de Vries LS. Management of post-hemorrhagic ventricular dilatation in the infant born preterm. J Pediatr. 2020;226:16–27. https://doi.org/10.1016/j.jpeds.2020.07.079.
24. Goeral K, Schwarz H, Hammerl M, Brugger J, Wagner M, Klebermass-Schrehof K, Kasprian G, Kiechl-Kohlendorfer U, Berger A, Olischar M. Longitudinal reference values for cerebral ventricular size in preterms born 23-27 weeks. J Pediatr. 2021;238:110–7. https://doi.org/10.1016/j.jpeds.2021.06.065.
25. Hollebrandse NL, Spittle AJ, Burnett AC, Anderson PJ, Roberts G, Doyle LW, Cheong JLY. School-age outcomes following intraventricular haemorrhage in infants born extremely preterm. Arch Dis Child Fetal Neonatal Ed. 2021;106(1):4–8. https://doi.org/10.1136/archdischild-2020-318989.
26. Tréluyer L, Chevallier M, Jarreau PH, Baud O, Benhammou V, Gire C, Marchand-Martin L, Marret S, Pierrat V, Ancel PY, Torchin H. Intraventricular hemorrhage in very preterm children: mortality and neurodevelopment at age 5. Pediatrics. 2023;151(4):e2022059138. https://doi.org/10.1542/peds.2022-059138.
27. Pascal A, Bruyn N, Naulaers G, Ortibus E, Hanssen B, Oostra A, Coen K, Sonnaert M, Cloet E, Casaer A, D'Haese J, Laroche S, Jonckheere A, Plaskie K, van Mol C, Bruneel E, van Hoestenberghe M, Samijn B, Govaert P, van den Broeck C. The impact of intraventricular hemorrhage and periventricular leukomalacia on mortality and neurodevelopmental outcome in very preterm and very-low-birthweight infants: a prospective population-based cohort study. J Pediatr. 2023;262:113600. https://doi.org/10.1016/j.jpeds.2023.113600.
28. Mukerji A, Shah V, Shah PS. Periventricular/intraventricular hemorrhage and neurodevelopmental outcomes: a meta-analysis. Pediatrics. 2015;136(6):1132–43. https://doi.org/10.1542/peds.2015-0944.
29. Tortora D, Martinetti C, Severino M, Uccella S, Malova M, Parodi A, Brera F, Morana G, Ramenghi LA, Rossi A. The effects of mild germinal matrix-intraventricular haemorrhage on the developmental white matter microstructure of preterm neonates: a DTI study. Eur Radiol. 2018;28(3):1157–66. https://doi.org/10.1007/s00330-017-5060-0.
30. Argyropoulou MI, Astrakas LG, Xydis VG, Drougia A, Mouka V, Goel I, Giapros V, Andronikou S. Is low-grade intraventricular hemorrhage in very preterm infants an innocent condition? Structural and functional evaluation of the brain reveals regional neurodevelopmental abnormalities. AJNR Am J Neuroradiol. 2020;41(3):542–7. https://doi.org/10.3174/ajnr.A6438.
31. Uccella S, Parodi A, Calevo MG, Nobili L, Tortora D, Severino M, Andreato C, Rossi A, Ramenghi LA; Eu-Brain Neonatal Group. Influence of isolated low-grade intracranial haemorrhages on the neurodevelopmental outcome of infants born very low birthweight. Dev Med Child Neurol. 2023. https://doi.org/10.1111/dmcn.15559. Online ahead of print.
32. Leijser LM, Miller SP, van Wezel-Meijler G, Brouwer AJ, Traubici J, van Haastert IC, Whyte HE, Groenendaal F, Kulkarni AV, Han KS, Woerdeman PA, Church PT, Kelly EN, van Straaten HLM, Ly LG, de Vries LS. Posthemorrhagic ventricular dilatation in preterm infants: when best to intervene? Neurology. 2018;90(8):e698–706. https://doi.org/10.1212/WNL.0000000000004984.
33. Cizmeci MN, de Vries LS, Tataranno ML, Zecic A, van de Pol LA, Alarcon A, Groenendaal F, Woerdeman PA. Intraparenchymal hemorrhage after serial ventricular reservoir taps in neonates with hydrocephalus and association with neurodevelopmental outcome at 2 years of age. J Neurosurg Pediatr. 2021;28(6):695–702. https://doi.org/10.3171/2021.6.PEDS21120.
34. Cizmeci MN, Groenendaal F, van der Aa NE, Vandewouw MM, Young JM, Han K, Benders MJNL, Taylor MJ, de Vries LS, Woerdeman PA. Corpus callosum injury after neurosurgical intervention for posthemorrhagic ventricular dilatation and association with neurodevelopmental outcome at 2 years. J Neurosurg Pediatr. 2022;30(1):1–8. https://doi.org/10.3171/2022.2.PEDS21577.
35. Soltirovska Salamon A, Groenendaal F, van Haastert IC, Rademaker KJ, Benders MJ, Koopman C, de Vries LS. Neuroimaging and neurodevelopmental outcome of preterm infants with a periventricular haemorrhagic infarction located in the temporal or frontal lobe. Dev Med Child Neurol. 2014;56(6):547–55. https://doi.org/10.1111/dmcn.12393.

36. Rademaker KJ, Groenendaal F, Jansen GH, Eken P, de Vries LS. Unilateral haemorrhagic parenchymal lesions in the preterm infant: shape, site and prognosis. Acta Paediatr. 1994;83(6):602–8. https://doi.org/10.1111/j.1651-2227.1994.tb13089.x.
37. Cizmeci MN, Groenendaal F, Liem KD, van Haastert IC, Benavente-Fernández I, van Straaten HLM, Steggerda S, Smit BJ, Whitelaw A, Woerdeman P, Heep A, de Vries LS, ELVIS study group. Randomized controlled early versus late ventricular intervention study in posthemorrhagic ventricular dilatation: outcome at 2 years. J Pediatr. 2020b;226:28–35. https://doi.org/10.1016/j.jpeds.2020.08.014.
38. Roze E, Benders MJ, Kersbergen KJ, van der Aa NE, Groenendaal F, van Haastert IC, Leemans A, de Vries LS. Neonatal DTI early after birth predicts motor outcome in preterm infants with periventricular hemorrhagic infarction. Pediatr Res. 2015;78(3):298–303. https://doi.org/10.1038/pr.2015.94.
39. de Bijl-Marcus K, Brouwer AJ, de Vries LS, Groenendaal F, Wezel-Meijler GV. Neonatal care bundles are associated with a reduction in the incidence of intraventricular haemorrhage in preterm infants: a multicentre cohort study. Arch Dis Child Fetal Neonatal Ed. 2020;105(4):419–24. https://doi.org/10.1136/archdischild-2018-316692.
40. Lai GY, Abdelmageed S, DeRegnier RO, Gaebler-Spira D, Dizon MLV, Lam SK. Degree of ventriculomegaly predicts school-aged functional outcomes in preterm infants with intraventricular hemorrhage. Pediatr Res. 2021a;91(5):1238–47. https://doi.org/10.1038/s41390-021-01631-2.
41. Lai GY, Chu-Kwan W, Westcott AB, Kulkarni AV, Drake JM, Lam SK. Timing of temporizing neurosurgical treatment in relation to shunting and neurodevelopmental outcomes in posthemorrhagic ventricular dilatation of prematurity: a meta-analysis. J Pediatr. 2021b;234:54–64.e20. https://doi.org/10.1016/j.jpeds.2021.01.030.
42. Park YS, Kotani Y, Kim TK, Yokota H, Sugimoto T, Nakagawa I, Motoyama Y, Nakase H. Efficacy and safety of intraventricular fibrinolytic therapy for post-intraventricular hemorrhagic hydrocephalus in extreme low birth weight infants: a preliminary clinical study. Childs Nerv Syst. 2021;37(1):69–79. https://doi.org/10.1007/s00381-020-04766-5.
43. Schaumann A, Bührer C, Schulz M, Thomale UW. Neuroendoscopic surgery in neonates—indication and results over a 10-year practice. Childs Nerv Syst. 2021;37(11):3541–8. https://doi.org/10.1007/s00381-021-05272-y.
44. Ahn SY, Chang YS, Sung SI, Park WS. Mesenchymal stem cells for severe intraventricular hemorrhage in preterm infants: phase 1 dose-escalation clinical trial. Stem Cells Transl Med. 2018;7(12):847–56. https://doi.org/10.1002/sctm.17-0219.

Cerebellar Hemorrhage

Gerda Meijler and Sylke J. Steggerda

Abbreviations

CBH   Cerebellar hemorrhage
MRI   Magnetic resonance imaging
NICU   Neonatal intensive care unit

G. Meijler (✉)
Department of Neonatology, Isala Women and Children's Hospital, Zwolle, The Netherlands
e-mail: gmeijler@gmail.com

S. J. Steggerda
Department of Pediatrics, Division of Neonatology, Willem-Alexander Children's Hospital,
Leiden University Medical Center (LUMC), Leiden, The Netherlands
e-mail: S.J.Steggerda@lumc.nl

© The Author(s) 2024
G. Meijler, K. Mohammad (eds.), *Neonatal Brain Injury*,
https://doi.org/10.1007/978-3-031-55972-3_4

4.1 For Parents

The cerebellum is also called the "little brain." It consists of two halves (the hemispheres), connected in the middle by a structure called the cerebellar vermis. It is positioned below the cerebrum and behind the brain stem (Fig. 4.1).

The mature cerebellum consists of less than 10% of the total brain volume. However, it contains more than 80% of all the brain's neurons (the brain cells that are connected to other neurons and that transmit information).

It is a very important brain structure for fine-tuning movements (balance and coordination). It also has an important role in many aspects of development, including behavior, emotions, learning, and language. The development of the cerebellum extends over a long period: it starts very early in fetal life and continues into infancy. In the second half of gestation, development is very fast, and during this rapid development, the cerebellum is especially vulnerable to injury. Therefore, children who are born prematurely have the highest risk of cerebellar injury.

4.1.1 How Will I Know If My Baby Has Symptoms of Cerebellar Injury?

Hemorrhage (or bleed) is the most common type of cerebellar injury. Hemorrhages can be small (so-called punctate cerebellar hemorrhages), larger (so-called limited

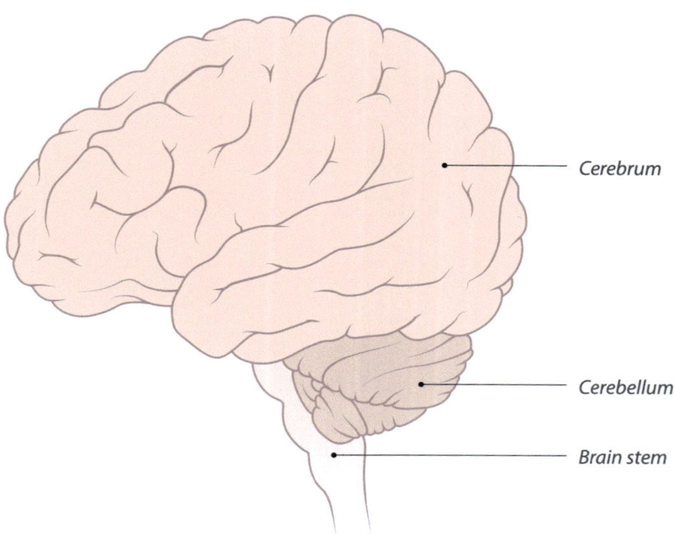

Fig. 4.1 The position of the cerebellum in relation to the cerebrum and brain stem. (© Amanda Gautier-Ronopawiro)

cerebellar hemorrhages), or even very large (also known as massive), involving much or most of the cerebellum.

Cerebellar hemorrhage mostly develops within the first 3 days after birth. The punctate and limited cerebellar hemorrhages usually cause no symptoms. The more rarely occurring massive cerebellar hemorrhages may cause symptoms such as agitation, apneic spells (short periods of absent or very superficial breathing), and blood pressure fluctuations. Cranial ultrasound scans are routinely performed in all babies born very prematurely. The limited and massive hemorrhages can be detected with cranial ultrasound. Cerebellar hemorrhages are recognized as more or less rounded white areas (whiter than the surrounding, healthy cerebellar tissue) within the cerebellar region. After a few weeks, these lesions tend to become darker than the surrounding, normal tissue. Even later, the affected part of the cerebellum may show signs of underdevelopment and impaired growth as compared to the unaffected tissue. Punctate hemorrhages are more difficult to detect with ultrasound but are often seen on MRI scans in preterm babies. These punctate hemorrhages can be a chance finding on MRI scans that are done for other reasons, such as neurological symptoms, other ultrasound abnormalities, or extreme prematurity. The punctate hemorrhages occur in around 20–25% of babies born before 28 weeks gestation. In infants with larger, ultrasound detected cerebellar hemorrhages, the neonatologist may recommend an MRI scan to obtain a more detailed view of cerebellar growth and development and of the rest of the brain.

4.1.2 Why Did My Baby Develop Cerebellar Hemorrhage?

As with most brain injuries in premature infants, there is no single cause for cerebellar hemorrhage. Doctors and other professionals therefore rather talk about risk factors.

Risk factors for cerebellar hemorrhage are prematurity as such: the more premature the baby, the higher the risk. In our experience, very premature infants who additionally are growth retarded (small for gestational age) have the highest risk. Other factors are a difficult delivery, respiratory problems needing artificial ventilation, unstable blood pressure, and serious infections. In all these circumstances, the very vulnerable and abundant small blood vessels at the cerebellar surface may rupture, thus causing hemorrhage within or around the cerebellar tissue.

4.1.3 What Is the Treatment If My Baby Is Diagnosed with Cerebellar Hemorrhage?

Except for gentle handling and individualized breathing support, which is applied in most NICUs, little can be done to prevent these cerebellar hemorrhages from occurring. And once they have occurred, there is no treatment for this complication.

It is, however, important to follow infants with larger cerebellar hemorrhages well into childhood and to give them individualized help and care such as physiotherapy or speech therapy and behavioral assessments and interventions if they develop problems. The earlier these interventions are started, the better, as the young brain can adapt very well.

4.1.4 What Will Happen to My Baby (Prognosis)?

If there are no other brain lesions, most infants with only punctate cerebellar hemorrhages or a limited cerebellar hemorrhage will have a favorable outcome. The infants with a massive cerebellar hemorrhage have a higher risk of developing motor, learning, and/or behavioral problems. Fortunately, these massive hemorrhages are rare. As mentioned before, close follow-up after discharge and early intervention with physiotherapy and other interventions, such as occupational therapy and speech therapy, may help to improve long-term outcome.

4.2 For Professionals

4.2.1 Development and Pathogenesis

The human cerebellum undergoes a protracted development, starting in the early embryonic period and extending into infancy [1, 2].

During the second half of gestation, the cerebellum is the fastest-growing structure in the human fetal brain. Between 24 and 40 weeks gestation, its volume increases fivefold [1, 3–5], and the transcerebellar diameter (TCD) doubles between 25 and 35 weeks gestation [6].

As a result of massive cell proliferation within the so-called external granular layer, which reaches a peak early in the third trimester of pregnancy, foliation increases exponentially during the fetal period (Fig. 4.2), and therefore the surface area of the cerebellar cortex increases more than 30-fold from 24 weeks gestation to term [1, 7, 8]. This is also a period of active migration and establishment of neuronal connectivity [1].

The external granular layer (a highly cellular and vascularized developmental layer of the cerebellum) is a transient structure that covers the complete cerebellar surface and is most prominent between 28 weeks gestation and 1–2 months post-term. From the external granular layer, granular cells proliferate and migrate inward to form the internal granular layer, and from there they connect with other cells both within and outside the cerebellum [1, 9, 10] Fig. 4.3.

Myelination starts much earlier (around 25 weeks gestation) in the cerebellum than in the supratentorial brain (around term age) [11–13].

Due to the combination of rapid growth and development during the fetal period and the presence of extensive, vulnerable layers (including the external granular layer), the immature cerebellum is very vulnerable to injury.

In preterm infants, cerebellar injury is mostly hemorrhagic [8, 14, 15].

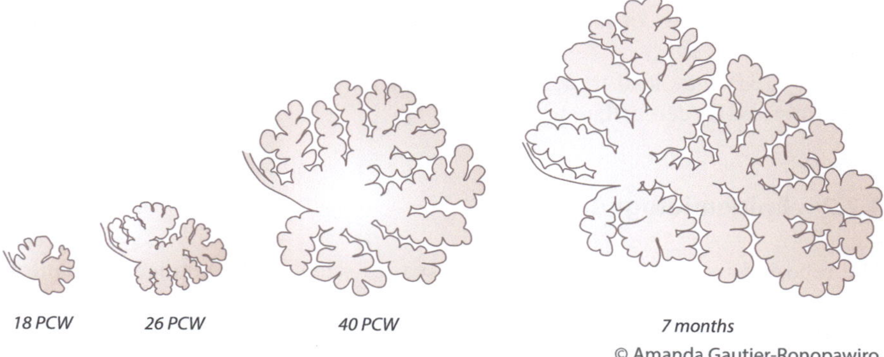

Fig. 4.2 The rapid increase of the cerebellar surface during the fetal period and infancy, due to extensive foliation. *PCW* postconceptional weeks (the last drawing represents the situation at 7 months postnatally). (© Amanda Gautier-Ronopawiro)

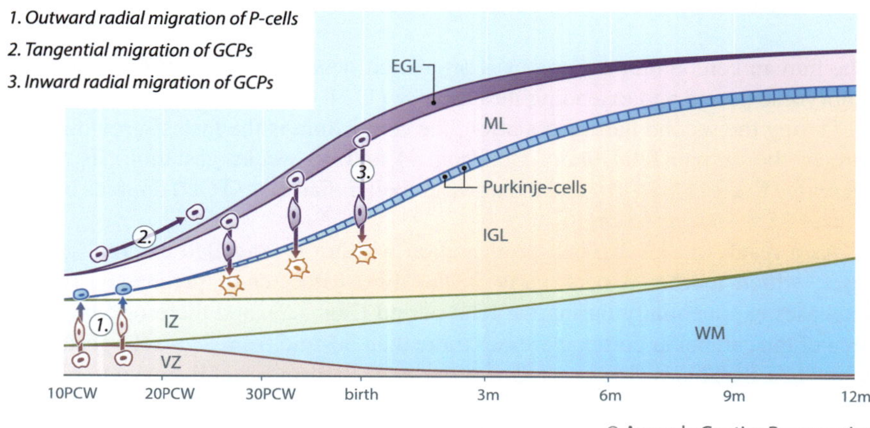

Fig. 4.3 Proliferation and migration from the cerebellar external granular layer. *P-cells* Purkinje cells, *GCPs* granule cell precursors, *IGL* internal granular layer, *ML* molecular layer, *EGL* external granular layer, *VZ* ventricular zone, *IZ* intermediate zone, *WM* white matter. (© Amanda Gautier-Ronopawiro)

Like supratentorial germinal matrix-intraventricular hemorrhage, preterm cerebellar hemorrhage (CBH) also originates from fragile developmental layers in the brain: the extensive external granular layer and/or the germinal matrix of the fourth ventricle and the rapidly developing internal granular layer [16]. Contributing factors are similar to those for supratentorial germinal matrix-intraventricular hemorrhage and include (extreme) prematurity and circulatory and respiratory failure [8, 17, 18].

In some cases CBH is caused by traumatic delivery through laceration of the cerebellum or rupture of the cerebellar bridging veins, which may lead to massive hemorrhage [17, 19].

Large CBH may lead to destruction of the cerebellar parenchyma and is thus often followed by cerebellar atrophy [15–17].

4.2.2 Epidemiology/Incidence

The reported incidence of preterm CBH varies widely. The youngest, smallest, and sickest infants are at greatest risk [14]. Small, punctate CBH are common in preterm infants [15, 20–23]. The incidence of larger, ultrasound detected CBH (see below) ranges between 3 and 9% in very low-birthweight infants [14, 21, 24, 24]. The largest and most destructive hemorrhages occur mainly in extremely preterm (<25 weeks gestation) and/or extremely low-birthweight (<750 g) infants, with reported incidences as high as 15% in these tiny infants [14, 24].

4.2.3 Clinical Signs and Diagnosis

CBH can be classified according to size (see below). The smallest, punctate (grade 1) lesions and the medium-sized, limited (grade 2) lesions rarely cause symptoms, although some infants may show some nonspecific symptoms such as restlessness or irritability and/or may have apneic spells. Grade 1 and 2 CBH are therefore mostly a chance ultrasound or MRI finding (Figs. 4.4 and 4.5). Large, massive (grade 3) CBH may cause serious symptoms, including respiratory and circulatory failure, irritability, and decreased consciousness [17].

Most CBH are diagnosed by neuro-imaging (ultrasound and/or MRI). Punctate CBH are not reliably detected by ultrasound and therefore generally a chance MRI finding [21, 22, 25–27]. The presence of punctate CBH can still be underestimated on conventional MRI. It is therefore recommended to add T2*-weighted or susceptibility-weighted sequences that improve the detection of these small lesions, as these sequences also show small hemosiderin depositions in tissue (Fig. 4.4) [28, 29]. Larger (grade 2 and 3) CBH can be visualized by ultrasound, especially when the mastoid fontanel is used as an additional acoustic window [21, 30, 27, 31] (Figs. 4.5 and 4.6).

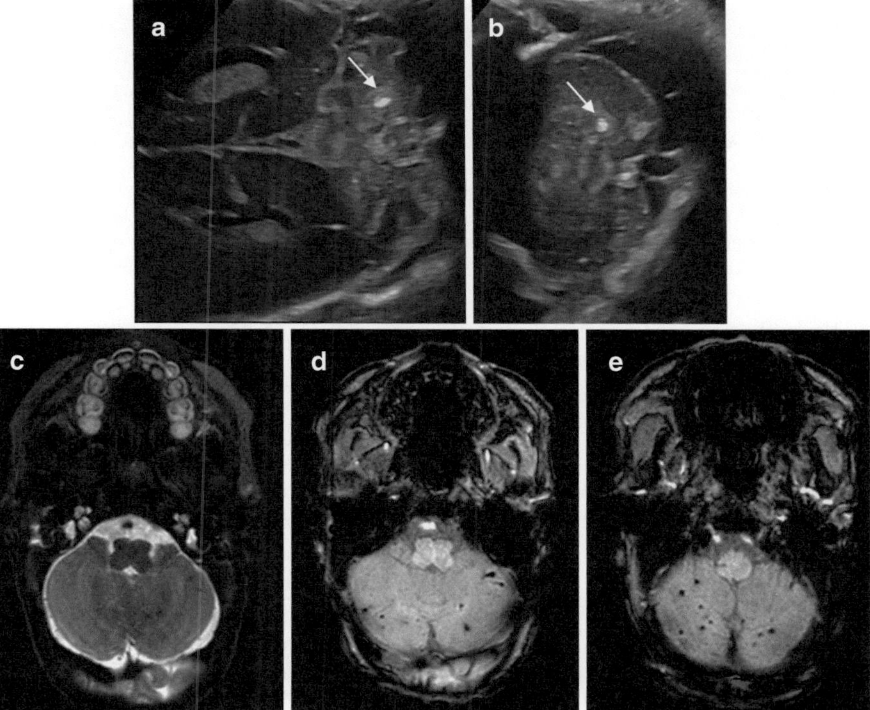

Fig. 4.4 Ultrasound images (**a** coronal, **b** axial) through mastoid fontanel of a likely punctate CBH (arrow) in a very preterm infant, scanned 1 week after birth. T2-weighted (**c**) and susceptibility weighted (**d, e**) transverse MR images performed at term equivalent age confirmed the presence of multiple punctate CBH (not all were visible on the initial ultrasound scan)

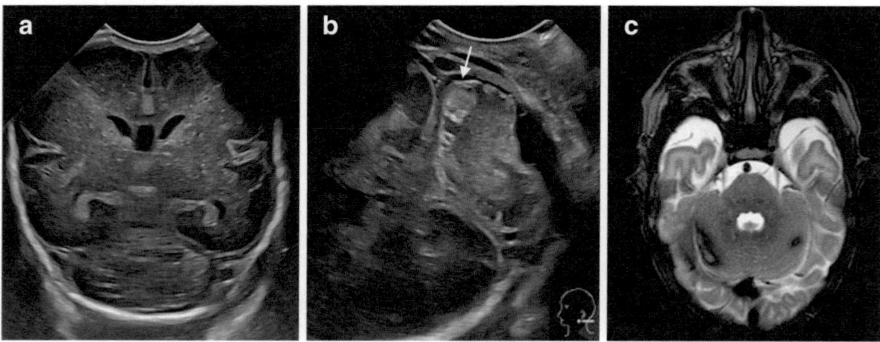

Fig. 4.5 Coronal ultrasound images (through anterior **a** and right mastoid fontanel **b**) at 3 days after birth and T2-weighted MRI image (**c**) at term equivalent age of grade 2 CBH on the right and smaller CBH on the left in in a preterm infant. The larger hemorrhage in the right cerebellar hemisphere (arrow) is visible from the right mastoid fontanel view (**b**) but not on the anterior fontanel view. The smaller hemorrhage in the left hemisphere was not detected on ultrasound

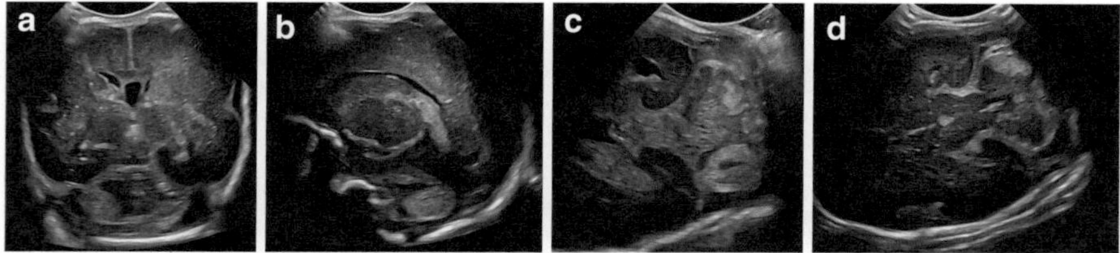

Fig. 4.6 Grade 3 CBH. Ultrasound images (**a** coronal, **b** para-sagittal, **c** and **d** coronal planes) at postnatal day 3 through anterior **a** and **b**, left mastoid fontanel **c**, and right mastoid fontanel **d** in an extremely preterm infant. The ultrasound images clearly show the large CBH in the right cerebellar hemisphere, which was already detected through the anterior fontanel. No MRI was performed

Recently we introduced a classification for CBH, depending on the size and extent [27, 32]:

- Grade 0: Normal echogenicity/signal intensity of the cerebellar vermis and hemispheres with normal anatomic features. No signs of destruction or atrophy.
- Grade 1: Small (<4 mm) focal, punctate lesion(s) in the cerebellar parenchyma. These punctate lesions are usually not detected by ultrasound but are a frequent finding on MRI performed in preterm infants. There is usually no atrophy on follow-up ultrasound or MRI (see Fig. 4.4).
- Grade 2: Limited CBH, larger than a punctate lesion (≥4 mm), but involving at the most one third of a cerebellar hemisphere. Usually, these lesions involve the lateral or inferior convexity of the cerebellar hemisphere(s). They can be detected by cranial ultrasound, especially when mastoid fontanel views are performed and proper settings are used. On follow-up scans focal cystic evolution or atrophy may be seen, involving again at the most one third of the affected cerebellar hemisphere (see Fig. 4.5).

- Grade 3: Extensive CBH, involving more than one third of the cerebellar hemisphere. They are easily detected with ultrasound. These lesions lead to obvious volume reduction of the cerebellar hemisphere on follow-up imaging (see Fig. 4.6).

4.2.4 Treatment

Preventive measures of CBH are similar to those of germinal matrix and intraventricular hemorrhage and consist of maintaining circulatory and respiratory stability, thus avoiding rapid fluctuations in cerebral blood flow. Antenatal administration of corticosteroids and magnesium sulfate may be protective [32]. Once CBH has developed, treatment is no longer possible, but maintaining stability is crucial to prevent further extension of the bleed. In the case of massive CBH and/or hemorrhage into the fourth ventricle, frequent follow-up imaging with cranial ultrasound is required to screen for the development of posthemorrhagic ventricular dilatation as this may have therapeutic consequences. Follow-up imaging is also important to assess possible subsequent cerebellar atrophy and/or destruction. Long-term follow-up of these infants is needed for the early detection of disabilities and to enable early interventions.

4.2.5 Prognosis (Table 4.1)

Cerebellar injury is increasingly recognized as a severe complication of preterm birth with possibly serious consequences for neurodevelopmental outcome [17, 24, 32, 34–37].

Table 4.1 Prognosis [17, 23, 30, 25, 31, 33–39]

cUS and/or MRI finding	Prognosis[a]
No abnormalities	Favorable if no supratentorial injury
Punctate (grade 1) CBH	Favorable if no cerebellar volume loss and no supratentorial injury
Limited (grade 2) CBH	Small risk of motor, cognitive, and/or behavioral problems, depending on location, laterality, vermis involvement, and size of lesion[a]
Massive (grade 3) CBH	High risk of motor and cognitive impairment and behavioral problems[a]
Cerebellar volume loss around TEA	Risk of motor and cognitive impairment and behavioral problems

[a]Prognosis depends on total volume and location of the cerebellar lesion(s), laterality and vermis involvement (higher risk of impairment with bilateral and/or vermis involvement), deeper extension of lesions into cerebellar tissue, volume loss of the cerebellar tissue, and on presence of supratentorial injury. Risks of impairments are influenced by multiple factors, such as lower gestational age and weight, prematurity-related morbidity, and required interventions. The table provides an indication, but risk needs to be assessed on an individual patient basis

Cerebellar injury may not only affect motor outcome but also cognitive and behavioral development [32, 35, 38, 39].

While grade 1 CBH in the absence of severe supratentorial injury is associated with favorable outcome [25, 26, 32, 40], grade 3 CBH (massive or extensive CBH) has a much less favorable prognosis even after correction for supratentorial injury and is associated with motor, cognitive, and behavioral problems [24, 32, 35, 38, 39, 41]. Involvement of the vermis carries a risk of behavioral problems and autism [35], while lesions in the medial anterior lobe are associated with motor impairment [24]. In a recent study, the outcome of infants with CBH was related to the above classification. Infants with grade 3 CBH had a high risk of abnormal outcome, while infants with grade 1 and 2 CBH had a comparable, generally more favorable outcome. The risk of abnormal outcome at 2 years corrected age increased with the size of the CBH [32]. In a systematic review, Hortensius et al. reported the highest incidence of abnormal outcome in infants with extensive bleeds and/or vermis involvement [38].

Estimation of prognosis in infants with CBH remains challenging, as there is often concomitant or associated supratentorial injury and as CBH mainly occurs in the sickest and smallest infants.

References

1. du Plessis AJ, Whitehead MT, Volpe JJ. Normal and abnormal development of the posterior fossa structures. Chapter 4 In: Volpe's Neurology of the Newborn. 7th edition, 2025
2. ten Donkelaar HJ, Lammens M, Wesseling P, Thijssen HO, Renier WO. Development and developmental disorders of the human cerebellum. J Neurol. 2003;250(9):1025–36.
3. Chang CH, Chang FM, Yu CH, Ko HC, Chen HY. Assessment of fetal cerebellar volume using three-dimensional ultrasound. Ultrasound Med Biol. 2000;26(6):981–8.
4. Limperopoulos C, du Plessis AJ. Disorders of cerebellar growth and development. Curr Opin Pediatr. 2006;18(6):621–7.
5. Clouchoux C, Guizard N, Evans AC, du Plessis AJ, Limperopoulos C. Normative fetal brain growth by quantitative in vivo magnetic resonance imaging. Am J Obstet Gynecol. 2012;206(2):173e171–8.
6. Triulzi F, Parazzini C, Righini A. MRI of fetal and neonatal cerebellar development. Semin Fetal Neonatal Med. 2005;10(5):411–20.
7. Rakic P, Sidman RL. Histogenesis of cortical layers in human cerebellum, particularly the lamina dissecans. J Comp Neurol. 1970;139(4):473–500.
8. Volpe JJ. Cerebellum of the premature infant: rapidly developing, vulnerable, clinically important. J Child Neurol. 2009;24(9):1085–104.
9. Ten Donkelaar HJ, Lammens M. Development of the human cerebellum and its disorders. Clin Perinatol. 2009;36(3):513–30.
10. Hadders-Algra M. Early human brain development: starring the subplate. Neurosci Biobehav Rev. 2018;92:276–90.
11. Gilles FH. Myelination in the neonatal brain. Hum Pathol. 1976;7(3):244–8.
12. Sie LT, van der Knaap MS, van Wezel-Meijler G, Valk J. MRI assessment of myelination of motor and sensory pathways in the brain of preterm and term-born infants. Neuropediatrics. 1997;28(2):97–105.
13. Counsell SJ, Maalouf EF, Fletcher AM, Duggan P, Battin M, Lewis HJ, Herlihy AH, Edwards AD, Bydder GM, Rutherford MA. MR imaging assessment of myelination in the very preterm brain. AJNR Am J Neuroradiol. 2002;23(5):872–81.

14. Limperopoulos C, Benson CB, Bassan H, Disalvo DN, Kinnamon DD, Moore M, Ringer SA, Volpe JJ, du Plessis AJ. Cerebellar hemorrhage in the preterm infant: ultrasonographic findings and risk factors. Pediatrics. 2005;116(3):717–24.
15. Steggerda SJ, Leijser LM, Wiggers-de Bruine FT, van der Grond J, Walther FJ, van Wezel-Meijler G. Cerebellar injury in preterm infants: incidence and findings on US and MR images. Radiology. 2009b;252(1):190–9.
16. Haines KM, Wang W, Pierson CR. Cerebellar hemorrhagic injury in premature infants occurs during a vulnerable developmental period and is associated with wider neuropathology. Acta Neuropathol Commun. 2013;1(1):69.
17. Limperopoulos C, du Plessis AJ, Volpe JJ. Cerebellar Hemorrhage. Chapter 27. In: Volpe's Neurology of the Newborn. 7th edition, 2025
18. Villamor-Martinez E, Fumagalli M, Alomar YI, Passera S, Cavallaro G, Mosca F, et al. Cerebellar hemorrhage in preterm infants: a meta-analysis on risk factors and neurodevelopmental outcome. Front Physiol. 2019;10:800.
19. van Steenis A, Fumagalli M, Kruit MC, Peeters-Scholte CMPCD, de Vries LS, Steggerda SJ. Cranial ultrasound is an important tool in the recognition of life-threatening Infratentorial hemorrhage in newborns. Neuropediatrics. 2021;52:170–8.
20. Kidokoro H, Neil JJ, Inder TE. New MR imaging assessment tool to define brain abnormalities in very preterm infants at term. AJNR Am J Neuroradiol. 2013;34(11):2208–14.
21. Parodi A, Rossi A, Severino M, Morana G, Sannia A, Calevo MG, Malova M, Ramenghi LA. Accuracy of ultrasound in assessing cerebellar haemorrhages in very low birthweight babies. Arch Dis Child Fetal Neonatal Ed. 2015;100:F289.
22. Neubauer V, Djurdjevic T, Griesmaier E, Biermayr M, Gizewski ER, Kiechl-Kohlendorfer U. Routine magnetic resonance imaging at term-equivalent age detects brain injury in 25% of a contemporary cohort of very preterm infants. PLoS One. 2017;12(1):e0169442.
23. Boswinkel V, Kruse-Ruijter MF, Nijboer-Oosterveld J, Nijholt IM, Edens MA, Mulder-de Tollenaer SM, Smit-Wu MN, Boomsma MF, de Vries LS, van Wezel-Meijler G. Incidence of brain lesions in moderate-late preterm infants assessed by cranial ultrasound and MRI: the BIMP-study. Eur J Radiol. 2021;136:109500.
24. Zayek MM, Benjamin JT, Maertens P, Trimm RF, Lal CV, Eyal FG. Cerebellar hemorrhage: a major morbidity in extremely preterm infants. J Perinatol. 2012;32(9):699–704.
25. Tam EW, Rosenbluth G, Rogers EE, Ferriero DM, Glidden D, Goldstein RB, Glass HC, Piecuch RE, Barkovich AJ. Cerebellar hemorrhage on magnetic resonance imaging in preterm newborns associated with abnormal neurologic outcome. J Pediatr. 2011;158(2):245–50.
26. Steggerda SJ, De Bruïne FT, van den Berg-Huysmans AA, Rijken M, Leijser LM, Walther FJ, van Wezel-Meijler G. Small cerebellar hemorrhage in preterm infants: perinatal and postnatal factors and outcome. Cerebellum. 2013;12:794.
27. Meijler G, Steggerda SJ. Neonatal cranial ultrasonography. Cham: Springer; 2019.
28. Benders MJ, Kersbergen KJ, de Vries LS. Neuroimaging of white matter injury, intraventricular and cerebellar hemorrhage. Clin Perinatol. 2014 Mar;41(1):69–82.
29. de Bruïne FT, Steggerda SJ, van den Berg-Huysmans AA, Leijser LM, Rijken M, van Buchem MA, van Wezel-Meijler G, van der Grond J. Prognostic value of gradient echo T2* sequences for brain MR imaging in preterm infants. Pediatr Radiol. 2014;44(3):305–12.
30. Steggerda SJ, Leijser LM, Walther FJ, van Wezel-Meijler G. Neonatal cranial ultrasonography: how to optimize its performance. Early Hum Dev. 2009a;85(2):93–9.
31. Sehgal A, El-Naggar W, Glanc P, Asztalos E. Risk factors and ultrasonographic profile of posterior fossa haemorrhages in preterm infants. J Paediatr Child Health. 2009;45(4):215–8.
32. Boswinkel V, Steggerda SJ, Fumagalli M, Parodi A, Ramenghi LA, Groenendaal F, Dudink J, Benders MN, Knol R, de Vries LS, van Wezel-Meijler G. The CHOPIn study: a multicenter study on cerebellar hemorrhage and outcome in preterm infants. Cerebellum. 2019;18(6):989–98.
33. Gano D, et al. Antenatal exposure to magnesium sulfate is associated with reduced cerebellar hemorrhage in preterm newborns. J Pediatr. 2016;178:68–74.

34. Dyet LE, Kennea N, Counsell SJ, Maalouf EF, Ajayi-Obe M, Duggan PJ, Harrison M, Allsop JM, Hajnal J, Herlihy AH, Edwards B, Laroche S, Cowan FM, Rutherford MA, Edwards AD. Natural history of brain lesions in extremely preterm infants studied with serial magnetic resonance imaging from birth and neurodevelopmental assessment. Pediatrics. 2006;118(2):536–54.
35. Limperopoulos C, Bassan H, Gauvreau K, Robertson RL Jr, Sullivan NR, Benson CB, Avery L, Stewart J, Soul JS, Ringer SA, Volpe JJ, duPlessis AJ. Does cerebellar injury in premature infants contribute to the high prevalence of long-term cognitive, learning, and behavioral disability in survivors? Pediatrics. 2007;120(3):584–93.
36. Messerschmidt A, Fuiko R, Prayer D, Brugger PC, Boltshauser E, Zoder G, Sterniste W, Weber M, Birnbacher R. Disrupted cerebellar development in preterm infants is associated with impaired neurodevelopmental outcome. Eur J Pediatr. 2008;167:1141.
37. Bednarek N, Akhavi A, Pietrement C, Mesmin F, Loron G, Morville P. Outcome of cerebellar injury in very low birth-weight infants: 6 case reports. J Child Neurol. 2008;23(8):906–11.
38. Brossard-Racine M, du Plessis AJ, Limperopoulos C. Developmental cerebellar cognitive affective syndrome in ex-preterm survivors following cerebellar injury. Cerebellum. 2015;14(2):151–64.
39. Hortensius LM, Dijkshoorn ABC, Ecury-Goossen GM, Steggerda SJ, Hoebeek FE, Benders M, Dudink J. Neurodevelopmental consequences of preterm isolated cerebellar hemorrhage: a systematic review. Pediatrics. 2018;142(5):e20180609.
40. Garfinkle J, Guo T, Synnes A, Chau V, Branson HM, Ufkes S, Tam EWY, Grunau RE, Miller SP. Location and size of preterm cerebellar hemorrhage and childhood development. Ann Neurol. 2020;88:1095–108.
41. Stoodley CJ. The cerebellum and neurodevelopmental disorders. Cerebellum. 2016;15(1):34–7.

White Matter Injury

5

Gerda Meijler and Lara M. Leijser

Abbreviations

cPVL	Cystic periventricular leukomalacia
cUS	Cranial ultrasound
MRI	Magnetic resonance imaging
NICU	Neonatal intensive care unit
Pre-Ols	Pre-myelinating oligodendrocytes
PVE	Periventricular echodensities
PWMLs	Punctate white matter lesions
TEA	Term equivalent age
WM	White matter
WMI	White matter injury

G. Meijler (✉)
Department of Neonatology, Isala Women and Children's Hospital, Zwolle, The Netherlands
e-mail: gmeijler@gmail.com

L. M. Leijser
Section of Newborn Critical Care, Department of Pediatrics, Cumming School of Medicine, University of Calgary, Calgary, AB, Canada
e-mail: lara.leijser@ucalgary.ca

© The Author(s) 2024
G. Meijler, K. Mohammad (eds.), *Neonatal Brain Injury*,
https://doi.org/10.1007/978-3-031-55972-3_5

5.1 For Parents

The brain consists of different tissues that each have a particular function. The tissue that forms the largest part of the brain is called white matter. This is made up of long fibers connecting one area of the brain to another forming the equivalent of an "electrical wiring" system in the brain. Each fiber originates from its nerve cell body and connects to other nerve cells. These nerve cell bodies together are called the gray matter of the brain (Fig. 5.1a). The fibers conduct electrical signals between cells. The fibers tend to group together in bundles making the conduction process more efficient. With time, a special insulating material called myelin covers the fiber bundles (Fig. 5.1b). Myelin protects the fiber bundles and increases the speed by which the electric signals can be transmitted. Much of the process of myelination of nerve fibers takes place in early infancy, and there is little myelin in the brain at term age (the due date of the baby) and even less in babies born too early (preterm, prematurely).

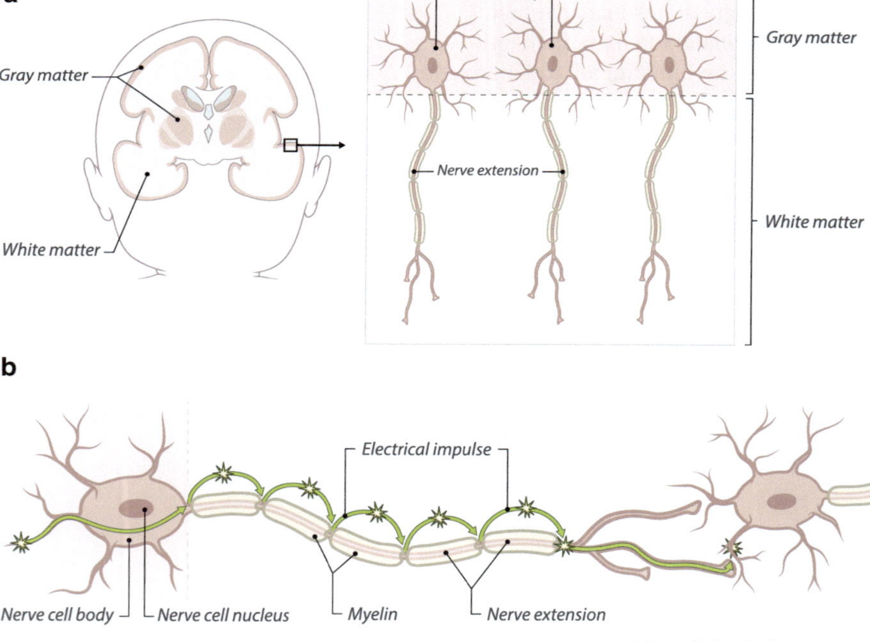

Fig. 5.1 (**a**) The brain white matter and gray matter. (**b**) Nerve cell extensions enveloped by myelin which increases the speed of signal conduction. (© Amanda Gautier-Ronopawiro)

5.1.1 How Will I Know If My Baby Has Symptoms of White Matter Injury?

In babies born too early (preterm, prematurely), injury to the white matter can develop anytime between birth and the due birth date, depending on the condition of the baby. Occasionally it may even develop before birth. White matter injury mostly develops gradually and rarely causes symptoms while the baby is still in the hospital. After a few weeks, babies may become somewhat restless, they may also show signs of abnormal muscle tone, and their movements may be less fluent than usual. Babies with more severe white matter injury may even develop seizures.

As most babies do not show symptoms, white matter injury is usually detected by imaging the brain using cranial ultrasound. Cranial ultrasound scans are routinely performed in all babies born very prematurely. On cranial ultrasound, changes in the white matter are seen as brighter areas (called echogenic) within an intermediate gray background of normally appearing white matter, looking like bright "clouds" (called abnormal echogenicities) within an otherwise clear light gray sky, and, when seen, scans are repeated more often to check if they remain visible. When they are present for only a short time (a few days), they are generally without consequence, but if they last longer, over weeks, or are patchy in appearance, some babies will develop small areas of damage or even small holes (cysts), resulting from the breakdown of the previously bright brain tissue. If the cysts are numerous and/or large, they cause reduced and disturbed brain growth.

In babies with persisting white matter abnormality on ultrasound scans, the neonatologist will probably also recommend an MRI scan of the brain, to get a more detailed view of the white matter changes and the brain growth and development. This MRI scan is typically performed around the time the baby was due to be born—this is frequently referred to as term-equivalent age.

5.1.2 Why Did My Baby Develop White Matter Injury?

In babies that are born too early, the cells that are responsible for making myelin are still immature. As a result, the nerve fibers do not yet have a myelin cover, and they function less efficiently and are more vulnerable to infection or a low oxygen content in the blood than the white matter of babies that are born full term. In addition, the blood vessels that run through the white matter and provide oxygen to the brain are still immature and fragile. If preterm babies are sick and unstable, there can be changes in the amount of blood and oxygen going to the brain. Infection, more frequently occurring in preterm than in full-term babies, can also cause injury to the developing white matter. Consequently, the brain of preterm babies, and especially the white matter, is vulnerable to injury.

5.1.3 What Is the Treatment If My Baby Is Diagnosed with White Matter Injury?

Unfortunately, there is as yet no specific treatment for white matter injury. As is also true for preterm babies without brain injury, the doctors and nurses want to keep the baby as stable as possible, to optimize and stabilize the blood and oxygen supply to the brain. They also prevent infections as much as possible and will treat infections promptly with antibiotics.

Restless babies may benefit from physical contact and/or swaddling, while babies who develop seizures will be treated with anti-seizure medicines. In babies with abnormal muscle tone, physiotherapy will be started early, even while the baby is still in the hospital. In some neonatal units, physiotherapy is even started based on the ultrasound findings, while there are no symptoms yet (see below).

5.1.4 What Will Happen to My Baby (Prognosis)?

Although a baby's development is also influenced by other factors, patchy abnormalities (the abnormal echogenicities) in the white matter that persist may have consequences later in life, such as motor (movement), learning, visual, and behavioral problems. These possible consequences depend on the extent and location of the injury within the white matter—something that is important to determine from the scans. Babies with many cysts are at the highest risk for problems later in life: they may develop cerebral palsy, visual impairment, learning and behavioral problems, and epilepsy. Fortunately, nowadays, cysts in the white matter are not commonly seen anymore.

When white matter injury is detected with ultrasound and/or MRI of the brain during the baby's stay in the NICU, interventions such as physiotherapy, occupational therapy or speech therapy can be started while the baby is still in the hospital or as soon as the baby is discharged home. Such early intervention can help babies develop as optimally as possible, leading to a better long-term outcome.

The interventions will usually be continued after discharge. Therefore, repeated ultrasound examinations of the brain are standard care when a preterm infant is admitted to the NICU and sometimes after discharge.

5.2   For Professionals

5.2.1   Pathogenesis

The white matter of preterm infants is vulnerable to injury, which is related to the brain's immaturity, pregnancy and birth complications, as well as early exposure to the extra-uterine environment. First, the immature vascularization of the white matter with arterial border zones in the periventricular area likely contributes to the susceptibility of the periventricular white matter to ischemia [1, 2]. Second, the immature oligodendrocytes (so-called pre-myelinating oligodendrocytes or pre-OLs) that are abundantly present in the immature white matter of preterm infants are susceptible to hypoxia-ischemia and inflammation. Ischemic or inflammatory insults may lead to injury or selective death of pre-OLs and, subsequently, to prohibit the maturation of pre-OLs to more mature oligodendrocytes. Mature oligodendrocytes are key to normal brain development, including myelination. Maturational arrest of pre-OLs may thus result in hypomyelination [1, [2]. Third, inflammation may lead to increased release of cytokines and activation of microglial cells. The cytokines are toxic to oligodendrocytes and neuronal lineage cells, while activated microglia may play a role in cortical dysmaturation [1, 3–5]. Finally, the immaturity of the autoregulation of the cerebral blood flow, thus the lack of compensation for changes in systemic blood pressure and flow, contributes to the vulnerability of the immature white matter.

Based on current knowledge, three forms of white matter injury (WMI) can be distinguished: focal (macroscopic) cystic necrosis, focal microscopic necrosis and diffuse non-necrotic injury [2, 4, 6–8]. All forms of WMI tend to be symmetrical. Focal cystic necrosis, representing cystic WMI, is the most severe form of WMI. Until recently, it was known as cystic periventricular leukomalacia (cPVL). Focal cystic necrosis is characterized by coagulation necrosis, degeneration of astrocytes and microglial activation [6, 9, 10]. The cystic lesions are generally bilateral and mostly symmetrical and most often seen at the trigones of the lateral ventricles and around the occipital horns but also in the frontal white matter [6, 11].

Focal microscopic WMI probably represents a milder form of WMI. The lesions are caused by focal necrosis, resulting from microglial and axonal degeneration, and often lead to areas of gliosis [6, 11].

Diffuse WMI is characterized by diffuse gliosis, without focal necrosis. The lesions are characterized by diffuse astrocytosis and microglial activation and relate to injury to the pre-OLs [6, 11, 12] (see also Chap. 1). Therefore, the distribution of vulnerable pre-OLs and timing of the insult in preterm infants seem crucial to the development of this form of WMI with relative sparing of other glial cell elements and axons [6, 11].

A clear distinction between the different forms of WMI, relevant to prognostication, cannot always be made. Brain pathology studies have shown that diffuse WMI and focal microscopic lesions are often seen in conjunction [11, 12]. Also, in very preterm infants (<32 weeks gestation), WMI is often associated with gray matter injury [4, 10, 13].

5.2.2 Epidemiology/Incidence

WMI (the now preferred terminology over periventricular leukomalacia) is the most frequently detected type of brain injury in very preterm infants. It is present in about 50% of infants born very prematurely and probably accounts for most of the motor, cognitive, and behavioral impairments encountered in this population [14]. Fortunately, macroscopic cystic WMI (cPVL), the form of WMI with the most severe implications for long-term outcome, is rarely seen nowadays [15–17]. The marked decrease in the incidence of cPVL is related to improvements in perinatal and neonatal care, such as the widespread use of antenatal corticosteroids to accelerate lung maturation and reducing inflammation, and less invasive, more individualized respiratory and hemodynamic support [15, 18, 19]. Applying neuroprotection care bundles also contributes to the prevention of severe brain injury in very preterm infants [20].

Non-cystic WMI is, however, seen more frequently in very preterm infants [2, 4, 13, 15, 21, 22]. It is detected in the vast majority of preterm infants with WMI as assessed with MRI [15, 17, 23, 24].

5.2.3 Clinical Signs and Diagnosis

WMI seldom causes symptoms during the neonatal period. However, infants with serious (cystic) WMI may be restless and irritable and/or may already show disturbances in tone or develop seizures. In most infants, the diagnosis is made with cUS. WMI mostly affects both hemispheres with a more or less symmetrical pattern (unlike hemorrhagic venous white matter infarction). Cystic WMI (or cPVL) is well detected with serial cranial ultrasound (cUS) (Chap. 14). It mostly starts with inhomogeneous increased echogenicity (also called abnormal flaring or abnormal periventricular echodensities [PVE]) of the periventricular white matter [15, 21, 25–28]. It should be noted that certain homogeneous PVE or flares represent normal maturational changes in the preterm infant's brain ([29, 30], Chap. 8).

Abnormal PVE may either resolve spontaneously over a variable period (thus representing transient changes or less severe WMI) or gradually evolve into cystic lesions over a period of 2–3 weeks and, in some cases with smaller focal cysts, up to 6 weeks. White matter cysts are well detected with cUS if the examinations are optimally timed and repeated sufficiently often (Fig. 5.2).

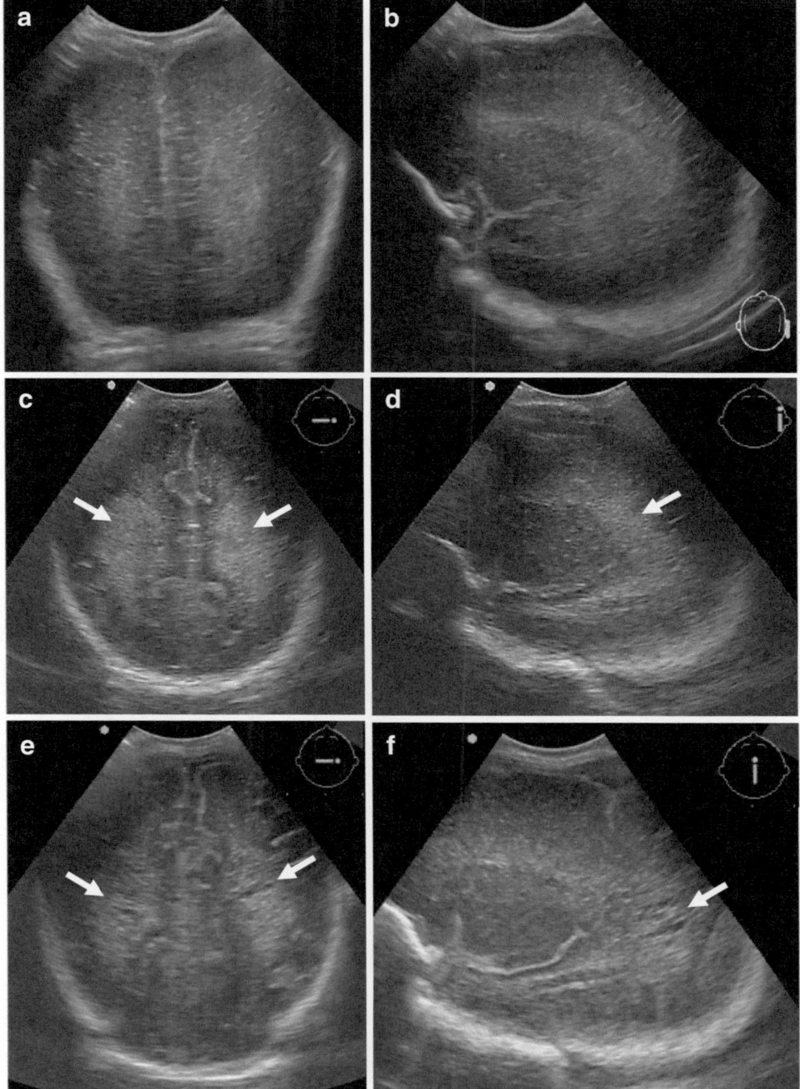

Fig. 5.2 (**a**) and (**b**) Coronal and parasagittal cUS images, respectively, performed in a very preterm infant, showing homogeneous, physiological echogenicity in the white matter. (**c–f**) cUS examination in a very preterm infant with postnatal infection and respiratory failure. (**c**) Coronal cUS image through the parieto-occipital lobes and (**d**) parasagittal image through the right hemisphere, showing mildly abnormal, inhomogeneous PVE in the parietal, occipital and temporal white matter (arrows). (**e**) Coronal and (**f**) parasagittal cUS images, performed 4 weeks later showing mostly symmetrical small cystic lesions (cystic WMI, cPVL; arrows). Also showing mild widening of the subarachnoidal space, representing white matter tissue loss. It is important to realize that extensive cystic WMI (cPVL) is a rare condition and that most abnormal PVE will either gradually disappear over time or will evolve into small, localized cystic lesions, as in this example. At 3 years corrected age, the child is microcephalic and has developed mild spastic diplegia (walking independently), is irritable with sleeping problems and has delayed speech development. Visual development is normal

However, if the cUS examinations are not well timed, the intervals between serial examinations are too long, or examinations are discontinued too early (before the natural evolution of cysts), the cystic stages of WMI may be missed. Fluid within the WM cysts is gradually absorbed over time, and small cysts mostly become invisible before term-equivalent age (TEA) [28, 31–33]. White matter volume loss will ensue, showing as irregularly shaped, (mildly) enlarged lateral ventricles (so-called ex vacuo ventricular dilatation), thinning of the corpus callosum, and widening of the subarachnoid spaces [15, 28, 32, 34, 35] (Fig. 5.3). Often the thalamic volume is also reduced. The signs of white matter volume loss are best seen around TEA, both on cUS and MRI. It should be noted that white matter volume loss can also occur in cases with WMI without cystic degeneration.

It is important to not confuse ex vacuo ventricular dilation with ventricular dilatation resulting from impaired drainage (outflow obstruction) and/or reabsorption of cerebrospinal fluid following an intraventricular hemorrhage or meningitis. In the latter, the shape of the lateral ventricles is more rounded, and the ventricular walls are less irregular (see Chap. 3).

In preterm infants WMI may develop at any time during the neonatal period, especially following complications such as sepsis, necrotizing enterocolitis,

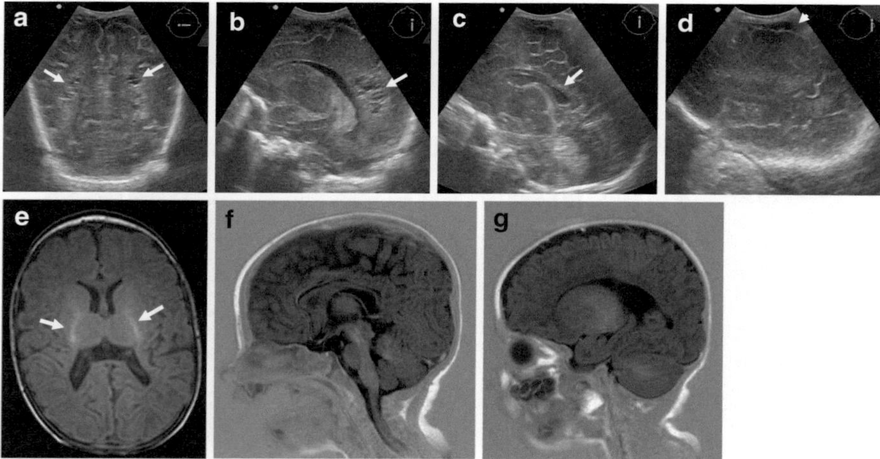

Fig. 5.3 (a) Coronal and (b) parasagittal cUS scan in very preterm and growth-restricted infant, scanned 4 weeks postnatally, showing extensive bilateral cystic lesions in the periventricular white matter (cWMI; arrows). (c) Midsagittal and (d) parasagittal cUS scan of the same infant scanned around TEA, showing wide subarachnoid space (arrowhead), irregular and thinned corpus callosum posteriorly (arrow), and coarse gyri due to volume loss. MRI performed around TEA in the same infant. (e) Axial, (f) midsagittal, and (g) parasagittal T1-weighted MR images of the same infant after TEA (2 months corrected age), showing irregular ventricular dilatation, thinning of the posterior part of the corpus callosum, wide subarachnoid spaces, and small thalami. The posterior limb of the internal capsules (PLIC) (arrows) is myelinated on both sides. At 2 years of age, the child has developed mild bilateral spastic cerebral palsy, but is able to walk independently. There are behavioral problems and cerebral visual impairment. The child is treated at a rehabilitation center

hemodynamic significant patent ductus arteriosus, and/or neonatal surgery. Therefore, serial cUS should be continued throughout the neonatal period, up to TEA, and be intensified after such complications.

Cystic WMI needs to be differentiated from the cystic stage of periventricular hemorrhagic infarction (see Chap. 3), which is mostly unilateral or evidently asymmetrical.

As mentioned above, abnormal PVE (Fig. 5.4) may also resolve over time (mostly days to weeks) without evolution into cystic lesions and no longer be detectable on cUS.

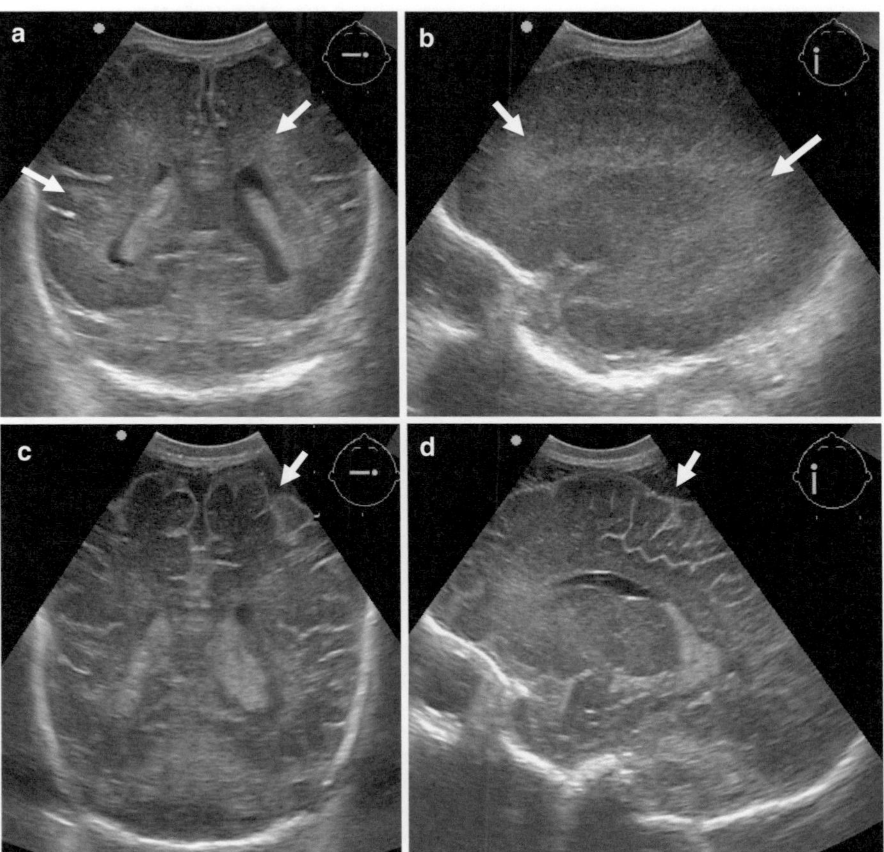

Fig. 5.4 cUS scans in very preterm infant with lung hypoplasia and respiratory failure. (**a**) and (**b**) Coronal and parasagittal scans, respectively, showing partially inhomogeneous PVE (arrows). cUS examinations were frequently repeated over the neonatal period. The abnormal PVE persisted over a longer period of time (>1 week), but cystic lesions were not detected. (**c**) and (**d**) Coronal and sagittal cUS, respectively, performed at TEA show wide subarachnoid spaces (arrows), mildly irregular shape of the lateral ventricle and coarse gyration, indicating WM volume loss. No parental consent for TEA MRI was obtained. At 5.5 years of age, the child has global psychomotor delay and behavioral problems, receives special education, and is enrolled in a rehabilitation program. The child did not develop cerebral palsy

Transient PVEs are considered a less severe form of WMI and probably represent focal microscopic necrosis [36]. When brain MRI is performed at the time inhomogeneous PVEs are seen on cUS, punctate white matter lesions (PWMLs) are often seen in the same areas [28, 32, 35]. PWMLs are small lesions in the white matter, often localized around the lateral ventricles, that tend to disappear over time [37] (Fig. 5.5). In some cases, PWMLs result in glial scarring that may be recognized at TEA with cUS, but are best seen with MRI and better on T1-than T2-weighted imaging [32, 35, 37] (Fig. 5.6).

In some preterm infants, serial cUS may be unremarkable, while MRI shows white matter changes, such as inhomogeneous signal intensity changes within the periventricular WM on T2-weighted images (Fig. 5.7) and/or PWML.

While smaller lesions can be detected with modern, high-quality ultrasound systems, cUS is not sensitive enough for reliable detection of diffuse or subtle WMI without punctate lesions or cysts [21, 28].

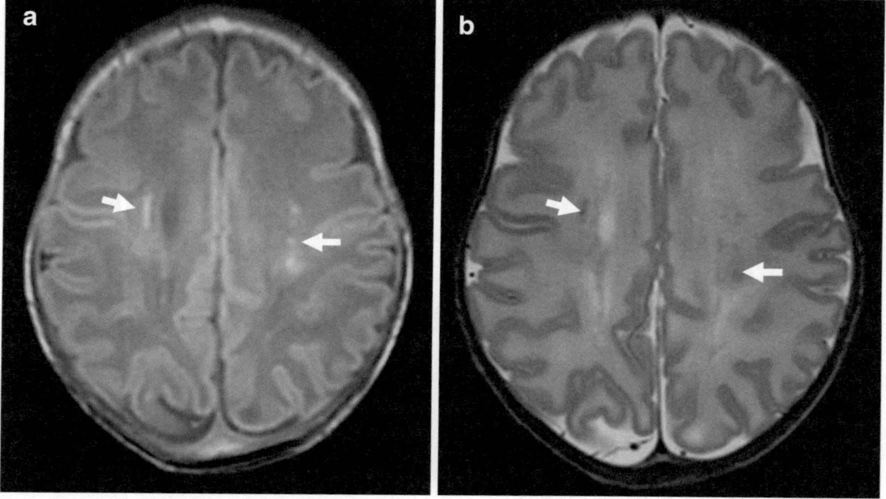

Fig. 5.5 Brain MRI performed around TEA in very preterm infant with chronic lung disease. cUS scans had shown patchy PVE. (**a**) Axial T1-weighted image at high ventricular level, showing small areas of increased signal intensity, representing punctate white matter lesions (PWMLs) (arrows). (**b**) Corresponding T2-weighted image, showing the same lesions as decreased signal intensity (arrows). PWMLs are mostly better depicted on T1-weighted images. There were no other abnormalities seen and the PLIC was normally myelinated. At 2 years corrected age, there was a mild fine motor delay, but the child was otherwise developing normally. Physiotherapy was started

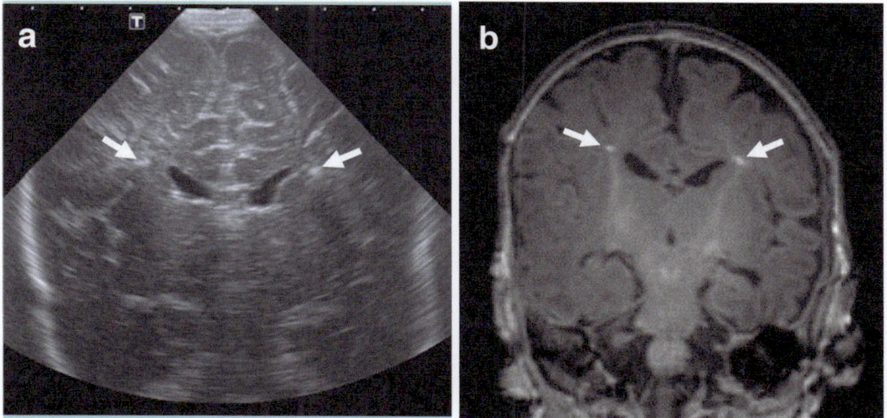

Fig. 5.6 (**a**) Coronal cUS and (**b**) coronal T1-weighted MRI scan in very preterm infant, scanned at TEA, showing mild gliosis (arrows) with both techniques. Myelination of the posterior limb of the internal capsules (PLIC) is somewhat poor but not absent. This child developed mild cerebral palsy and is walking independently

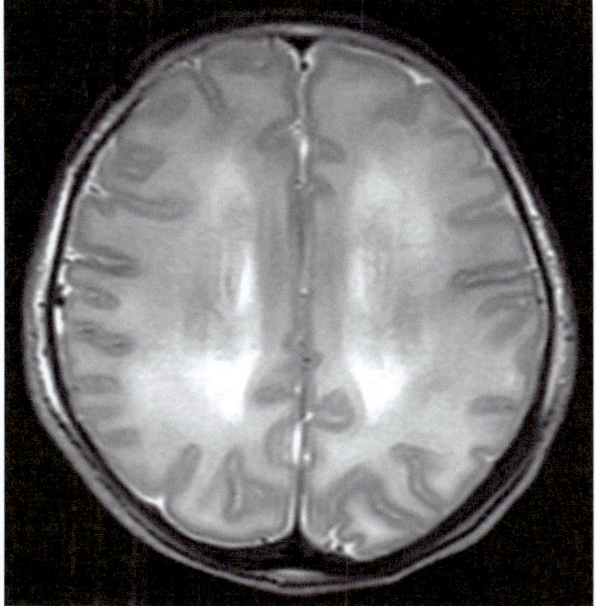

Fig. 5.7 T2-weighted axial MR image at a high ventricular level in a late preterm infant with hypoxic-ischemic encephalopathy. MRI scan performed at 39 weeks postmenstrual age shows increased signal intensity in the white matter, mainly around the trigones of the lateral ventricles and in the frontal white matter. At 2 years of age, the child has a mild motor delay

5.2.4 Treatment

Although trials of stem cell and erythropoietin treatment are being undertaken, at present no treatment is known to reduce WMI [15, 38]. Therefore, the focus of neuroprotective strategies in preterm infants lies on the prevention of WMI through avoidance of sudden changes in cerebral blood flow, hypocarbia, neuroinflammation, hypoglycemia, and hypoxic-ischemic events [15, 20]. This can be achieved with measures such as maintaining the infant hemodynamically and respiratory stable, prevention of maternal and neonatal infections, prompt treatment of infections, hypoglycemia, and apneic spells, and application of neonatal care bundles [20].

Optimizing nutrition and pain management also contribute to the prevention of (further deterioration of) this condition [8, 15].

Symptoms, such as irritability and seizures, should be treated accordingly. Early interventions, including physiotherapy and speech therapy, may improve functional outcome [15, 39].

5.2.5 Prognosis (Table 5.1)

Severe WMI is strongly associated with adverse long-term outcomes, and the presence and severity of disabilities are related to the severity and extent of the white matter changes. Infants with extensive cystic WMI, leading to significant white matter volume loss, almost invariably develop severe motor problems (e.g. spastic diplegia), often combined with cognitive and behavioral problems, epilepsy, and visual impairment later in life [15, 18, 19, 40–42, 44–48]. Infants with small, more localized WMI, including only a few small cysts, may also develop cerebral palsy. However, the incidence and severity of cerebral palsy in these infants are considerably less than in infants with extensive WMI [15, 17, 36, 37, 43, 44, 49–52].

While infants with subtle or diffuse WMI may experience later cognitive and/or behavioral problems, they may also have a normal outcome [14, 36, 53–57]. Prognostication remains uncertain on an individual basis, especially for babies with milder forms of WMI.

Table 5.1 Prognosis [15, 36, 40–43]

cUS finding	Conjunctive MRI finding (Look at site and extension of lesions and PLIC myelination)	Prognosis[a]
No WM abnormalities	No WM abnormalities	Favorable
No WM abnormalities or inhomogeneous PVE	<6 PWMLs	Up to 10% risk of CP and/or mild motor delay
Inhomogeneous PVE	≥6 PWMLs	Up to 10% risk of CP and/or mild motor delay (especially if PLIC not well myelinated and/or lesions adjacent to the CST)[b]
Persistent, inhomogeneous PVE, followed by small, focal cystic lesions	Small, focal cystic lesions	60–80% risk of (mostly mild) CP (especially if PLIC not well myelinated and/or lesions adjacent to the CST)[b]. CP unlikely if lesions only present in frontal white matter ±50% risk of (mild) cognitive impairment
Small, focal periventricular WM cystic lesions	Small, focal periventricular cystic WM lesions or ex vacuo dilation and/or punctate glial scars	High (up to 80%) risk of (mostly mild) CP (especially if PLIC not well myelinated and/or lesions adjacent to the CST)[b], ± 50% risk of (mild) cognitive impairment
More extensive cystic WM lesions with volume loss at TEA	More extensive cystic WM lesions with volume loss at TEA	High (up to 90%) risk of more severe CP[b]; high risk of cognitive, behavioral, and/or visual impairment
Extensive cystic lesions, also in the deep white matter	Extensive cystic lesions, also in the deep white matter	Very high risk of CP and severe cognitive, behavioral, and visual impairments

WM white matter, *PWML* punctate white matter lesion, *CP* cerebral palsy, *CST* corticospinal tract, *SI* signal intensity, *PVE* periventricular echodensities, *TEA* term-equivalent age

[a]Noted risks are based on the average occurrence of deficits across the very preterm population. However, risks are influenced by multiple factors, such as lower gestational age and weight, prematurity-related morbidity, and required interventions. The severity of deficits can span the spectrum from mild to severe. The table thus provides an indication, but risk needs to be assessed on an individual patient basis

[b]If cysts do not involve the corticospinal tracts and myelination is normal in the posterior limb of the internal capsule (PLIC) at term age, there is a high chance of a normal motor outcome [41]

References

1. Back SA and Volpe JJ. Encephalopathy of Prematurity: Pathophysiology. Chapter 19. In Volpe's Neurology of the Newborn. 7th edition, 2025
2. Khwaja O, Volpe JJ. Pathogenesis of cerebral white matter injury of prematurity. Arch Dis Child Fetal Neonatal Ed. 2008;93:F153–61.
3. Verney C, Pogledic I, Biran V, et al. Microglial reaction in axonal crossroads is a hallmark of noncystic periventricular white matter injury in very preterm infants. J Neuropathol Exp Neurol. 2012;71:251–64.
4. Back SA, Miller SP. Brain injury in premature neonates: a primary cerebral dysmaturation disorder? Ann Neurol. 2014;75:469–86.

5. Volpe JJ. Dysmaturation of premature brain: importance, cellular mechanisms, and potential interventions. Pediatr Neurol. 2019;95:42–66.
6. Encephalopathy of Prematurity: Neuropathology. Chapter 18. In: Volpe's Neurology of the Newborn. 7th Edition, 2025
7. Schneider J, Miller SP. Preterm brain injury: white matter injury. Handb Clin Neurol. 2019;162:155–72.
8. Guillot M, Miller SP. The dimensions of white matter injury in preterm infants. Semin Perinatol. 2021;45:151469.
9. Banker BQ, Larroche JC. Periventricular leukomalacia of infancy. A form of neonatal anoxic encephalopathy. Arch Neurol. 1962;7:386–410.
10. Pierson CR, Folkerth RD, Billiards SS, et al. Gray matter injury associated with periventricular leukomalacia in the premature infant. Acta Neuropathol. 2007;114:619–31.
11. Back SA. White matter injury in the preterm infant: pathology and mechanisms. Acta Neuropathol. 2017;134(3):331–49.
12. Buser JR, Maire J, Riddle A, et al. Arrested preoligodendrocyte maturation contributes to myelination failure in premature infants. Ann Neurol. 2012;71:93–109.
13. Volpe JJ. Brain injury in premature infants: a complex amalgam of destructive and developmental disturbances. Lancet Neurol. 2009a;8:110–24.
14. Volpe JJ. The encephalopathy of prematurity—brain injury and impaired brain development inextricably intertwined. Semin Pediatr Neurol. 2009b;16(4):167–78.
15. Inder TE and Volpe JJ. Encephalopathy of the Preterm-Clinical Aspects. Chapter 20. In: Volpe's Neurology of the Newborn. 7th Edition, 2025
16. Hintz SR, Barnes PD, Bulas D, et al. Neuroimaging and neurodevelopmental outcome in extremely preterm infants. Pediatrics. 2015;135:e32–42.
17. Guo T, Duerden EG, Adams E, et al. Quantitative assessment of white matter injury in preterm neonates: association with outcomes. Neurology. 2017;88:614–22.
18. Hamrick SE, Miller SP, Leonard C, et al. Trends in severe brain injury and neurodevelopmental outcome in premature newborn infants: the role of cystic periventricular leukomalacia. J Pediatr. 2004;145:593–9.
19. van Haastert IC, Groenendaal F, Uiterwaal CSPM, et al. Decreasing incidence and severity of cerebral palsy in prematurely born children. J Pediatr. 2011;159:86–91.
20. Murthy P, Zein H, Thomas S, et al. Neuroprotection care bundle implementation to decrease acute brain injury in preterm infants. Pediatr Neurol. 2020;110:42–8.
21. Leijser LM, de Bruïne FT, van der Grond J, et al. Is sequential cranial ultrasound reliable for detection of white matter injury in very preterm infants? Neuroradiology. 2010;52(5): 397–406.
22. Leijser LM, Srinivasan L, Rutherford MA, et al. Frequently encountered cranial ultrasound features in the white matter of preterm infants: correlation with MRI. Eur J Paediatr Neurol. 2009b;13(4):317–26.
23. Gano D, Andersen SK, Partridge JC, et al. Diminished white matter injury over time in a cohort of premature newborns. J Pediatr. 2015;166(1):39–43.
24. Wagenaar N, Chau V, Groenendaal G, et al. Clinical risk factors for punctate white matter lesions on early magnetic resonance imaging in preterm newborns. J Pediatr. 2017;182:34–40.
25. de Vries LS, Eken P, Dubowitz LM. The spectrum of leukomalacia using cranial ultrasound. Behav Brain Res. 1992;49(1):1–6.
26. Sie LT, van der Knaap MS, van Wezel-Meijler G, et al. Early MR features of hypoxic-ischemic brain injury in neonates with periventricular densities on sonograms. AJNR Am J Neuroradiol. 2000;21(5):852–61.
27. van Wezel-Meijler G, de Bruïne FT, Steggerda SJ, et al. Ultrasound detection of white matter injury in very preterm neonates: practical implications. Dev Med Child Neurol. 2011;53:29–34.
28. Agut T, Alarcon A, Cabañas F, et al. Preterm white matter injury: ultrasound diagnosis and classification. Pediatr Res. 2020;87(Suppl 1):37–49.
29. Leijser LM, de Bruine FT, Steggerda SJ, et al. Brain imaging findings in very preterm infants throughout the neonatal period: part I. Incidences and evolution of lesions, comparison between ultrasound and MRI. Early Hum Dev. 2009a;85:101–9.

30. Meijler G, Steggerda SJ. Maturational changes of the neonatal brain. Chapter 8. In: Meijler G, Steggerda SJ, editors. Neonatal cranial ultrasonography. 3rd ed. Berlin: Springer; 2019a. p. 195–217.
31. Sarkar S, Shankaran S, Laptook AR, et al. Cranial imaging at multiple time points improves cystic periventricular leukomalacia detection. Am J Perinatol. 2015;32(10):973–9.
32. de Vries LS, Benders MJ, Groenendaal F. Imaging the premature brain: ultrasound or MRI? Neuroradiology. 2013;55(Suppl 2):13–22.
33. Meijler G, Steggerda SJ. Timing of ultrasound examinations. Chapter 5. In: Meijler G, Steggerda SJ, editors. Neonatal cranial ultrasonography. 3rd ed. Berlin: Springer; 2019b. p. 85–136.
34. Horsch S, Muentjes C, Franz A, Roll C. Ultrasound diagnosis of brain atrophy is related to neurodevelopmental outcome in preterm infants. Acta Paediatr. 2005;94(12):1815–21.
35. Benders MJ, Kersbergen KJ, de Vries LS. Neuroimaging of white matter injury, intraventricular and cerebellar hemorrhage. Clin Perinatol. 2014;41(1):69–82.
36. Inder TE, de Vries LS, Ferriero DM, et al. Neuroimaging of the preterm brain: review and recommendations. J Pediatr. 2021;237:276–87.
37. Kersbergen KJ, Benders MJ, Groenendaal F, et al. Different patterns of punctate white matter lesions in serially scanned preterm infants. PLoS One. 2014;9(10):e108904.
38. Vaes JEG, Vink MA, De Thije CGM, et al. The potential of stem cell therapy to repair white matter injury in preterm infants: lessons learned from experimental models. Front Physiol. 2019;10:540.
39. Spittle A, Orton J, Anderson PJ, et al. Early developmental intervention programmes provided post hospital discharge to prevent motor and cognitive impairment in preterm infants. Cochrane Database Syst Rev. 2015;2015:CD005495.
40. de Vries LS, van Haastert IL, Rademaker KJ, et al. Ultrasound abnormalities preceding cerebral palsy in high-risk preterm infants. J Pediatr. 2004;144(6):815–20.
41. Martinez-Biarge M, Groenendaal F, Kersbergen K, et al. Neurodevelopmental outcomes in preterm infants with white matter injury using a new MRI classification. Neonatology. 2019;116:227–35.
42. Rees P, Callan C, Chadda KR, et al. Preterm brain injury and neurodevelopmental outcomes: a meta-analysis. Pediatrics. 2022;150:e2022057442.
43. Cayam-Rand D, et al. Predicting developmental outcomes in preterm infants. A simple white matter injury imaging rule. Neurology. 2019;93:e1231–40.
44. de Vries LS, Eken P, Groenendaal F, et al. Correlation between the degree of periventricular leukomalacia diagnosed using cranial ultrasound and MRI later in infancy in children with cerebral palsy. Neuropediatrics. 1993;24(5):263–8.
45. Wilkinson I, Bear J, Smith J, et al. Neurological outcome of severe cystic periventricular leukomalacia. J Paediatr Child Health. 1996;32(5):445–9.
46. Leijser LM, Liauw L, Veen S, et al. Comparing brain white matter on sequential cranial ultrasound and MRI in very preterm infants. Neuroradiology. 2008;50(9):799–811.
47. de Vries LS, van Haastert IC, Benders MJ, Groenendaal F. Myth: cerebral palsy cannot be predicted by neonatal brain imaging. Semin Fetal Neonatal Med. 2011;16(5):279–87.
48. Skiöld B, Hallberg B, Vollmer B, et al. A novel scoring system for term-equivalent-age cranial ultrasound in extremely preterm infant. Ultrasound Med Biol. 2019;45(3):786–94.
49. Resch B, Vollaard E, Maurer U, et al. Risk factors and determinants of neurodevelopmental outcome in cystic periventricular leucomalacia. Eur J Pediatr. 2000;159(9):663–70.
50. Pierrat V, Duquennoy C, van Haastert IC, et al. Ultrasound diagnosis and neurodevelopmental outcome of localised and extensive cystic periventricular leucomalacia. Arch Dis Child Fetal Neonatal Ed. 2001;84(3):F151–6.
51. Sarkar S, Shankaran S, Barks J, et al. Outcome of preterm infants with transient cystic periventricular leukomalacia on serial cranial imaging up to term equivalent age. J Pediatr. 2018;195:59–65.
52. de Bruïne FT, van den Berg-Huysmans AA, Leijser LM, et al. Clinical implications of MR imaging findings in the white matter in very preterm infants: a 2-year follow-up study. Radiology. 2011;261(3):899–906.

53. van Wezel-Meijler G, van der Knaap MS, Oosting J, et al. Predictive value of neonatal MRI as compared to ultrasound in premature infants with mild periventricular white matter changes. Neuropediatrics. 1999;30(5):231–8.

54. Sie LT, Hart AA, van Hof J, et al. Predictive value of neonatal MRI with respect to late MRI findings and clinical outcome. A study in infants with periventricular densities on neonatal ultrasound. Neuropediatrics. 2005;36(2):78–89.

55. Woodward LJ, Anderson PJ, Austin NC, et al. Neonatal MRI to predict neurodevelopmental outcomes in preterm infants. N Engl J Med. 2006;355(7):685–94.

56. Dyet LE, Kennea N, Counsell SJ, et al. Natural history of brain lesions in extremely preterm infants studied with serial magnetic resonance imaging from birth and neurodevelopmental assessment. Pediatrics. 2006;118(2):536–48.

57. Woodward LJ, Clark CA, Bora S, Inder TE. Neonatal white matter abnormalities an important predictor of neurocognitive outcome for very preterm children. PLoS One. 2012;7(12):e51879.

Arterial Infarction in Preterm Infants

6

Sylke J. Steggerda and Frances M. Cowan

Abbreviations

Baby CIMT	Constraint-induced movement therapy for babies
CP	Cerebral palsy
GMAs	General Movements Assessment
HINE	Hammersmith Infant Neurological Examination
NAIS	Neonatal arterial ischemic stroke
MCA	Middle cerebral artery
PAIS	Perinatal arterial ischemic stroke
PLIC	Posterior limb of the internal capsule
RCT	Randomized controlled trial
TEA	Term-equivalent age

S. J. Steggerda
Department of Pediatrics, Division of Neonatology, Willem-Alexander Children's Hospital,
Leiden University Medical Center (LUMC), Leiden, The Netherlands
e-mail: S.J.Steggerda@lumc.nl

F. M. Cowan (✉)
Department of Paediatrics, Imperial College London, London, UK
e-mail: f.cowan@imperial.ac.uk

© The Author(s) 2024
G. Meijler, K. Mohammad (eds.), *Neonatal Brain Injury*,
https://doi.org/10.1007/978-3-031-55972-3_6

6.1   For Parents

Arterial infarction, often referred to as a "stroke," is a term used to describe a localized area of tissue damage in the brain, usually but not necessarily on one side of the brain. Strokes can occur at any age, most often in older adults. But strokes can also occur in babies before birth when they are still in the womb, around the time of birth, and afterwards both in babies born at term (when expected) and those born early (preterm). They occur more commonly in some groups of babies, e.g. those with heart problems or infection or in identical twins. The term "stroke" is mainly used to mean an area of damage to brain tissue in a region that gets its blood supply from one arterial blood vessel that becomes blocked—also called perinatal or neonatal arterial ischemic stroke (PAIS and NAIS). The term stroke can also be used for brain injury associated with thrombosis in a vein or hemorrhage.

Strokes occurring around the time of birth were thought to be less common in babies born early than in babies born at term, though a recent study suggests this is not actually the case. Stroke in preterm babies is often detected on routine brain imaging done using cranial ultrasound during their stay on the neonatal unit. The stroke may appear to have occurred recently perhaps in relation to severe illness—but it also may look as if it could have occurred before birth. Most often the baby does not show any specific signs or symptoms of stroke at this time.

6.1.1   Why Did My Baby Develop a Stroke?

Few studies exist on stroke in preterm infants. One study found that having a low blood sugar was a risk factor. An abnormal heart rate pattern before birth was also a risk factor. Identical twins who share a placenta can be affected by a condition known as twin-to-twin transfusion syndrome and they are also more at risk. Stroke detected in the days and weeks after birth may occur in relation to sickness, infection, having some thrombosis (clots) or surgery. Very often we do not know exactly why the strokes happen. As with term-born babies, strokes in preterm babies seldom occur again.

6.1.2   What Will Happen to My Baby?

The long-term effects (outcome) of stroke depend on which part(s) of the brain are affected and whether there are other problems present that may occur in babies born early. Strokes in preterm babies tend to occur on one side and in the central parts of the brain, but they may also affect other areas, as happens in babies born when expected. As well as regular early cranial ultrasound scanning, it is important to have good magnetic resonance (MR) brain imaging at least when the baby reaches term age to enable the best prediction for the future.

6.1.3   What Is the Treatment?

If the scans suggest that problems with movements are expected, early physiotherapy may be helpful rather than a "wait and see" approach. Importantly most babies with a stroke on one side will walk independently even if they have a problem with movement and most attend mainstream school. If the scan does not suggest that movement problems will occur, this is reassuring, though problems in other areas of development may still occur and the scan may also help in predicting these—for example, whether there is an increased risk of difficulties with learning, vision, or behavior and whether seizures (epilepsy) might occur later. Early referral for assessment by therapists should be made, as well as arrangements for long-term follow-up and support for the child and the family, well into school age.

6.2   For Professionals

Take-Home Points

Focal ischemic stroke in preterm infants
1 There is still relatively little data. Most stroke registry studies focus on full-term infants, and preterm infants are often excluded or their data is not given separately
2 The onset of the stroke in preterm infants is often later in relation to the time of birth than in full-term infants, and the onset is often asymptomatic, so easily missed
3 Awareness of the possibility of stroke in preterms especially around times of sickness, infection, and surgery is needed together with regular cranial ultrasound scanning for prompt detection
4 MRI scanning at term age gives the optimum information for prognosis

Perinatal stroke may affect the fetus, preterm, and term-born infant and be a cause of serious long-term disability. Its early and accurate detection is increasingly important because of the development of treatment options both in the neonatal period and in infancy and in a few cases because of genetic implications. Although the term "stroke" may be used to include lesions associated with cerebral sinovenous thrombosis (CSVT, see Chap. 11) and even periventricular hemorrhagic (venous) infarction (see Chap. 3), this chapter is limited to addressing ischemic stroke occurring within an arterial territory in preterm infants.

6.2.1   Incidence of Stroke in Preterm Infants

As with full-term infants, stroke in preterms may have occurred antenatally or may occur around the time of birth or during the neonatal period. In preterm infants occurrence sometime during the postnatal period is commonest, but some strokes are clearly present and established at birth. They are mostly referred to as perinatal arterial ischemic stroke (PAIS), but by definition this term covers a period starting at 20 weeks of pregnancy, lasting till day 7 after birth, and neonatal arterial ischemic stroke (NAIS) covers the period from birth to 28 days or up to term age in preterm infants.

The prevalence of stroke in preterm infants is not well studied [1], but in one tertiary referral center in the Netherlands, stroke was diagnosed in 7 per 1000 preterm infants born <34 weeks gestation [2]. A recent study [3] indicates that stroke in preterm infants is actually more common than in term infants (32/100,000 preterm vs. 21/100,000 term). Very often the diagnosis is made from routine cranial ultrasound examination, or if the baby has unexplained apneas and not because of seizures [3–5], unlike in full-term infants. It may occur and be detected several weeks after birth in relation to surgery, thrombosis, or the presence of long venous or arterial catheters or postnatal infection [3, 6].

6.2.2 Risk Factors and Investigations

Risk factors for neonatal stroke in preterm infants are twin-to-twin-transfusion syndrome (Fig. 6.1), abnormal intrapartum fetal heart rate pattern, neonatal hypoglycemia [2, 4, 7], and sepsis [3]. The presence of catheters and evidence of placental inflammation increase the risk of stroke, as does the presence of thrombosis (Fig. 6.2). It is recommended that cranial ultrasound scans are obtained pre- and

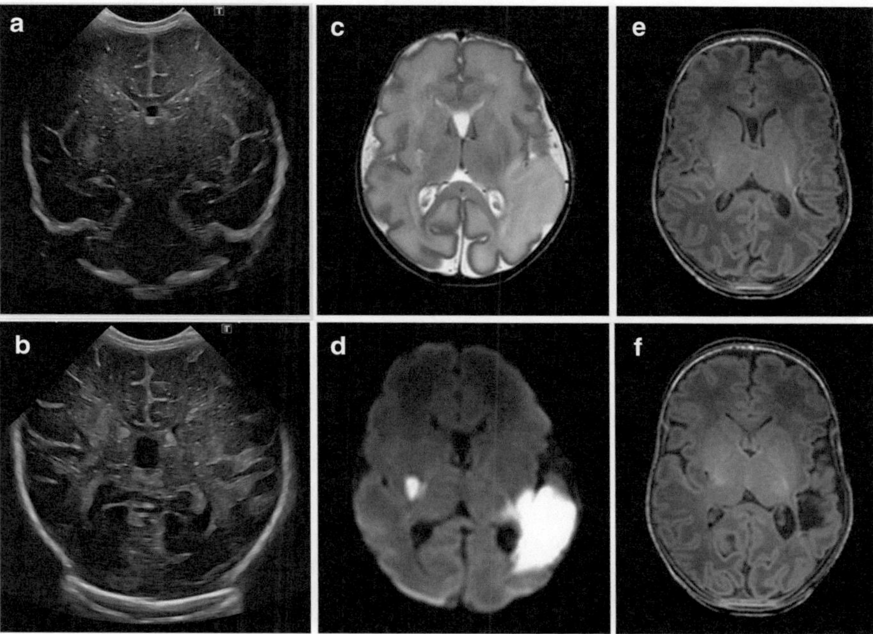

Fig. 6.1 Monochorionic twin pregnancy affected by twin-twin transfusion syndrome treated with laser ablation at the beginning of the second trimester. The twins were delivered by caesarian section at 30 weeks gestation. Apgar scores and cord pH were good. CPAP was needed only briefly and there were no neurological symptoms. Cranial ultrasound on day 4 (**a**) shows a small focus of increased echogenicity on the right in the posterior basal ganglia and (**b**) bilateral white matter echogenicity particularly on the left extending out toward the cortex. The MRI on day 5 (**c**) T2-W axial and (**d**) axial diffusion-weighted image, shows a small acute infarction in the posterior right basal ganglia adjacent to the posterior limb of the internal capsule (PLIC) which also shows abnormal signal. There is a larger stroke in the posterior left MCA territory extending to the cortex but not affecting the central gray matter or the PLIC on the T2-W image and only the very posterior part of the PLIC with minimal change in the thalamus on the diffusion-weighted image. The MRI at term-equivalent age (**e**, **f**, axial T1-W images) shows the smaller stroke on the right with tissue loss in the posterior basal ganglia and poor myelination of the PLIC predicting a left-sided hemiplegia. The lesion on the left has evolved with white matter tissue loss but relative preservation of the cortex and a normal appearance to the left PLIC and thalamus. There is tissue loss alongside the ventricle adjacent to the left optic radiation. This child developed a clear asymmetry of motor function with abnormal signs on the left quite early on, likely related to the smaller lesion on the right which was affecting the motor pathway. This child is also at risk of some asymmetry of visual field development and later epilepsy

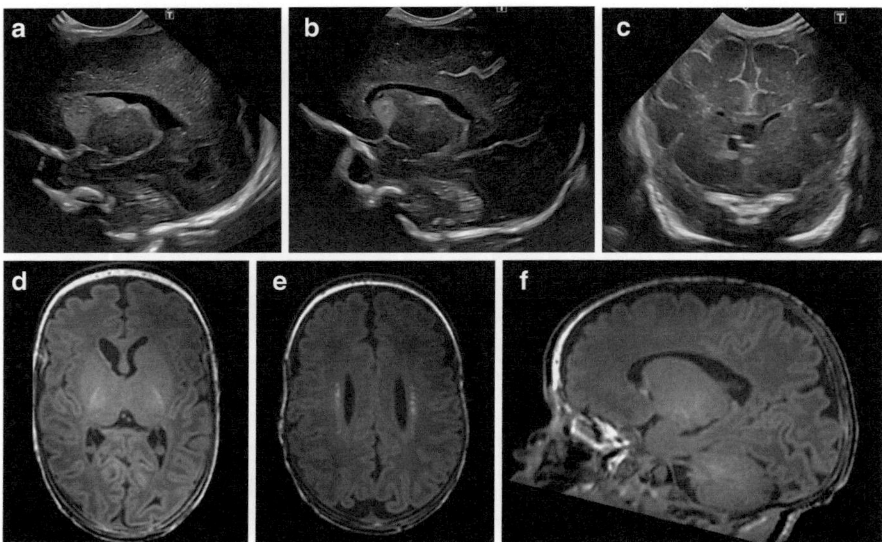

Fig. 6.2 A lenticulostriate (perforator) stroke in the right caudate nucleus in a very preterm infant, first seen on cranial ultrasound (**a**) around 2 weeks of age and 6 days after an umbilical venous cannula was removed. Cardiac evaluation showed a large thrombus in the right atrium, and low molecular weight heparin therapy was begun. The lesion became more defined at 4 weeks, (**b**), and by term-equivalent age (TEA) (**c**) a cyst had formed at the site of the stroke. The MRI at TEA (**d–f**; lower row, 2 axial and 1 sagittal T1-W images) showed atrophy at the site of the stroke, but otherwise normal basal ganglia and a normal posterior limb of the internal capsule (PLIC) on both sides, predicting a good motor outcome. However there were additional bilateral periventricular punctate white matter lesions (PWMLs) (**e**) with mild ventricular dilatation at the trigone (**f**) not uncommon in preterm infants, that might lead to a mild motor deficit. This is an example of the importance of imaging the brain at TEA, not only to assess the known lesion but also to detect other unsuspected problems that may influence outcome. This child has developed, at a relatively young age, increased tone in both lower limbs, findings likely related to the bilateral PWMLs.

post-surgery especially in infants with cardiac problems. Strokes were not more common in males in the study from Benders et al. [5], but Sorg et al. [3] found a male predominance as seen in term-born infants. Stroke is reported to be more common after recreational drug use in pregnancy [8].

Isolated causes of stroke are seldom found. Review of the placenta in infants with a stroke clearly of antenatal onset (Fig. 6.3) and a cardiac ultrasound to look for thrombus (Fig. 6.2) in those with a postnatal onset and to exclude congenital heart disease are recommended. Although in general routine thrombophilic testing is no longer recommended in cases of stroke [9], if the stroke is of antenatal onset, of an unusual pattern, associated with hemorrhage or congenital developmental abnormality on the MRI and/or ultrasound scan or there is a positive family history, one should consider both thrombophilic and genetic testing, e.g. testing for Col4A1/2 variants.

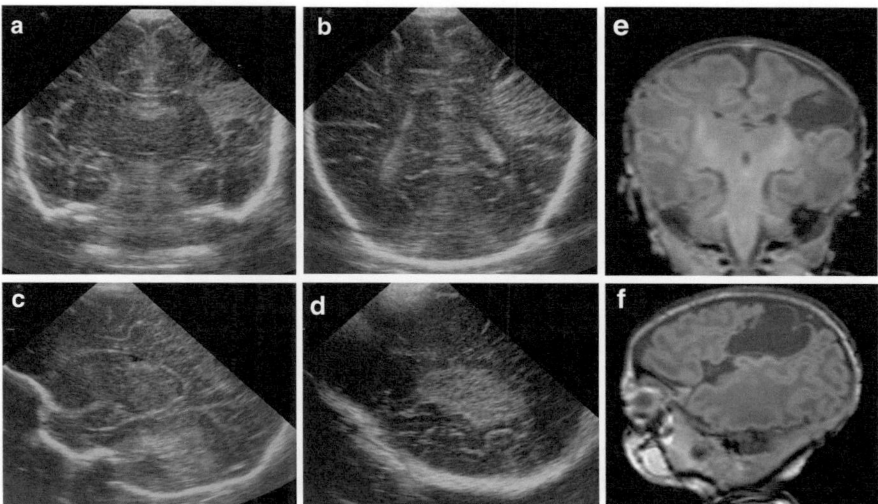

Fig. 6.3 Cranial ultrasound images (**a–d**) obtained soon after birth in a late preterm growth-retarded infant. No seizures were seen but the infant was jittery. There is a clearly defined area of increased echogenicity in the left hemisphere (**a, b, d**) in the territory of the middle cerebral artery but no involvement of the basal ganglia (**a, c**). There is no overt evidence of atrophy, and the appearances suggest an onset of stroke a week or so before birth. An MRI (T1-W coronal and parasagittal images (**e, f**) done 4 weeks later confirms a stroke and shows complete atrophy of the region but preservation of the basal ganglia and posterior limb of the internal capsule. Such rapid tissue atrophy occurs typically in newborn infants with stroke

6.2.3 Site of Stroke

An MRI brain scan is the best method for fully defining the type and extent of the stroke. If only one MRI scan is feasible then, it is best done at term-equivalent age when myelin can be seen in the posterior limb of the internal capsule (PLIC) and the cerebral peduncle in the mesencephalon. As in the term infant, it is important to determine which tissue is involved, particularly the central gray matter and the cortico-spinal tract [10]. Strokes in preterm infants are more common in the central gray matter and are often referred to as lenticulostriate or perforator strokes (Fig. 6.2), but they can occur anywhere in the brain. An isolated perforator stroke is usually easily identified using cranial ultrasound as it is in the center of the imaging field, but here too defining the site accurately is important as primary involvement of the basal ganglia and the adjacent PLIC is likely to lead to the development of a contralateral hemiplegia, whereas perforator stroke in other areas generally has a good outcome in all domains. If there is uncertainty about the extent of tissue involvement, especially the cortico-spinal tracts, a repeat MRI scan at 3 post-term months is recommended [11]. It is also important to record whether the stroke affects the optic radiation or the visual cortex [12].

In the very preterm infant, there may be preservation of a cortical rim around the area of stroke (Fig. 6.1), which is not usually seen in more mature infants. It is probably due to the stage of cerebral vascular development at the time of the insult [13]. Unfortunately this cortical sparing does not seem to confer neurodevelopmental benefit.

Stroke in the cerebellum is rare. It may be that earlier reports of cerebellar stroke in preterm infants, usually with imaging some time after the occurrence of the lesion, mainly described cases with primary cerebellar hemorrhage and secondary cystic degeneration and/or atrophy in the cerebellum rather than ischemic stroke [14] (see Chap. 4).

6.2.4 Prognosis

Similar principles in predicting outcomes to those used in term-born infants apply to the preterm—see Wagenaar et al. [10] and Chap. 9, but with the need to take into account additional effects of prematurity and other lesions the infant may sustain (Fig. 6.2).

Infants with a middle cerebral artery (MCA) territory infarction and PLIC/peduncle involvement (Fig. 6.1) will develop a hemiplegia, and about a quarter will develop epilepsy by 2 years [15]. Despite this almost all children with a unilateral stroke will walk independently, albeit a little later than usually expected, unless they have additional complications leading to other difficulties [16].

In one comparative study [5], preterm infants with larger strokes did less well on cognitive outcome testing at 2 years than full-term infants with stroke though the difference was not found significant (perhaps due to small numbers). For other small MCA strokes and strokes in other sites, the overall developmental quotient (DQ) was in the lower normal range and best for small isolated perforator strokes (Fig. 6.2). Preterm infants had more problems with language development—this may more be due to their prematurity than their stroke—and further studies need to be done to address this issue. Infants with posterior cerebral artery territory stroke and those with more posterior MCA stroke affecting the optic radiation need referral for assessment of their visual abilities.

6.2.5 Treatment

No specific acute treatments are currently available for preterm stroke. Management is as for full-term infants: paying attention to maintaining normothermia, normoglycemia, and normotension and avoiding hypocapnia. If the baby is having seizures or symptoms such as apneas suggestive of seizures than monitoring with EEG or aEEG should be done. Seizures should be treated quickly and aEEG monitoring continued till the seizures have stopped. There is no evidence to support the long-term continuation of anti-seizure medications.

Additionally, none of the non-acute therapeutic interventions has been especially trialed in preterm infants. It is sensible to make an early referral for physiotherapy assessment, especially if a hemiplegia is likely to ensue, in addition to the routine follow-up for infants born preterm. Physiotherapy could be started on the neonatal unit if the infant is still an inpatient for a long time after the diagnosis is made and a motor deficit is anticipated.

An assessment of general movements (GMAs) at 3–4 months post-term age (age corrected for prematurity) together with a Hammersmith Infant Neurological Examination (HINE) score will help in assessing the likelihood of developing cerebral palsy (CP). Preterm infants with absent fidgety movements but a HINE score >50 at 3 months are highly likely to develop a hemiplegia, while those with absent fidgety movements and HINE scores <50 are most likely to develop bilateral CP [17]. Asymmetries in hand function can be quantified using the HAI (Hand Assessment for Infants) from 3 months post-term age [18].

For infants with asymmetries of limb function, encouraging bimanual activities and also, in some cases, constraint therapy (Baby CIMT) of the unaffected limb for periods of the day have been shown to improve early motor function [19], and a clinical trial of this therapy is underway in Australia [20]. A study is ongoing to assess the effects of focused therapy for lower limb function in infants with hemiplegia with encouraging early results, but the findings from the full RCT are yet to be published [21]. While there are data to support early interventions, long-term effects and sustained improvements are yet to be established.

If the visual pathway appears affected (Fig. 6.1), visual assessment and support for visual development are needed [22].

Follow-up plans should include long-term cognitive, language, and behavioral review and monitoring for later seizure occurrence as well as support for the family [23–25].

Readily accessible information and support for parents and carers are available from, for example, Hemihelp in the UK (https://contact.org.uk/help-for-families/information-advice-services/hemihelp/), and similar associations in Europe and the USA (http://chasa.org) have greatly increased both professional and public knowledge of the condition.

6.3   Conclusion

Arterial infarction is more common in preterm infants than generally recognized. Diagnosis is often made from cranial ultrasound scans performed regularly during the neonatal period.

It is especially important to think of this diagnosis around times of illness, in relation to surgeries and in infants affected by twin-to-twin transfusion syndrome. MRI scanning is the best method for defining exactly the tissues involved and for prognosis. Early referral for physiotherapy and planning long-term follow-up and parental/carer support are very important.

References

1. Roy B, Walker K, Morgan C, et al. Epidemiology and pathogenesis of stroke in preterm infants: a systematic review. J Neonatal Perinatal Med. 2021;15:11. https://doi.org/10.3233/NPM-200597.
2. Benders MJNL, Groenendaal F, Uiterwaal CS, et al. Maternal and infant characteristics associated with perinatal arterial stroke in the preterm infant. Stroke. 2007;38:1759–65.
3. Sorg AL, von Kries R, Klemme M, et al. Incidence estimates of perinatal arterial ischemic stroke in preterm- and term-born infants: a National Capture-Recapture Calculation Corrected Surveillance Study. Neonatology. 2021;118:727. https://doi.org/10.1159/000514922.
4. Ecury-Goossen GM, Raets MM, Lequin M, et al. Risk factors, clinical presentation, and neuroimaging findings of neonatal perforator stroke. Stroke. 2013;44:2115–20.
5. Benders MJNL, Groenendaal F, de Vries LS. Preterm arterial stroke. Semin Fetal Neonatal Med. 2009;14(5):272–7.
6. Bhat R, Kumar R, Kwon S, et al. Risk factors for neonatal venous and arterial thromboembolism in the neonatal intensive care unit-a case control study. J Pediatr. 2018;195:28–32.
7. Golomb MR, Garg BP, Edwards-Brown M, et al. Very early arterial ischemic stroke in premature infants. Pediatr Neurol. 2008;38:329–34.
8. Srivastava R, Dunbar M, Shevell M, Oskoui M, Basu A, Rivkin MJ, Shany E, de Vries LS, Dewey D, Letourneau N, Hill MD, Kirton A. Developmental and validation of a prediction model for perinatal arterial ischemic stroke in term neonates. JAMA Netw Open. 2022;5(6):e2219203. https://doi.org/10.1001/jamanetworkopen.2022.19203.
9. Curtis C, Mineyko A, Massicotte P, Leakerr M, Jiang XY, Kirton A. Thrombophilia risk is not increased in children after perinatal stroke. Blood. 2017;129(20):2793–800. https://doi.org/10.1182/blood-2016-11-750893.
10. Wagenaar N, Martinez-Biarge M, van der Aa NE, van Haastert IC, Groenendaal F, Benders MJNL, Cowan FM, de Vries LS. Neurodevelopment after perinatal arterial ischemic stroke. Pediatrics. 2018;142(3):e20174164. https://doi.org/10.1542/peds.2017-4164.
11. van der Aa N, Leemans A, Northington FJ, et al. Does diffusion tensor imaging-based tractography at 3 months of age contribute to the prediction of motor outcome after perinatal arterial ischemic stroke? Stroke. 2011;42(12):3410–4.
12. van der Aa NE, Dudink J, Benders MJNL, et al. Neonatal posterior cerebral artery stroke: clinical presentation, MRI findings, and outcome. Dev Med Child Neurol. 2013;55(3):283–90.
13. van der Aa NE, Benders MJNL, Nikkels PG, et al. Cortical sparing in preterm ischemic arterial stroke. Stroke. 2016;2016(47):869–71. https://doi.org/10.1161/STROKEAHA.115.011605.
14. Mercuri E, Hu J, Curati WL, Dubowitz LMS, Cowan FM, Bydder GM. Cerebellar infarction and atrophy in infants and children with a history of premature birth. Pediatr Radiol. 1997;27:139–43.
15. Ecury-Goossen GM, van der Haer M, Smit LS, et al. Neurodevelopmental outcome after neonatal perforator stroke. Dev Med Child Neurol. 2016;58(1):49–56.
16. Steggerda SJ, de Vries LS. Neonatal stroke in premature infants. Semin Perinatol. 2021;45(7):151471. https://doi.org/10.1016/j.semperi.2021.151471.
17. Romeo DMM, Guzzetta A, Scoto M, Cioni M, Patusi P, Mazzone D, Romeo MG. Early neurologic assessment in preterm-infants: integration of traditional neurologic examination and observation of general movements. Eur J Paed Neurol. 2008;12:183–9.
18. Ryll UC, Krumlinde-Sundholm L, Verhage CH, Sicola E, Sgandurra G, Bastiaenen CHG, Eliasson AC. Predictive validity of the hand assessment for infants at risk of unilateral cerebral palsy. Dev Med Child Neurol. 2021;63(4):436–43. https://doi.org/10.1111/dmcn.14739.
19. Eliasson AC, Nordstrand L, Ek L, Lennartsson F, Sjöstrand L, Tedroff K, Krumline-Sundholm L. The effectiveness of baby-CIMT in infants younger than 12 months with clinical signs of unilateral-cerebral palsy; an explorative study with randomized design. Res Dev Disabil. 2018;72:191–201.

20. Boyd RN, Ziviani J, Sakzewski L, et al. REACH: study protocol of a randomised trial of rehabilitation very early in congenital hemiplegia. BMJ Open. 2017;7(9):e017204.
21. Hurd C, Livingstone D, Brunton K, et al. Early intensive lower extremity rehabilitation show preliminary efficacy after perinatal stroke; results of a pilot randomised controlled trial. Neurorehabil Neural Repair. 2022;36(6):360–70.
22. Fazzi E, Micheletti S, Calza S, Merabet L, Rossi A, Galli J, Early Visual Intervention Study Group. Early visual training and environmental adaptation for infants with visual impairment. Dev Med Child Neurol. 2021;63:1180–93.
23. Kirton A, deVeber G. Life after perinatal stroke. Stroke. 2013;44:3265–71.
24. Peterson RK, Williams T, Dlamini N, Westmacott R. Parent experiences and developmental outcomes following neonatal stroke. Clin Neuropsychol. 2021;35(5):973–87.
25. Khan U, Watson R, Pearse JE, Irwin L, Rapley T, Basu AP. Grappling with uncertainty—experiences of parents of infants following perinatal stroke. Res Dev Disabil. 2022;124:104201. https://doi.org/10.1016/j.ridd.2022.104201.

Hypoxic-Ischemic Encephalopathy in Preterm Infants

7

Miriam Martinez-Biarge and Frances M. Cowan

Abbreviations

BGT	Basal ganglia and thalami
CTG	Cardiotocography
CP	Cerebral palsy
DWI	Diffusion weighted imaging
GA	Gestational age
HIE	Hypoxic ischemic encephalopathy
MRI	Magnetic resonance imaging
NICU	Neonatal intensive care unit
PEG	Percutaneous gastrostomy
STL	Symmetrical thalamic lesions

M. Martinez-Biarge (✉)
Department of Paediatrics, Imperial College Healthcare NHS Trust, London, UK
e-mail: miriam.martinez-biarge@nhs.net

F. M. Cowan
Department of Paediatrics, Imperial College London, London, UK
e-mail: f.cowan@imperial.ac.uk

© The Author(s) 2024
G. Meijler, K. Mohammad (eds.), *Neonatal Brain Injury*,
https://doi.org/10.1007/978-3-031-55972-3_7

7.1   For Parents

Before birth, your baby receives a constant supply of nutrients and oxygen from the mother through the placenta which is connected to the baby by the umbilical cord. Birth is a stressful event for any baby. If the labor is particularly difficult or there are problems that lead to the baby being born early, these may affect the supply of nutrients and oxygen necessary for the baby's brain to function normally. If, e.g. the cord appears before the baby or there is bleeding from the placenta, the baby's blood supply may diminish greatly. However, such dramatic events are not necessary for a baby to suffer a lack of oxygen. Infection, which may be a reason for labor to start early, may also make the baby very susceptible to a lack of oxygen. Sometimes we do just not know why this happens.

As preterm babies usually need some help with breathing shortly after birth and they may not feed well because their suck has not yet developed and they do not move as much or respond as quickly as babies born at term age, it can be difficult to tell by looking at the baby alone whether they are seriously affected or not. Measuring the acidity in the blood in the cord is useful as is recording the brain waves (EEG) to see if there are seizures as these are not always obvious. Imaging the brain regularly over the first days using ultrasound and getting an MRI as soon as the baby can be safely taken to the scanner will be the most help in trying to know whether the brain is injured and what will happen.

There are no specific treatments for this problem in preterm babies. In older babies we use cooling down to 33.5 °C for 3 days to reduce the demands of brain cells while they try to recover, but small preterm babies do not tolerate this treatment well, and a recent study did not show improvements. We try to keep the baby as stable as possible to prevent any further damage and treat any signs of infection or seizures.

Often the results of brain imaging are the best way to tell if there has been any permanent damage. The type of injury seen and the places in the brain where it is tell us a lot about how the baby will progress in the future. If the central parts of the brain have been affected, then the future can be very difficult particularly in terms of moving independently and feeding but also in many other areas of development and some babies may not survive. If the brain looks normal or only mildly affected, even if the baby has been very sick, usually future progress will be good. For all babies we suggest regular follow-up to check on this well into school age. Early intervention programs (such as physiotherapy, rehabilitation, speech therapy) help the young, still resilient brain to overcome or to lessen developmental problems.

7.2 For Professionals

7.2.1 Epidemiology

The true incidence of HIE in preterm infants is difficult to determine, and different definitions have been used [1]. Salhab and Perlman found, over a 10-year period, that 61 infants (1%) of all preterm babies (31–36 weeks GA) admitted to their NICU had an umbilical cord blood pH <7 but only 8 of the 61 infants were described as being encephalopathic—of these 8, 3 died and the others had abnormal neonatal outcomes [2]. Chalak et al. [3] identified 9 of 1305 (0.7%) infants of 33–35 weeks GA, with HIE, but only 3 had a poor outcome. An incidence of 0.9% of 1325 pre-terms of 32–36 weeks GA was reported by Schmidt and Walsh in 2010. Of these infants, 52 had a 5-min Apgar score <6, but only 12 also had a cord or initial blood pH <7 or base deficit >15 mmol/L, experienced a sentinel event and had seizures and hypotonia taken as evidence of encephalopathy; 7 of these 12 infants had a poor outcome [4]. In a study by Logitharajah et al. of 55 preterm infants ≤36 weeks GA, all were diagnosed with HIE and had an MRI, and the main criteria used for inclusion were an Apgar score <5 at 1 min and <7 at 5 min and the need for major resuscitation (pH was not available in many infants). Additional supporting evidence came from a sentinel event, abnormal intrapartum CTG, meconium staining, cord pH <7, multiorgan failure, and seizures [5]. In the Preemie RCT (NCT 01793129: https://clinicaltrials.gov/study/NCT01793129?tab=results) of hypothermia for pre-term infants of 33–35 weeks gestation, criteria were severe acidosis and/or resuscitation at birth as well as moderate or severe encephalopathy.

Placental abruption was the commonest identifiable antecedent in all the studies that examined antenatal and perinatal factors [1, 2, 4–7]. Other intrapartum complications (abnormal fetal heart rate, cord abnormalities) have also been described [1, 2, 5, 6]. In the Preemie randomized trial of hypothermia (2023) study, 10% of infants had a cord-related event, 45% a placental problem, and 75% an abnormal CTG [8].

7.2.2 Clinical Signs and Diagnosis

Encephalopathy in preterm infants, who often have low muscle tone, need ventilating and assisted feeding because of their immaturity may be difficult to recognize, and the more so, the more immature they are—indeed there are no studies of clinical neurological signs in extremely preterm infants [1]. The frequency of seizures is very variable between studies (35–82%) [1, 5, 6], and EEG monitoring has not been routinely used in preterm infants. It is well documented however that after an acute and severe hypoxic insult, preterm infants may develop a similar pattern of injury to that seen in term infants (see Chap 8).

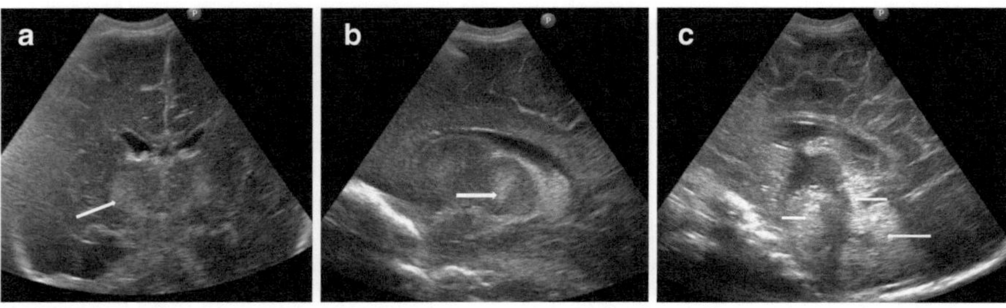

Fig. 7.1 Cranial US scan of a 33 weeks gestation infant with hypoxic-ischemic encephalopathy showing increased echogenicity in the thalami ((**a**) coronal plane, (**b**) parasagittal view) and in the tectum and tegmentum of the brainstem (two shorter arrows) and vermis (longer arrow) ((**c**) mid-sagittal plane)

In an MRI study of 55 infants of 26–37 weeks GA, median 35 weeks, referred to a tertiary center with evidence of HIE, Logitharajah et al. [5] found that sites of injury were similar to the full-term infant, being the basal ganglia and thalami (70%, >50% being severe), white matter (89%), brainstem (44%), and cortex (58%) though the cortex was relatively spared, increasingly so in younger infants, as formerly reported [9]. The patterns of injury seen were not typical of the injury seen in the preterm population in general as described in other chapters (see Chaps. 3, 4, and 5). Few infants had intraventricular hemorrhage, cystic white matter injury or cerebellar hemorrhage though of course these may co-occur. In a very recent study of 80 preterm infants with evidence of perinatal asphyxia, including a great number of younger GA infants, more hemorrhage was seen in the extremely-very preterm and WM injury in the moderate-late preterm infants [10].

As in full-term infants, signs of injury can be recognized 12–24 h after the acute event on cranial ultrasound as focal areas of increased echogenicity within the basal ganglia and/or thalami (Fig. 7.1). This part of the brain is not usually the focus of attention in preterm infants who are more susceptible to intraventricular hemorrhage and white matter injury, emphasizing the importance of looking specifically at the central gray matter in all preterm babies.

The severity of the central gray matter injury may not be recognized in preterm infants until it becomes difficult to wean them from a ventilator or not possible to establish feeding, and contractures resulting from lack of movement may become apparent. This combination of symptoms may lead to extensive investigations for neuromuscular or metabolic disorders [1]. Early appropriate investigation and diagnosis help avoid this difficult and distressing situation.

7.2.3 Treatment

There is currently no specific treatment for preterm infants with HIE. Good general management is of course mandatory. Care needs to be taken to keep blood gases, avoiding any hypocapnia, and blood pressure in the normal range. Preterm infants are particularly susceptible to hyperglycemia as well as hypoglycemia and also thrombocytopenia, clotting derangements, and hemorrhage which may complicate management.

Unlike in term infants where therapeutic hypothermia is standard treatment (see Chap. 8), there are considerable concerns about the use of hypothermia in small and immature infants because cooling may have a deleterious effect on hemodynamic and physiological stability [7, 11], with the risk of causing or worsening any brain injury they already have. Herrera et al. treated 30 preterm infants with hypothermia, and 50% of those with known outcomes either died or had a moderate to severe neurodevelopmental impairment. A randomized control trial of cooling was undertaken in the USA (Preemie Hypothermia for Neonatal Encephalopathy) in preterm infants with signs of HIE, enrolling 168 infants between 33 and 35 weeks GA and weighing more than 1500 g. The trial, completed in 2022 with follow-up at 18–22 months, showed no benefit of the cooling treatment [8].

7.2.4 Outcome and Prognosis

The prognosis after HIE in preterm infants seems to be poorer than in term infants. The early mortality rate is high (25–33%), partly related to the high incidence of central gray matter and brainstem injury and also to the associated multiorgan failure, and most survivors develop some degree of developmental impairment [1, 2, 5, 11]. In the recent Preemie RCT, death or disability occurred in 35% of cooled infants and 29% of non-cooled infants.

In the study by Logitharajah et al., neurodevelopmental outcomes were predictable from the pattern of injury (Fig. 7.2), with severe injury to the basal ganglia-thalami and brainstem leading to death or severe quadriplegia in 95%. Normal scans were associated with normal 2-year outcomes (corrected age) in all cases. While white matter injury was common, in general it was mild, only three infants developing cystic changes; ten infants had some hemorrhage, but these were mostly small punctate lesions. Intraventricular hemorrhage was only seen in four infants, none developing post-hemorrhagic ventricular dilatation. In the recent study [10] with 80 preterm infants who had early and/or term-age MRI, 44% of infants had an adverse outcome, and deep gray matter abnormalities and a low Kidokoro score [12] were strongly associated with adverse neurodevelopmental outcomes. Smit et al report on 6 late cooled preterm infants - none died but two had a poor outcome [13].

There are no longer-term studies of preterm infants with HIE, but it is reasonable to presume that the data showing more subtle problems affecting memory, learning, behavior and motor skills becoming apparent at early school age in the term-born population would apply to the preterm population (see Chap. 8). Long-term follow-up is therefore recommended.

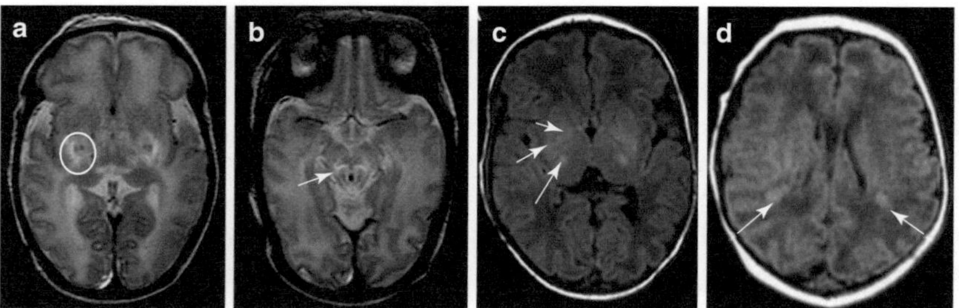

Fig. 7.2 Prediction of outcome from the pattern of injury on neonatal MRI in preterm infants with HIE. *Severe BGT lesions* (same infant as shown in Fig. 7.1) are in most cases associated with brainstem injury and white matter involvement. These are clearly seen on these axial T2-W images at the level of (**a**) the lower BGT and (**b**) the mesencephalon. Outcome is uniformly poor: almost all infants have severe neurodevelopmental impairment affecting all developmental domains, with a high incidence of feeding problems or they do not survive the first few months. (**c**) *Mild-moderate BGT lesions* in a 36 weeks GA infant, shown on this axial T1-W image at the level of the BGT. In most cases this is associated with a normal-looking brainstem and normal white matter or only mild injury. Outcomes are variable, ranging from normal (50%) to severe impairment and death (30–40%). (**d**) *Isolated white matter injury* in a 35 weeks GA infant with normal BGT and brainstem (axial T1-W image). Most infants with isolated white matter injury have normal assessments at 2–3 years; mild developmental impairment may occur in a few. *BGT* basal ganglia and thalami, *GA* gestational age

7.3 Symmetrical Thalamic Lesions (Fig. 7.3)

This is a poorly understood condition also affecting both preterm and full-term infants, often with a history of early rupture of membranes, polyhydramnios, reduced fetal movements, and antenatal maternal blood loss. The infants usually have marked hypotonia at birth but may have contractures and often poor oromotor control. They quite quickly go on to develop limb spasticity with persisting central hypotonia. The condition is typified by symmetrical thalamic lesions (STLs). Often the brainstem is also involved, and the pattern of injury and outcome overlaps with that described by Logitharajah et al. [5] in preterm infants with HIE.

Cranial ultrasound scans usually show abnormal thalamic echogenicity immediately after birth, and these changes can be more obvious than abnormalities seen on MRI. MRI changes are most marked on T1-weighted images, and acute DWI changes are rarely seen suggesting that the injury is of antenatal onset. Outcome is almost uniformly very poor in relation to the severe injury pattern (see [14]).

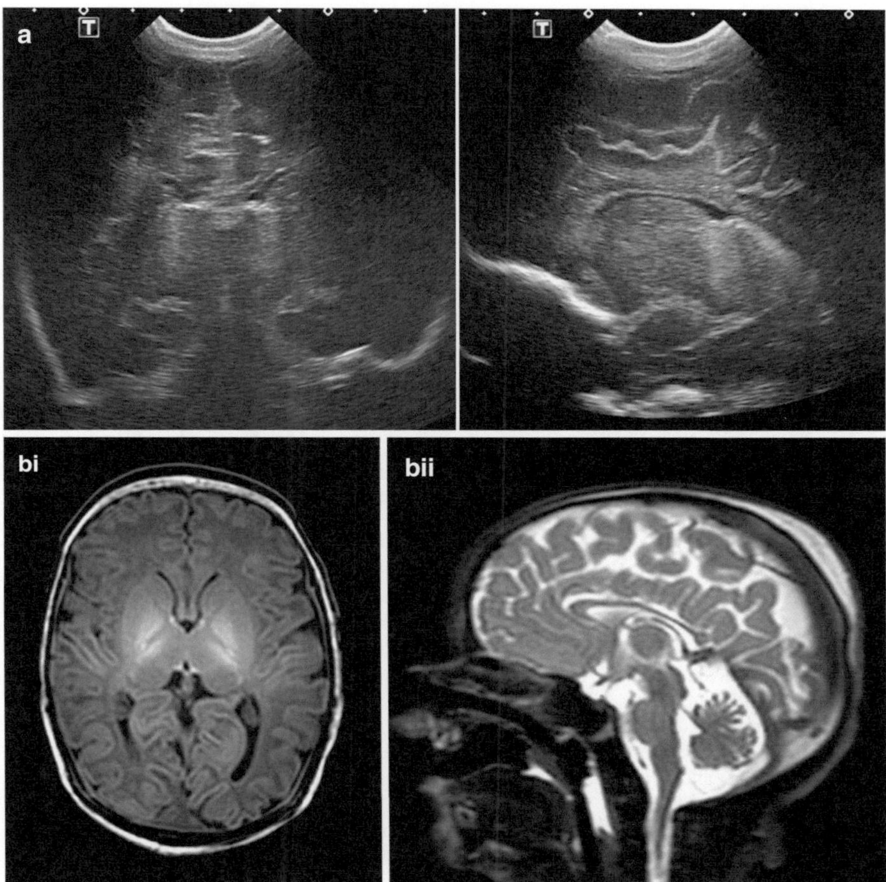

Fig. 7.3 Symmetrical thalamic lesions. Baby born by breech delivery at 39 weeks GA. Apgar scores 3/6/8. Normal cord gases. After brief resuscitation she breathed spontaneously for a few hours but needed ventilation again till day 10. She had contractures at the knees, hips, and elbows, and she did not swallow and had a facial diplegia. Her cUS shows marked bilateral thalamic echogenicities (**a**), coronal and parasagittal). MRI (**bi**, axial T1-W at BGT level), shows abnormal signal in the thalami and posterior limbs of the internal capsules and to some extent in the globus pallidi. These findings were most obvious on the T1-W imaging shown. **bii** mid-sagittal T2-W image shows a thin corpus callosum and open sulci of the vermis suggesting some atrophy already present at birth, consistent with an antenatal insult. No acute changes were seen on DWI. Outcome: Poor suck, continued need for suctioning, aspiration. PEG insertion. CP (axial hypotonia and 4-limb hypertonia). Severe hearing loss. At 2 years she had poor facial expression and poor head control; she could roll and remain in a sitting position, but not get herself into sitting. *BGT* basal ganglia and thalami, *CP* cerebral palsy, *cUS* cranial ultrasound scan, *DWI* diffusion weighted imaging, *GA* gestational age, *PEG* percutaneous gastrostomy

References

1. Gopagondanahall KV, Li J, Fahey MC, Hunt RW, Jenkin G, Meiller SL, Malhotra A. Preterm hypoxic–ischemic encephalopathy. Review. Front Pediatr. 2016;4:114. https://doi.org/10.3389/fped.2016.00114.
2. Salhab WA, Perlman JM. Severe fetal acidemia and subsequent neonatal encephalopathy in the larger premature infant. Pediatr Neurol. 2005;32(1):25–9.
3. Chalak LF, Rollins N, Morriss MC, Brion LP, Heyne R, Sanchez PJ. Perinatal acidosis and hypoxic-ischemic encephalopathy in preterm infants of 33 to 35 weeks' gestation. J Pediatr. 2012;160(3):388–94.
4. Schmidt JW, Walsh WF. Hypoxic-ischemic encephalopathy in preterm infants. J Neonatal Perinatal Med. 2010;3:277–84.
5. Logitharajah P, Rutherford MA, Cowan FM. Hypoxic-ischemic encephalopathy in preterm infants: antecedent factors, brain imaging, and outcome. Pediatr Res. 2009;66(2):222–9.
6. Garfinkle J, Wintermark P, Shevell MI, Oskoui M. Children born at 32 to 35 weeks with birth asphyxia and later cerebral palsy are different from those born after 35 weeks. J Perinatol. 2017;37(8):963–8.
7. Rao R, Trivedi S, Vesoulis Z, Liao SM, Smyser CD, Mathur AM. Safety and short-term outcomes of therapeutic hypothermia in preterm neonates 34-35 weeks gestational age with hypoxic-ischemic encephalopathy. J Pediatr. 2017;183:37–42.
8. Faix R, Laptook A, Shankaran S, Eggleston B, Wusthoff C, Das A, Tyson J, Pedroza C, Sanchez P, Laughon M, Heyne R, Sonifacio S, Preemie Hypothermia Sub-Committee of the Neonatal Research Network. Randomised trial of targeted temperature management with whole body hypothermia for moderate and severe encephalopathy in premature infants 33-35 weeks gestation—a Bayesian study. PAS Abstr. 2023.
9. Barkovich AJ, Sargent SK. Profound asphyxia in the premature infant: imaging findings. AJNR Am J Neuroradiol. 1995;16(9):1837–46.
10. Parmentier CEJ, de Vries LS, Verhagen EA, el Bakkali L, Steggerda SJ, de Haan TR, Alderliesten T, Lequin M, Benders MJNL, KoopmanEsseboom C, Groenendaal F. Brain injury patterns and neurodevelopmental outcome in preterm infants with perinatal asphyxia. jENS. 2023:517.
11. Herrera TI, Edwards L, Malcolm WF, et al. Outcomes of preterm infants treated with hypothermia for hypoxic-ischemic encephalopathy. Early Hum Dev. 2018;125:1–7.
12. Kidokoro H, Neil JJ, Inder TE. New MR imaging assessment tool to define brain abnormalities in very preterm infants at term. AJNR Am J Neuroradiol. 2013;34(11):2208–14.
13. Smit E, Liu X, Jary S, Cowan F, Thoresen M. Cooling neonates who do not fulfil the standard cooling criteria—short- and long-term outcomes. Acta Paediatr. 2015;104:138–45.
14. Pols T, de Vries LS, Salamon AS, et al. Symmetrical thalamic lesions in the newborn: a case series. Neuropediatrics. 2019;50(3):152–9.

Part III

Brain Injury in the (Near) Term Neonate

Hypoxic-Ischemic Encephalopathy (HIE) in Term and Near-Term Infants

8

Khorshid Mohammad ⓘD, Linda S. de Vries ⓘD, Gerda Meijler ⓘD, and Frances M. Cowan

Abbreviations

ADC	Apparent diffusion coefficient
aEEG	Amplitude-integrated electroencephalography
BGT	Basal ganglia and thalamus
BSID	Bayley Scales of Infant Development
cUS	Cranial ultrasound
DWI	Diffusion-weighted imaging
HIE	Hypoxic-ischemic encephalopathy
MRI	Magnetic resonance imaging
NICU	Neonatal intensive care unit
PAIS	Perinatal arterial ischemic stroke
PLIC	Posterior limb of the internal capsule

K. Mohammad
Section of Newborn Critical Care, Department of Pediatrics, Alberta Children's Hospital and University of Calgary, Calgary, AB, Canada
e-mail: mkhorshi@ucalgary.ca

L. S. de Vries
Divison of Pediatrics, Department of Neonatology, Willem-Alexander Hospital, Leiden University Medical Center (LUMC), Leiden, The Netherlands
e-mail: l.s.de_devries@lumc.nl

G. Meijler
Department of Neonatology, Isala Women and Children's Hospital, Zwolle, The Netherlands
e-mail: gmeijler@gmail.com

F. M. Cowan (✉)
Department of Paediatrics, Imperial College London, London, UK
e-mail: f.cowan@imperial.ac.uk

© The Author(s) 2024
G. Meijler, K. Mohammad (eds.), *Neonatal Brain Injury*,
https://doi.org/10.1007/978-3-031-55972-3_8

PVL   Periventricular leukomalacia
PWMLs   Punctate white matter lesions
ROS   Reactive oxygen species
TH   Therapeutic hypothermia
TTNT   Time to normal trace

8.1   For Parents

Before birth, the baby receives a constant supply of nutrients and oxygen from its mother through the placenta which is connected to the baby by the umbilical cord. Birth is a stressful event and complications can happen during this process. Some complications may cause an interruption to the blood supply to the baby. This lack of blood supply will affect the delivery of essential nutrients and oxygen to your baby and may affect the brain and cause your baby not to be normally active after birth. When this happens a condition called hypoxic-ischemic encephalopathy develops - often shortened to HIE.

8.1.1   How Will I Know If My Baby Has Symptoms of HIE?

Certain key information helps us make this diagnosis:

- A sudden event close to the time of birth such as cord prolapse (when the umbilical cord exits before the baby) or placental abruption (when the placenta detaches before birth).
- A low Apgar score—an Apgar score is a summary measure of your baby's health condition shortly after birth and includes breathing and heart rate as well as your baby's general activity and color—these are scored on a scale of 0–10, 0 being the most worrisome. Apgar scores are recorded for all babies at 1, 5, and often 10 minutes after birth. We also do tests on the blood from the umbilical cord to look for signs of stress (known as the cord gases).
- The presence of certain symptoms within the first 6 hours after birth such as lethargy (being sleepy and not crying vigorously), weakness or absent spontaneous activity, having floppy arms and legs, a weak or absent suck, weak or interrupted breathing, twitching or jerky movements (seizures), and/or coma. Combinations of these symptoms is what is called hypoxic-ischemic encephalopathy (HIE).

8.1.2   What Is the Treatment If My Baby Is Diagnosed with HIE?

Treatment is aimed at preventing any further damage following the reduced blood supply and low oxygen levels. This includes, for example, keeping the blood pressure and oxygen levels as stable as possible and within the normal range, avoiding a high temperature and being prompt to treat seizures. Your baby may qualify for a treatment called therapeutic hypothermia. Therapeutic hypothermia means the baby is cooled, using a "cooling" blanket that the baby is either laid on or wrapped in (see Picture 8.1). Cooling limits the damage to the brain after a low blood supply/oxygen event by slowing the metabolism in the affected brain cells. This is a bit like hibernation for the brain, so it can try to recover. The hypothermia treatment usually will last for 72 hours, and your baby will be cooled until the body temperature is down to 33.5°C; then your baby will slowly be rewarmed to a normal temperature. Your baby will be monitored for pain or discomfort on a regular basis, and anti-pain

Picture 8.1 Baby wrapped in a cooling blanket in an incubator. The baby has two tubes, one for help with breathing and one in the mouth so any air in the stomach can be removed

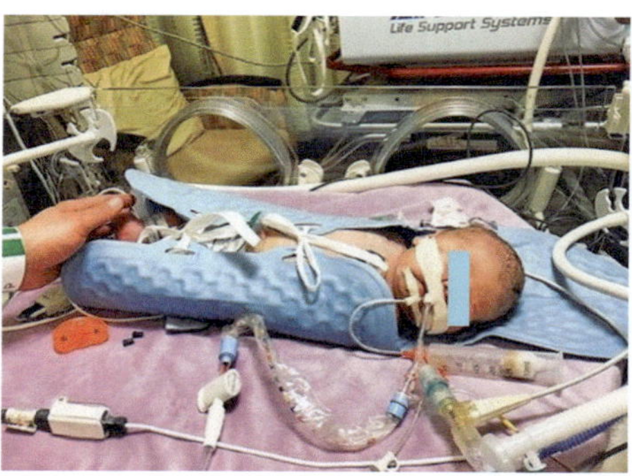

medication and/or a sedative will be given as needed. Because of your baby's problem and also the cooling and medication, your baby will move less than usual, and so the skin will be frequently checked for pressure effects.

Careful feeding is important because of decreased blood flow to your baby's stomach and bowels around the time of delivery. In the beginning nutrition will be started through an intravenous (IV) line, so your baby can receive the nutrients it cannot get through drinking. As soon as possible, your baby will receive small amount of fresh breast milk (if available) or formula administered through a gastric tube to stimulate the gut even while being cooled. If your baby is stable enough, you may be helped to hold your baby while wrapped in the cooling blanket.

There are other interventions that possibly improve outcomes such as gentle handling, music, massage therapy, reading, holding, etc. For these interventions, the evidence as yet is not strong, so ask your baby's doctor for information about this.

8.1.3 What Will Happen to My Baby (Prognosis)?

HIE is divided into three stages (or grades): mild, moderate, and severe. Outcome i.e. the future for your baby, depends (among other things) on the severity of HIE.

Some babies with very severe HIE may not survive. Fortunately, most babies will survive, but a small number of babies with HIE will develop a motor (movement) disability such as cerebral palsy.

Outcomes have improved, i.e., later problems have lessened considerably since the introduction of therapeutic hypothermia in the first decade of this century, and nowadays more babies with moderate and severe HIE do well, developing and behaving as their peers. However, there remains a risk of some long-term problems, such as learning disorders, delayed development, memory problems, or milder motor problems. Most infants with milder HIE have a good outcome, but still we recommend longer-term follow-up well into school age to ensure they are doing well with learning and memory and with developing their social skills. The neonatal brain is more resilient than the adult brain, as it is still developing and making new connections. Parents play a key role in improving the outcome regardless of the severity of the brain injury as they provide essential stimulation to their baby's brain. Follow-up with a developmental specialist after discharge will be important to assess your baby's progress and to support your baby and you.

Your child will be followed up and assessed closely by a specialized team for hearing, vision, motor, speech and language, cognitive function, and the possible development of epilepsy. The goal is to ensure that your child remains healthy and to identify problems early, so your child can be treated and enrolled in early intervention programs. These early intervention programs (such as physiotherapy, rehabilitation, speech therapy) help the young, still resilient brain to overcome or to lessen any developmental problems.

8.2 For Professionals

8.2.1 Incidence, Risk Factors, and Pathogenesis

The incidence of HIE varies depending on the country of birth. In high-income countries, the incidence of perinatal asphyxia is 1–4/1000 live births [1], while it is up to 10–20/1000 live births in low- and middle-income countries [2, 3].

Although often no causation is found, there are many risk factors for perinatal asphyxia [4]; some are listed below:

- Maternal health and conditions: Primiparity, advanced age, pre-pregnancy weight, pregnancy-induced hypertension, and gestational diabetes.
- Newborn related: Advanced gestational age, large for gestational age, and small for gestational age.
- Delivery related: Induced labor, breech presentation, need for instrumental delivery (forceps or vacuum), perinatal inflammation, cord prolapse, uterine rupture, or placental abruption [5–8].

The pathophysiology of HIE is complex and a process over time. The key processes are ischemia-reperfusion phases and primary and secondary energy failure. The primary energy failure occurs during the ischemic phase which involves ATP pump failure and entrapment of ions inside cells followed by water diffusion and restriction of its movement across membranes. Following the ischemic/primary energy failure, reperfusion and energy restoration occur with influx of reactive oxygen species (ROS), toxins, and an inflammatory cascade. During the reperfusion phase, some cells may get "overwhelmed" and undergo secondary energy failure, apoptosis, necroptosis, or inflammation. The role of inflammation or infection is unclear in HIE but may be important particularly in lower-income settings. The goal of therapeutic hypothermia, sedation, and minimal handling initiated in the early reperfusion phase is to slow down the reperfusion and inflammation process to allow cells to recover. A tertiary phase when gliosis and impaired oligodendrocyte maturation occur can last years [9]

8.2.2 Diagnosis

The staging of severity of HIE was introduced by Dr. Sarnat in 1976 (see Table 8.1) [10] and was based on careful physical examination, vital signs, and EEG findings. It is very important to make a diagnosis of HIE and determine as soon as possible the eligibility for therapeutic hypothermia (TH). Infants must be of certain gestational age (usually ≥ 35 weeks at birth) and birth weight (usually >1800 g). Furthermore, a baby must fulfill criteria A and B:

Table 8.1 The major categories and sub-categories for assessing the severity of neonatal encephalopathy (adapted from Sarnat encephalopathy staging) [10]

Encephalopathy	Normal	Mild	Moderate	Severe
1. Level of consciousness	☐ Normal	☐ Hyperalert	☐ Lethargy	☐ Stupor/coma
2. Spontaneous activity	☐ Active	☐ Active	☐ Decreased activity	☐ No activity
3. Posture	☐ Normal	☐ Mild distal flexion	☐ Strong distal flexion of arms and extension of legs	☐ Strong extension of arms and legs
4. Tone	☐ Normal	☐ Hypertonia	☐ Hypotonia	☐ Flaccid
5. Deep tendon reflexes	☐ Normal	☐ Brisk	☐ Brisk	☐ Absent
6. Primitive reflexes				
Suck	☐ Normal	☐ Weak	☐ Weak/absent	☐ Absent
Moro	☐ Complete	☐ Strong/ Jittery	☐ Incomplete	☐ Absent
7. Autonomic system				
Pupils	☐ Equal & reactive	☐ Dilated	☐ Constricted	☐ Variable and/ or poorly reactive, often unequal
Heart rate (HR)	☐ Normal	☐ Tachycardia	☐ Bradycardia	☐ Variable HR
Respirations	☐ Normal	☐ Normal	☐ Periodic breathing	☐ Apnea
8. Seizures (clinical or electrographic)	☐ No	☐ No	☐ Yes	☐ Yes

Criteria A: a combination of fetal acidosis (cord arterial blood gas pH ≤7 and base excess (BE) ≤−16) and need for resuscitation (Apgar score ≤5 and need for respiratory support at 10 min after birth) [11–15]

Criteria B: the presence of seizures or abnormal findings in three of six categories (level of consciousness, spontaneous activity, posture, tone, primitive reflexes, and autonomic system) [14].

The Thompson HIE score (see Table 8.2) was developed to assess the severity of perinatal asphyxia. This score was shown to be predictive of short- and long-term outcomes. A Thompson score of >7 is used as an indication for TH treatment [16–18].

8.2.3 Brain Monitoring

Some form of brain monitoring (commonly amplitude integrated EEG (aEEG) or EEG) is used in HIE for seizure monitoring during cooling and the rewarming phase. It is essential to monitor infants with moderate to severe HIE by aEEG or continuous video EEG for seizures. EEG background activity, particularly time to

Table 8.2 Thompson scoring system

	Score				Day		
Sign	0	1	2	3	1	2	3
Tone	Normal	Hypertonia	Hypotonia	Flaccid			
Conscious state	Normal	Hyper alert, stare	Lethargic	Comatose			
Fits	None	Infrequent <3/day	Frequent >2/day				
Posture	Normal	Fisting/cycling	Strong, distal flexion	Decerebrate			
Moro reflex	Normal	Partial	Absent				
Grasp reflex	Normal	Poor	Absent				
Suck	Normal	Poor	Absent ± bites				
Respiration	Normal	Hyperventilation	Brief apnea	IPPV (apnea)			
Fontanel	Normal	Full not tense	Tense				
	Total score per day						

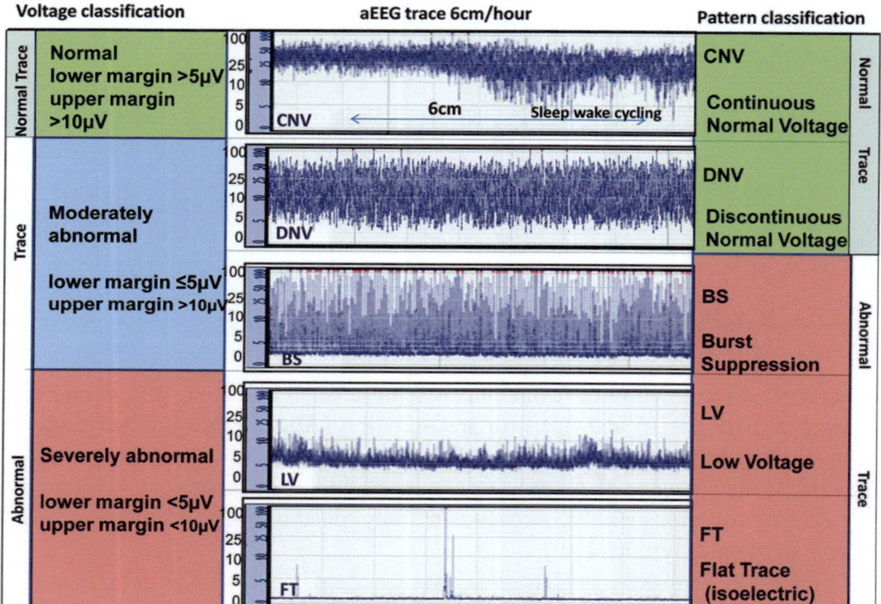

Fig. 8.1 Classification of five example traces using the pattern recognition method (right) and voltage method (left) to assess the aEEG background at 3 to 6 hours after birth (from [19]). (*Publisher acknowledges that the material will be published in an OA publication*)

normal trace, can be helpful in prognostication and assessment of brain recovery (see Chap. 16 for more details).

aEEG background can be classified based on the voltage and pattern (Fig. 8.1) [19].

8.2.4 EEG/aEEG Background and Prognosis

During therapeutic hypothermia (TH), the recovery time taken to achieve a normal background pattern (time-to-normal-trace or TTNT) is the best predictor of good and poor outcomes. Among infants who never gain a normal trace, all had poor outcomes and 72% died [19]. Furthermore, combining longitudinal background analysis with a sleep-wake cycling score may improve the predictive value of aEEG [20] (see Chap. 16).

8.2.4.1 Presence of Seizures and Prognosis

Short and focal seizures may be missed using aEEG, and cEEG (continuous EEG monitoring) is therefore recommended, but this is not possible in all centers especially over a long period. High electrographic seizure burden (>40 min) is associated with abnormal long-term outcomes, independent of HIE severity or TH [21, 22]. Seizures occurring during rewarming are also associated with a poor outcome and are seen in infants who have a poor background activity during TH [23].

Early seizure detection and treatment within 1 hour are critical in achieving seizure control and decreasing seizure burden [24].

Continuous brain monitoring can improve seizure detection and decrease anti-seizure medication burden [25].

8.2.5 Neuroimaging

8.2.5.1 Cranial Ultrasound (cUS)

Cranial ultrasound (cUS) (including Doppler) is the primary neuroimaging modality in neonates including infants with HIE (see Fig. 8.2) and plays an important role in determining non-HIE causes of neonatal encephalopathy as well as assessing the timing and evolution of hypoxic-ischemic brain injury, the effects of TH treatment (i.e., basal ganglia changes improving over time during TH), and prognostication [26–28]. A scoring system based on white/gray matter differentiation, size of the ventricles, and echogenicity of the periventricular and subcortical white matter (Table 8.3 and Fig. 8.2) was predictive of long-term neurodevelopmental outcomes [29]. cUS needs to be performed on admission and repeated at least twice in the first week to assess the progress of any injury. With an acute insult, the initial scan may well appear normal, and this, in itself, is important information but does not exclude an evolving injury pattern.

8.2.5.2 MRI

Brain MRI is the gold standard for detecting and defining the extent of acute injury after perinatal asphyxia. Brain MRI is usually done shortly after rewarming to help with counseling families as soon as possible; the MRI is either done between days 4–6 in order to take advantage of information from diffusion-weighted imaging (DWI) (see Chap. 15 "MRI") and then into the second week to see maximum injury

Table 8.3 Cranial ultrasound (cUS) scoring system for brain injury in HIE

	Item	Normal-mildly abnormal (0)	Moderately abnormal (1)	Severely abnormal (2)	Total points
White matter items	Edema: Impaired white/gray matter differentiation and/or slit-like ventricles	Normal differentiation between gray and white matter and open ventricles	Reduced differentiation between gray and white matter and/or slit-like ventricles	No differentiation between gray and white matter and slit-like ventricles	
	Echogenicity periventricular white matter	Normal echogenicity or minor hyperechogenicity	Moderate or focal hyperechogenicity, but not as white as the choroid plexus.	Severe and diffuse hyperechogenicity, as white as the choroid plexus	
	Echogenicity subcortical white matter	Normal echogenicity or minor hyperechogenicity	Focal hyperechogenicity of the subcortical white matter. Moderate differentiation between white and (subcortical) gray matter	Clear "tramlines" sign: hyperechogenicity of the subcortical white matter similar to that of the sulci with intervening hyposignal of the cortex	
Gray matter items	Echogenicity of the thalami	Normal echogenicity or minor hyperechogenicity	Moderate or focal hyperechogenicity of the thalami	The hyperechogenicity is severe and diffuse	
	Echogenicity of the putamina	Normal echogenicity or minor hyperechogenicity	Moderate or focal hyperechogenicity of the putamina	The hyperechogenicity is severe and diffuse	
		Absent (0)	**Present (1)**		
	Four-column sign	Normal echogenicity or minor hyperechogenicity	On the coronal cUS plane the four-column sign is apparent caused by moderate or severe bilateral hyperechogenicity of the thalami and putamina		
	Visibility of the posterior limb of the internal capsule (PLIC)	The PLIC is not visible as a hypo-echogenic line between the putamen and thalamus	The PLIC is clearly visible as a hypo-echogenic line between the hyperechogenic thalamus and putamen		
Scoring	White matter involvement is the sum of edema, periventricular, and subcortical white matter damage (0–6 points) Gray matter involvement includes hyperechogenicity of the thalami, putamen, visibility of the PLIC, and four-column sign (0–6 points)				

Adapted from Annink KV et al. Pediatric Research 2020;87 (Suppl 1):59–66 [29]
PLIC posterior limb of internal capsule

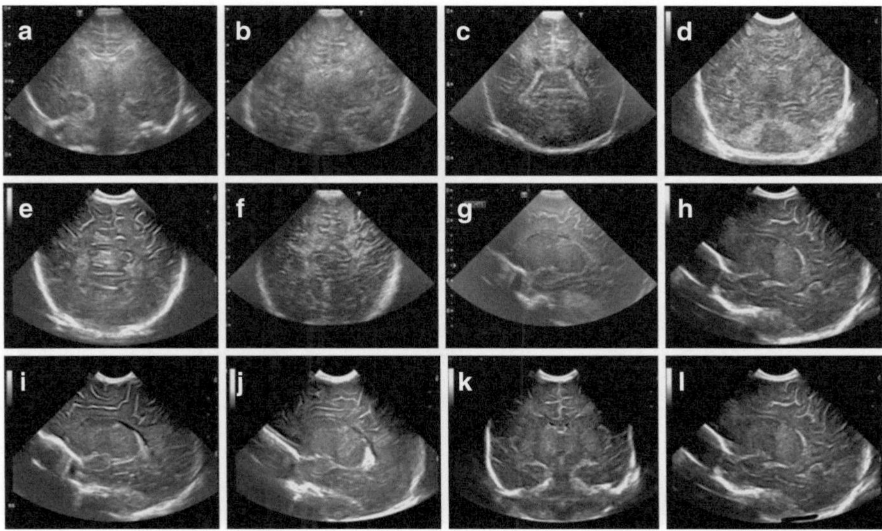

Fig. 8.2 Examples of scored brain injury in HIE using cUS: (**a**) moderate cerebral edema (1 point), (**b**) severe cerebral edema (2 points), (**c**) moderate periventricular white matter (1 point), (**d**) severe periventricular white matter (2 points), (**e**) moderate subcortical white matter (1 point), (**f**) severe subcortical white matter (2 points), (**g**) moderate thalamus (1 point), (**h**) severe thalamus (2 points), (**i**) moderate putamen and thalamus (1 point), (**j**) severe putamen and thalamus (2 points), (**k**) "four-column sign" which means that both left and right thalamus and putamen are visible on coronal view as four columns (1 point), (**l**) visibility of the PLIC on parasagittal view (1 point). For the scoring sheet and definitions, see Table 8.3 [29].

on conventional MRI. If one MRI examination is done, the preferred timing is between day 4 and 6.

Acute ischemic brain injury due to HIE detected by cUS and MRI can be divided into the following:

A. *Central/Basal Ganglia—Thalamus (BGT) Predominant Pattern* (Fig. 8.3): This pattern is characterized by injury to the gray matter of the BGT and cerebral cortex, usually localized to the perirolandic region, and is often referred to as the cerebrocortical-deep nuclear pattern on neuropathology. The pattern is typically bilateral and symmetric. The predominant neuropathological features include selective neuronal necrosis in the basal ganglia and thalamus and perirolandic cortex as well as the hippocampus (pyramidal neurons) [30]. On neuroimaging, the predominant features include injury to the BGT (Fig. 8.4a) and perirolandic cortex. Hippocampal injury is more difficult to detect unless the MRI is done within the DWI window [31, 32]. Nevertheless, it may be detected chronically as reduced volume by quantitative morphometry [33]. Clinically, the central/BGT pattern is commonly observed following perinatal sentinel events [34, 35] and moderate to severe, relatively prolonged insults [30].

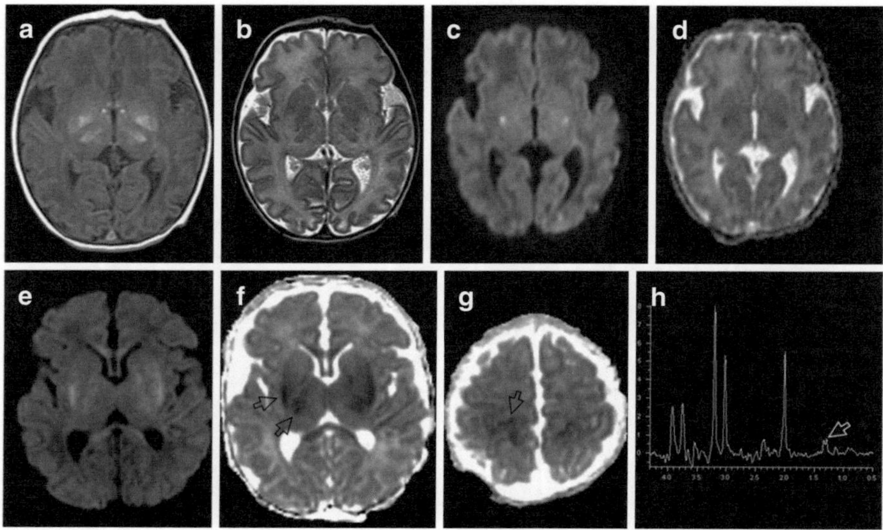

Fig. 8.3 Central basal ganglia—thalamus (BGT). (**a–d**) MR scan performed 1 day after birth in a full-term infant with neonatal encephalopathy and no clear history of perinatal depression. Axial T1-weighted (**a**), axial T2-weighted (**b**), axial diffusion-weighted imaging (DWI) (**c**), and axial apparent diffusion coefficient (ADC) (**d**) MRI images. There is bilateral and symmetric injury to the BGT with T1 hyperintense and T2 hyperintense signal. There are only small areas of involvement that have concomitant restricted diffusion with hyperintensity on DWI and hypointensity on ADC. The established signal alteration on the T1- and T2-weighted sequences on MR imaging 1 day after birth supports an antenatal timing of injury in this infant. (**e–h**) MR scan performed 3 days after birth in a full-term infant with clinical encephalopathy, respiratory distress, and perinatal depression at delivery. Axial diffusion-weighted imaging (DWI) (**e**), axial apparent diffusion coefficient (ADC) (**f, g**) MRI images, and single voxel MR spectroscopy (**h**). Bilateral and symmetric injury to the BGT and perirolandic cortex is identified from areas of restricted diffusion (open arrows). MR spectroscopy sampling of the left BGT, using a single voxel and long echo time (TE 270), revealed elevated cerebral lactate (doublet peak at 1.3 ppm, white outlined arrow) from anaerobic metabolism

B. *Deep Gray Nuclei—Brainstem* (Fig. 8.4): This pattern is characterized by injury to the basal ganglia, thalamus, and brainstem (mesencephalon, pons, and medulla). The predominant neuropathological features include selective neuronal necrosis in the BGT and select brainstem nuclei. Injury to these areas may be visualized on neuroimaging, in particular on MRI; while this pattern is well documented on neuropathology, in neuroimaging studies, isolated injury to the deep nuclear gray and brainstem is relatively rare; more commonly, there is also injury to the cerebral cortex (see paragraph above) [36]. Experimental studies in primates suggest that injury to the deep nuclear gray and brainstem results from an acute total hypoxic-ischemic event [30].

C. *Global Pattern* (Fig. 8.5): The global pattern, also referred to as "near total brain injury," is the most severe, characterized by diffuse brain injury. The predominant neuropathological feature is widespread neuronal necrosis across essentially all levels of the neuraxis (cortex, deep gray nuclei, brainstem). On neuroimaging, the global pattern is characterized by diffuse signal

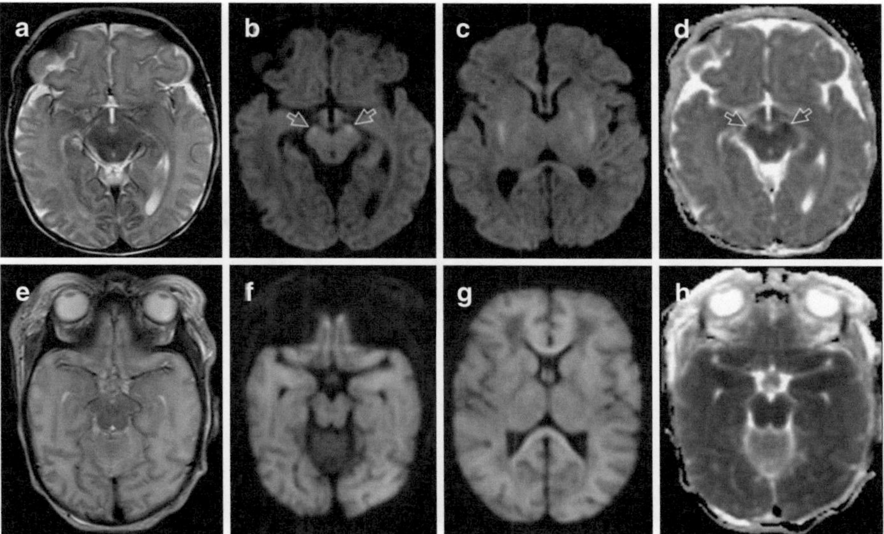

Fig. 8.4 Brainstem injury. (**a–d**) MR scan performed 3 days after birth in a full-term infant with clinical encephalopathy, respiratory distress, and perinatal depression at delivery (same case as shown in BGT figure above, (**e–h**) Axial T2-weighted (**a**), axial diffusion-weighted imaging (DWI) (**b, c**), and axial apparent diffusion coefficient (ADC) (**d**) MRI images. Small symmetric focal lesions in the cerebral peduncles of the midbrain (white arrows) have restricted diffusion with hyperintensity on DWI and hypointensity on ADC. The focal (<50%) brainstem injury was associated with injury to the BGT in this infant. (**e–h**) MR scan performed 4 days after birth in a full-term infant with clinical encephalopathy and severe prolonged asphyxia. Axial T2-weighted (**e**), axial DWI (**f, g**), and axial ADC (**h**) MRI images. The midbrain has diffuse restricted diffusion and its extensive (>50%) injury was associated with the global HIE in this infant (referred as white brain) [31]. Of note the cerebellum appeared relatively spared in this case

abnormalities in the BGT, cortex, brainstem, and white matter. The cerebellum may appear relatively normal, though quantitative imaging metrics (e.g., apparent diffusion coefficient) may be abnormal [37]. Clinically, the global pattern has been associated with very severe and prolonged insults and experimentally with prolonged asphyxia [30, 38].

D. *Parasagittal/Watershed Pattern* (Fig. 8.6): The parasagittal pattern is characterized by injury to the cerebral cortex and/or subadjacent white matter in a parasagittal distribution along the vascular border zone between the major cerebral arteries (for this reason, this pattern is also referred to as the watershed or border zone pattern). The injury is typically bilateral, although it may be asymmetric. The predominant neuropathological feature is selective neuronal necrosis involving cortical neurons along the parasagittal convexity [30]. Neurons in deeper cortical layers and, in particular, localized in the depths of sulci are especially affected [39]. In the most severe cases, the area of necrosis extends across the entire parasagittal convexity; however, more commonly, it is localized to posterior parietal-occipital regions. This pattern is among the least common observed at autopsy, especially in isolation; however, it is among the more

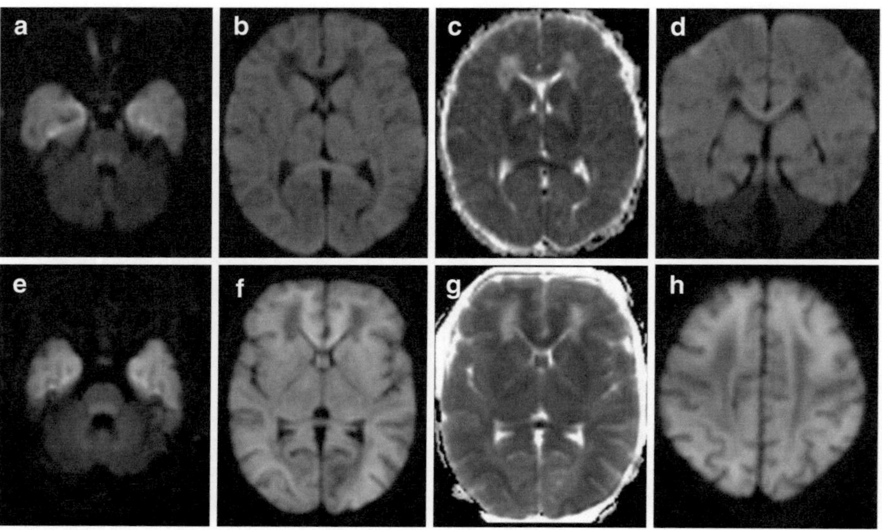

Fig. 8.5 Global injury pattern. (**a–d**) MR scan performed 4 days after birth in a full-term infant transferred to our NICU from outside hospital following emergency C-section for persistent fetal heart rate decelerations. Severe neonatal encephalopathy. Axial diffusion-weighted imaging (DWI) (**a, b**), axial apparent diffusion coefficient (ADC) (**c**), and coronal DWI (**d**). MRI images. Extensive signal abnormalities and restricted diffusion involve the BGT, posterior pons, cortex, and cerebral white matter with hyperintensity on DWI and hypointensity on ADC. The cerebellum appears relatively spared. (**e–h**) MR scan performed 4 days after birth in a full-term infant with severe prolonged asphyxia delivered by emergency C-section. Axial DWI (**e, f, h**) and axial ADC (**g**) MRI images. Global pattern of restricted diffusion with more extensive brainstem involvement than in the example above. The cerebellum again appears generally spared

common patterns observed on neuroimaging, with the observed differences likely attributed to the fact that most infants with this pattern of injury that does not include injury to the central gray matter survive long term. In clinical and experimental studies, parasagittal injury is associated with hypotension [30, 39].

E. *White Matter Injury Pattern* (Fig. 8.7): White matter injury may be primary or secondary, such as Wallerian degeneration. The primary white matter injury patterns are characterized by injury to the parasagittal white matter (described above) and the periventricular white matter. On neuropathology, this periventricular white matter injury is characterized by focal necrotic lesions in the periventricular white matter surrounded by larger areas of diffuse reactive gliosis. On neuroimaging, these are often referred to as predominant punctate white matter lesions (PWMLs) and may be visualized on cranial ultrasound, or more often on MRI, as punctate foci of high signal on T1-weighted imaging with or without concomitant restricted diffusion. This pattern is relatively common, in particular, among premature infants and (near)term infants with a milder degree of encephalopathy [40]. Clinically, white matter injury in term infants with HIE has been associated with chorioamnionitis, decreased placental maturation [41], and hypoglycemia [42] as well as pathological genetic mutations [43]. Experimental studies in primates suggest that white matter injury, including

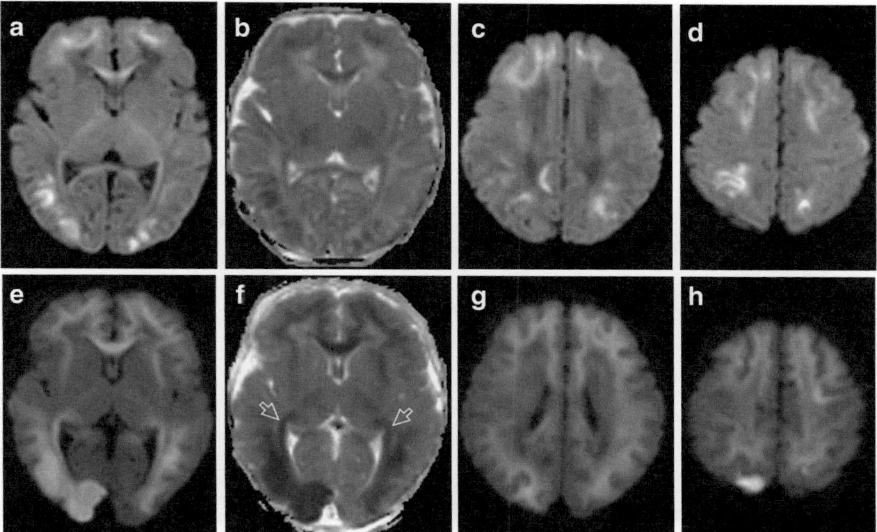

Fig. 8.6 Watershed injury pattern in two infants with neonatal encephalopathy. Both infants were delivered by emergency C-section due to decreased fetal movements and bradycardia. (**a–d**) MR scan performed 4 days after birth in a full-term infant. Axial diffusion-weighted imaging (DWI) (**a, c, d**) and axial apparent diffusion coefficient (ADC) (**b**) MR images. Predominant restricted diffusion involves the cortex and subcortical white matter in the watershed zones. The basal ganglia and thalami are generally spared. Note also low ADC in the genu and splenium of the corpus callosum in (**b**). (**e–h**) MR scan performed 4 days after birth in a full-term infant. Axial DWI (**e, g, h**) and axial ADC (**f**) MR images. A similar injury pattern involves the cerebral cortex and subcortical white matter in a parasagittal distribution along the vascular border zone between the major cerebral arteries. The basal ganglia and thalami are generally spared. Note also low ADC in the optic radiations (black arrows) and genu of the corpus callosum. Additional perinatal arterial ischemic strokes involve the right occipital and right parietal lobes

PVL, results from clinical circumstances that lead to hypoxia, but without a significant degree of acidosis [38].

F. *Perinatal Arterial Ischemic Stroke Pattern* (Fig. 8.8): Perinatal asphyxia is one of the many risk factors for perinatal arterial ischemic stroke (PAIS), which is characterized by an acute ischemic lesion localized within a cerebral artery distribution, most commonly the middle cerebral artery. It is not a common pattern seen with HIE and more commonly occurs in the absence of HIE (see Chap. 9). Infants with a large stroke are encephalopathic. On neuroimaging, these lesions appear as acute on early scans (i.e., first week), indicating they were acquired in the perinatal period and are readily recognized due to their wedge-like shape and localization in a vascular distribution (Fig. 8.8).

G. *Cerebellar Injury Pattern* (Fig. 8.9): Cerebellar injury has been largely under-recognized in infants with HIE. Although experimental studies in primates and neuropathological studies in infants have both demonstrated that cerebellar neurons are vulnerable to hypoxia-ischemia [30, 44], this insult has received less attention in clinical studies. However, recent studies have demonstrated

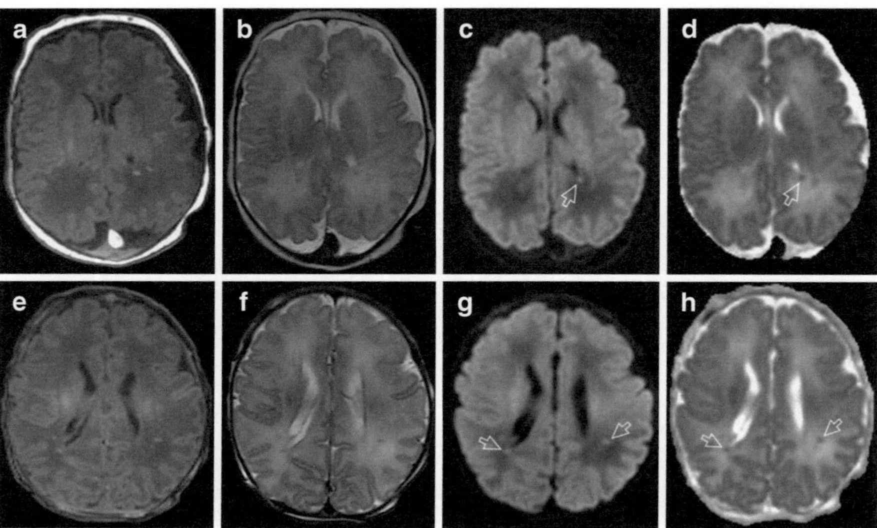

Fig. 8.7 Predominant white matter injury (**a–d**). MR scan performed 11 days after birth in a full-term infant with neonatal encephalopathy post therapeutic hypothermia. Axial T1-weighted (**a**), T2-weighted (**b**), diffusion-weighted imaging (DWI) (**c**), and apparent diffusion coefficient (ADC) (**d**) MRI images. There are multiple punctate foci of T1-weighted hyperintense and T2-weighted hypointense signal (PWMLs) in the periventricular white matter. Some foci have concomitant restricted diffusion with hyperintensity on DWI and hypointensity on ADC (arrows). An earlier MR scan performed 4 days after birth showed fewer and less conspicuous PWMLs. Images also show a trace volume of subdural blood layering along the left side of the posterior interhemispheric falx. (**e–h**) MR scan performed 4 days after birth in a full-term infant with clinical encephalopathy. Axial T1-weighted (**e**), T2-weighted (**f**), DWI (**g**), and ADC (**h**) MRI images show similar punctate foci of high signal on T1-weighted imaging with or without concomitant restricted diffusion (white arrows)

cerebellar abnormalities on cUS and MRI as well as a correlation between these abnormalities and microglia activation on neuropathology among infants with HIE [37, 45–47].

H. *Mamillary bodies* (Fig. 8.10): Recent studies have demonstrated acute injury to the mammillary bodies in HIE [48] even after TH, best seen on thin T2-W axial images but also, though less often, on diffusion weighted images. This injury may co-occur with other patterns discussed above or can occur in isolation even after treatment with TH. Noting injury to the mammillary bodies is important as it is associated, even independent of hippocampal injury, with significant memory problems at early school age and later imaging shows atrophy of the tissue [49, 50]. In order to access the mammillary bodies neonatally it is necessary to include thin (2mm) T2W axial slices in the neonatal HIE imaging protocol.

I. *Other Injury Patterns* (Fig. 8.11): In addition to the hallmark patterns described above, other injury patterns have been identified by neuroimaging in infants with HIE. These include hemorrhages, focal ischemic lesions, venous infarcts, and sinovenous thrombosis (see Chap. 11).

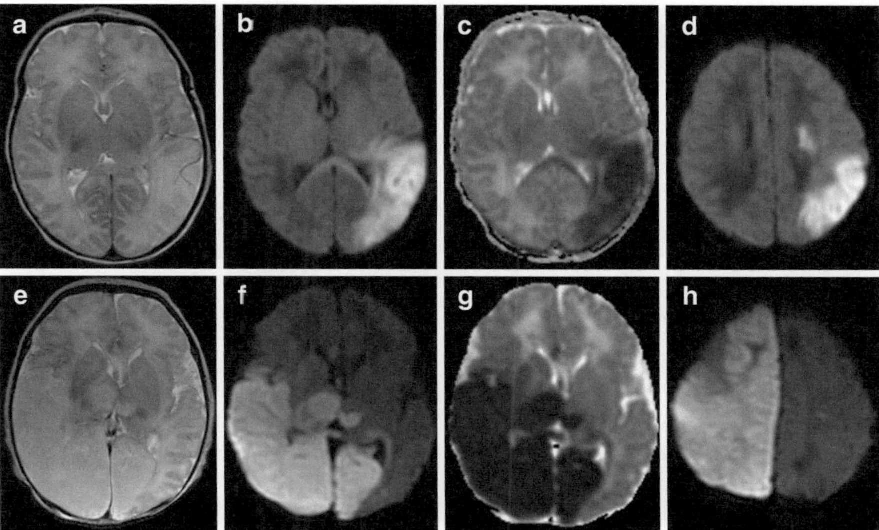

Fig. 8.8 Perinatal arterial ischemic stroke. (**a–d**) MR scan performed 3 days after birth in a full-term infant born asphyxiated and treated with therapeutic hypothermia. The baby had thrombocytopenia and left cerebral hemisphere focal onset seizures. Axial T2-weighted (**a**), diffusion-weighted imaging (DWI) (**b, d**), and apparent diffusion coefficient (ADC) (**c**) MRI images. Acute left middle cerebral artery infarct affecting mainly the posterior distribution area, with T2 hyperintense signal and restricted diffusion (hyperintensity on DWI and hypointensity on ADC map) in the white matter and cortex. The posterior limb of the internal capsule and basal ganglia appear minimally involved. Secondary changes are seen in the pulvinar of the left thalamus and crossing the splenium of the corpus callosum. (**e–h**) MR scan performed 1 day after birth in an asphyxiated full-term infant with severe neonatal encephalopathy for possible redirection of care. Axial T2-weighted (**e**), DWI (**f, h**), and ADC (**g**) MRI images. Extensive bilateral perinatal arterial ischemic stroke involved multiple arterial territories in the anterior, middle, and posterior cerebral circulation with bilateral thalamic and brainstem (not shown) involvement. Congruent ADC hypointensity of the infarcts is consistent with injury caused by a single embolic shower event. Restricted diffusion typically occurs within 30–120 min after cerebral infarction, pseudonormalising by 10–14 days

8.2.6 Treatment

Efforts should focus on effective resuscitation in the first hour after birth to allow optimal transition from fetal to neonatal circulation and restore perfusion and oxygenation and glycemia as quickly and effectively as possible as well as the avoidance of hyperoxia, hypocarbia, and hyperthermia. Clinical and electrical seizures should be treated quickly and effectively, and this means that continuous EEG or aEEG monitoring needs to be instituted. Evidence suggestive of infection should be sought (e.g. prolonged rupture of membranes, maternal fever, chorioamnionitis either from the history and directly in the baby) and treated until proven negative. Therapeutic hypothermia (TH) is so far the only proven effective evidenced-based intervention as shown by multiple well-designed RCTs [51]. For TH to be effective, it needs to be initiated as early as possible (preferably 1–2 hours but up to 6 hours

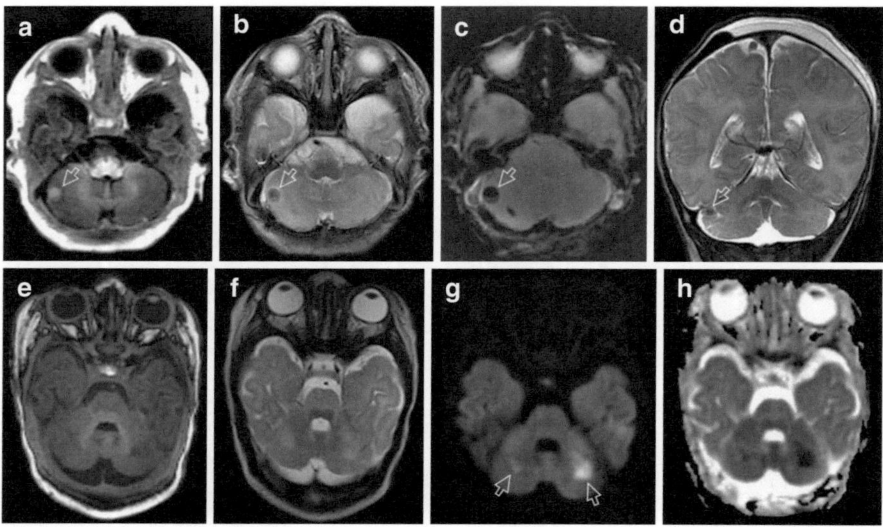

Fig. 8.9 Cerebellar injury. (**a–d**) MR scan performed 4 days after birth in a full-term infant with clinically suspected hypoxic-ischemic encephalopathy and limited right cerebellar hemorrhage (arrows). Axial T1-weighted (**a**), T2-weighted (**b**), T2* gradient-echo weighted (GRE) (**c**), and coronal T2-weighted (**d**) MRI images. The signal characteristics of the blood (T1 hyperintense, T2 hypointense, and very dark on T2* GRE) are consistent with intracellular methemoglobin and an early subacute stage (>3 days to 1 week) of intraparenchymal hemorrhage. No other parenchymal lesions were seen in this infant. A subgaleal hemorrhage is also visible on the coronal T2-weighted image. (**e–h**) MR scan performed 4 days after birth in a full-term infant with clinical encephalopathy. Axial T1-weighted (**e**), T2-weighted (**f**), diffusion-weighted imaging (DWI) (**g**), and apparent diffusion coefficient (ADC) (**h**) MRI images. MR imaging shows acute bilateral cerebellar infarcts that have subtle T1 hypointense and mild T2 hyperintense signal but have more conspicuous restricted diffusion with hyperintensity on DWI (arrows) and hypointensity on ADC. Additional supratentorial cerebral infarcts of similar age (not shown) were present in a watershed distribution

from birth), although some suggest that it can still be effective up to 8–12 hours of age [52]. Many adjunct therapies (e.g., erythropoietin, stem cells, xenon, melatonin) to TH are being studied but as yet none with strong evidence supporting [53–56].

It is important to keep infants undergoing TH well sedated and to avoid noxious stimuli. Morphine is currently the opioid of choice and extensively studied. If the infant is hemodynamically unstable, then fentanyl is an option. If, despite opioid sedation, the infant is still restless or uncomfortable, midazolam (as sedative) can be added.

There is an increasing interest in a multi-intervention bundled approach using quality improvement methodology to prevent neonatal brain injury. Neuroprotection bundles may target reducing acute brain injury or reinforcing neuroplasticity. The key concepts in the acute brain injury prevention bundles are early identification and referral, prevent fluctuations in physiologic parameters (such as pCO_2, blood pressure, temperature, etc.), minimal handling and pain management, early seizure diagnosis and treatment, early nutrition, normoglycemia, treatment of acidosis, and optimizing fluid and electrolyte balance including calcium [57–61]. Implementing

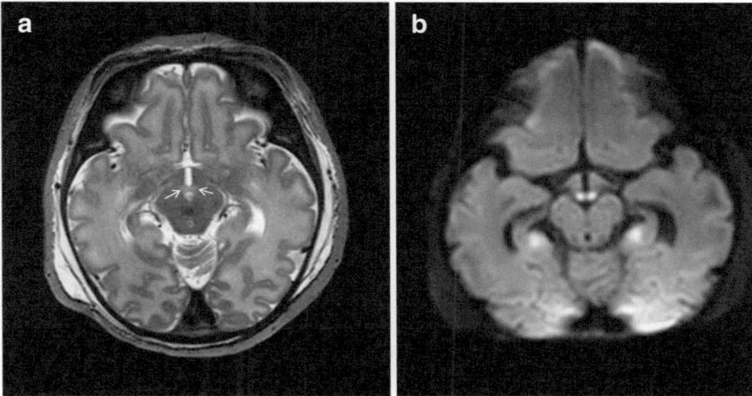

Fig. 8.10 Abnormal high signal and swelling is seen in both mammillary bodies on a thin 2mm T2-W axial image (**a**) with abnormal high signal on the diffusion-weighted image (**b**) in a term infant with perinatal asphyxia, treated with therapeutic hypothermia. The infant was imaged toward the end of the first postnatal week. Abnormal signal is also seen in both hippocampi in this instance. No other lesions were seen on this infant's scan

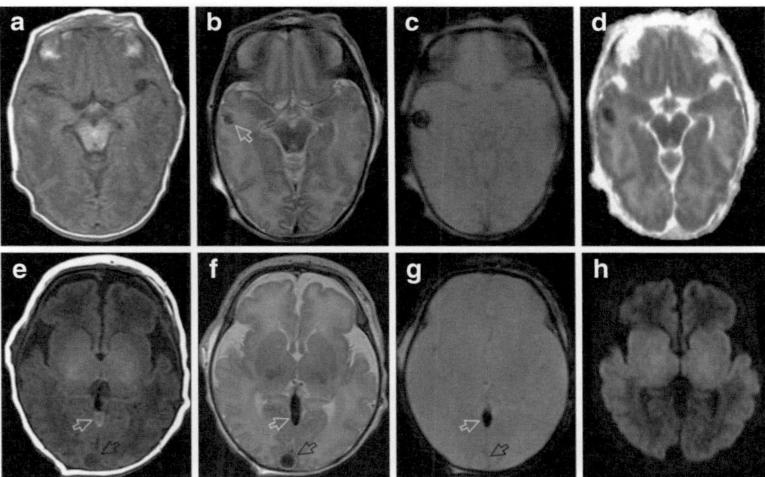

Fig. 8.11 Other injury. (**a–d**) MR scan performed 3 days after birth in a full-term infant with a small right temporal lobe hemorrhage. Axial T1-weighted (**a**), T2-weighted (**b**), T2* gradient echo (GRE) (**c**), and apparent diffusion coefficient (ADC) (**d**) MRI images. The signal characteristics of the blood (T1 mild hyperintense, T2 hypointense, dark on ADC, and "blooming" on T2* GRE) are consistent with deoxyhemoglobin and an acute stage (1–3 days) of intraparenchymal hemorrhage. The mechanism is most likely venous because the lesion is within the (sub)cortex and hemorrhagic. (**e–h**) MR scan performed 5 days after birth in a full-term infant with neonatal encephalopathy and cerebral sinovenous thrombosis of the straight sinus (open white arrows). Axial T1-weighted (**e**), T2-weighted (**f**), T2* GRE (**g**), and diffusion weighted (DWI) (**h**) MRI images. On the T2-weighted sequence, the dark signal of acute sinovenous thrombosis (white arrows) mimics normal intrasinus "flow void" that is seen within the patent superior sagittal sinus (black arrows). However, clues to the presence of an acute clot in the straight sinus are its moderately enlarged size ("fat sinus" sign) and, compared to the superior sagittal sinus, its differential mildly hyperintense T1 signal (**e**) compared to brain and its profoundly hypointense signal ("blooming") on T2* GRE (**g**). The straight sinus thrombosis was believed non-occlusive, and no ischemic changes were seen in the venous drainage territories

neuroprotection bundle approach has proven to be effective in improving HIE identification (through outreach educational programs) and preventing short-term morbidities and brain injury, anti-seizure medication burden, use of boluses and inotropes, temperature fluctuation, and overall hospital length of stay [25, 62–66].

Neuroplasticity bundles, unlike those aiming to prevent acute brain injury, target potential brain injury and brain growth well beyond the first few days of birth and after discharge [67]. Key elements in such bundles are as follows:

- Empowering families through family-centered care model (FICARE) [68].
- Optimizing nutrition [69].
- Developmental care [70].
- Skin to skin care and massage therapy [71, 72].
- Positive stimulating sounds such as music therapy, reading programs [73].
- Parental voice [74, 75].
- Minimizing disturbing noises [76].
- Enhancing physiologic sleep-wake cycles [77].
- Encouraging positive social interaction [78].

These neuroplasticity interventions may improve long-term cognitive and motor outcomes [71–73].

8.2.7 Other Diagnoses That Mimic HIE

It is important to keep in mind other conditions that can present with acute encephalopathy at birth such as vascular conditions, congenital anomalies, neuromuscular and metabolic diseases, and genetic conditions (Table 8.4).

8.2.8 Prognosis and Follow-Up

Fortunately, with the advances in neonatal care, long-term neurodevelopmental outcomes have improved for infants receiving TH for HIE. However, infants are still at risk of adverse neurodevelopmental outcomes even when the encephalopathy is mild or after they received TH [80]. Moreover, in many clinical settings, TH is not available and might even be detrimental especially in the context of infection [81].

Normal serial clinical neurological exams during the first week after birth, normal aEEG/cEEG background recovery within 24 hours of birth, and normal brain imaging are good predictors of normal neurodevelopmental outcomes. However more recent studies have shown that children with neonatal brain imaging and other findings considered normal or near normal and who are functioning within the normal range at 2–3 years may still have problems later with higher executive functions, memory, more subtle motor development, and social interactions at early and mid-school age [82, 83].

Unfortunately, some children will have unfavorable long-term outcomes though fewer than before the introduction of TH. Although the most discussed outcome is

Table 8.4 Features distinguishing HIE from other causes of neonatal encephalopathy [79]; originally published in Seminars in Fetal and Neonatal Medicine, 2021, https://doi.org/10.1016/j.siny.2021.101272, all rights reserved

	Suggestive of HIE	Suggestive of other NE
History	– Sentinel event during labor or immediately before/during birth	– IUGR
	– Fetal heart rate abnormalities consistent with an acute event	– Oligohydramnios or polyhydramnios
	– Need for resuscitation at birth	– Maternal infection
	– Apgar <5 at 5 and 10 min	– Maternal medication or substance use
	– Encephalopathy evident immediately from birth	– Family history of genetic disorders, neonatal illness, or seizures
		– Delayed onset of symptoms after birth
Exam	– Abnormal Sarnat exam in isolation	Abnormal Sarnat exam in association with: – Congenital anomalies – Microcephaly – Macrocephaly – Contractures – Spasticity – Absent deep tendon reflexes ± hypotonia – Hepatosplenomegaly – Rashes/signs of infection
Blood tests	– Cord pH or blood gas with acidosis (pH < 7.0)	– Severe and/or persistent electrolyte derangements (hypoglycemia, hypermagnesemia, elevated lactate)
	– Elevated lactate	– Elevated WBC count, inflammatory markers
	– Evidence of multisystem end-organ dysfunction (abnormal CK, BUN/Cr, LFTs, troponin, LDH)	– Positive urine or meconium toxicology screens
	– Bleeding/clotting abnormalities	– Hyperammonemia, hypouricemia
Imaging	– cUS or MRI showing pattern of brain injury consistent with HIE	– cUS or MRI with evidence of chronic injury (e.g., cystic changes, atrophy) soon after birth
		– cUS or MRI with other brain abnormality or injury (brain malformations, sub-ependymal or other cysts and/or calcifications, hemorrhage, lenticulostriate vasculopathy (on cUS))
		– Normal MRI
Other studies	– Acute/subacute placental lesions on placental pathology, with or without chronic changes	– Chronic placental lesions on placental pathology

BUN/Cr Blood Urea Nitrogen/Creatine, *CK* creatine kinase, *cUS* cranial ultrasound, *IUGR* Intrautering growth restriction, *LDH* Lactate Dehydrogenase, *LFTs* Liver Function Tests, *WBC* White blood cells

cerebral palsy, there are many other problems that may ensue including cognitive, speech and language, visual and/or hearing impairments, feeding difficulties, milder motor problems, memory problems, behavioral problems, later seizures/epilepsy, and abnormal higher executive functions [84, 85]. As a rule of thumb, injuries isolated to the deep gray matter put infants at risk of motor more than cognitive disabilities. On the other hand, injury to the watershed areas with normal central gray matter increases the risk for cognitive impairment that may only be first recognized at school age together with other non-motor impairments [86]. Most studies classify children into good/poor outcome categories, but this binary approach does not take into account the range of issues that may occur. It is important to try to make as precise a prognosis as possible to inform and empower parents and to put in place early intervention programs, including early support for feeding and communication issues [87].

A good guide published pre-TH is that of Martinez Biarge et al. for babies with any injury to the central gray matter and for those without central gray matter injury but different grades of white matter injury [42, 87–89]. These studies relate different grades of injury seen on MRI to a range of outcomes at 2–3 years, e.g., most infants with severe injury to the central gray matter will in addition to their motor problems have significant feeding difficulties including the need for PEG placement and also speech and communication problems that need to be addressed early.

While outcomes have improved with TH, the relationship between imaging findings and outcomes remains unclear especially between mild to moderate central gray matter injury and motor deficits. In the post-TH era, scoring systems assessing different regions of the brain have been validated for predicting outcomes but still with a binary approach to outcome [90, 91]. So while low MRI scores predict good 2-year outcomes, higher scores encompass a range of problems. However a recent study published by van Steenis et al. has shown that individualized neuroprognostication in HIE is possible and accurate, in the era of TH, not just for the motor domain but also for mortality, cognition, epilepsy, central visual impairment and feeding across a range of severities [92], confirming the earlier work of Martinez-Biarge et al.

It is also important to try to assess early how much parents wish to know. In most cases parents appreciate having the wider picture and being made aware of potential problems. This means providing parental support and enrolling the infant in a follow-up and early-intervention program with a pro-active rather than "wait and see" approach. It is crucial to follow these babies closely, frequently, and long term till at least to school age. It is also important to provide early and ongoing parental support at a very difficult time.

For a guide to outcomes at 2 years in relation to brain imaging, please see Figs. 8.12, 8.13, 8.14, and 8.15 and Table 8.5. Figures 8.12, 8.13, and 8.14 give information on a range of outcome domains in infants with mild, moderate and severe basal ganglia/thalamic injury including whether the posterior limb of the internal capsule (PLIC) and other tissues are involved. Whilst this data was obtained in the pre-cooling era there is no definite evidence that the relationship between MRI findings in HIE and 2-year outcomes has changed significantly since cooling was introduced.

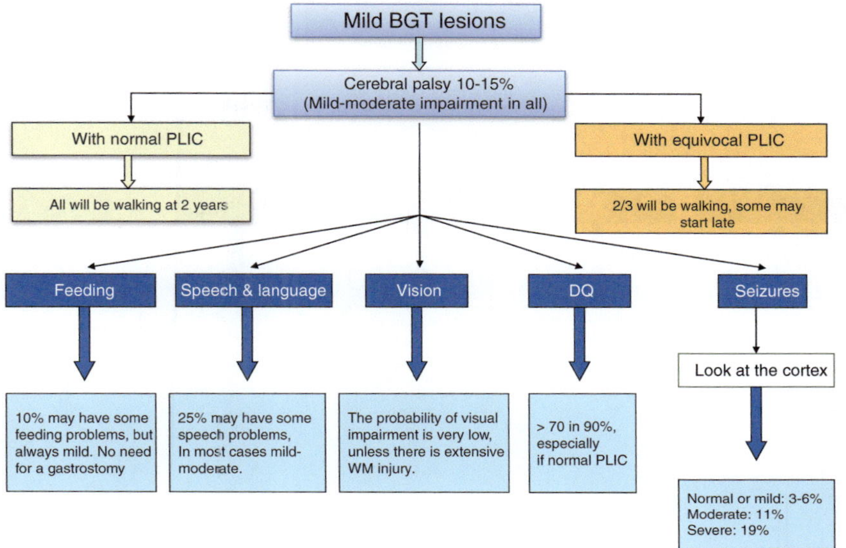

Fig. 8.12 Flow chart showing patterns of outcomes with mild basal ganglia/thalamic (BGT) injury. (Martinez-Biarge et al. Originally published in Early Human Development. 2010. https://doi.org/10.1016/j.earlhumdev.2010.08.013. All rights reserved). PLIC Posterior limb of the internal capsule and other tissues are involved [89]

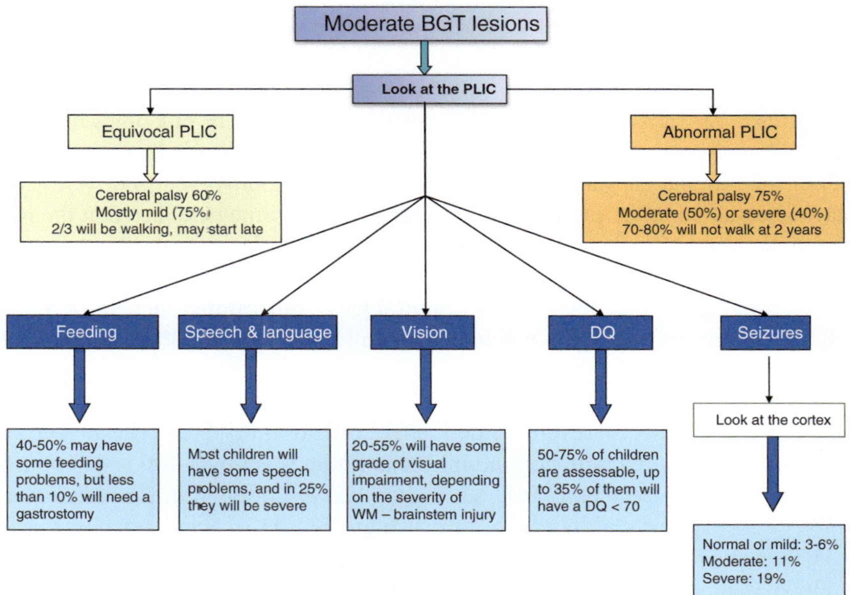

Fig. 8.13 Flow chart showing patterns of outcomes with moderate basal ganglia/thalamic (BGT) injury. (Martinez-Biarge et al. Originally published in Early Human Development. 2010. https://doi.org/10.1016/j.earlhumdev.2010.08.013. All rights reserved). PLIC Posterior limb of the internal capsule

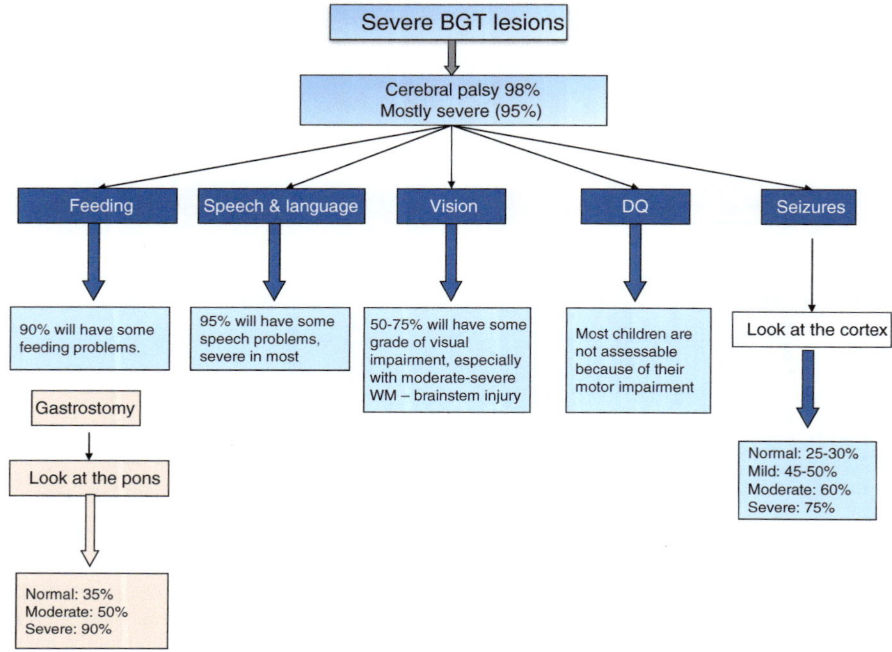

Fig. 8.14 Flow chart showing patterns of outcomes with severe basal ganglia/thalamic (BGT) injury. (Martinez-Biarge et al. Originally published in Early Human Development. 2010. https://doi.org/10.1016/j.earlhumdev.2010.08.013. All rights reserved). PLIC Posterior limb of the internal capsule

Figures 8.12, 8.13, and 8.14 give information on a range of outcomes in infants with mild, moderate, and severe basal ganglia injury including whether the posterior limb of the internal capsule (PLIC) and other tissues are involved [89]. While this data was obtained in the pre-cooling era, there is no definite evidence that the relationship between MRI findings and 2-year outcomes has changed significantly since cooling was introduced.

Figure 8.15 gives outcomes (death, cerebral palsy, other impairments) for infants with central gray matter injury defined as present or not in two cohort of infants all of whom were cooled for their HIE [91].

Table 8.5 gives outcomes for infants with normal looking central gray matter, but no or mild, moderate, or severe white matter/cortical injury [42]. The 2-year DQ values here for children with normal/mild scan findings are over 100 and similar to those reported by Weeke et al. [91] but higher than those found in the recent study by Wu et al. [56] for children with normal scans (BSID-III mean cognitive score 93.5). Reasons for this difference are unclear. One speculation could be the heterogeneity of diagnoses under the umbrella of HIE and differences in early intervention programs between cohorts.

Acknowledgements The authors of this chapter are grateful to Dr. James Scott (james.scott@ahs.ca) for giving permission to use (Figs. 8.3, 8.4, 8.5, 8.6, 8.7, 8.8, 8.9, and 8.11).

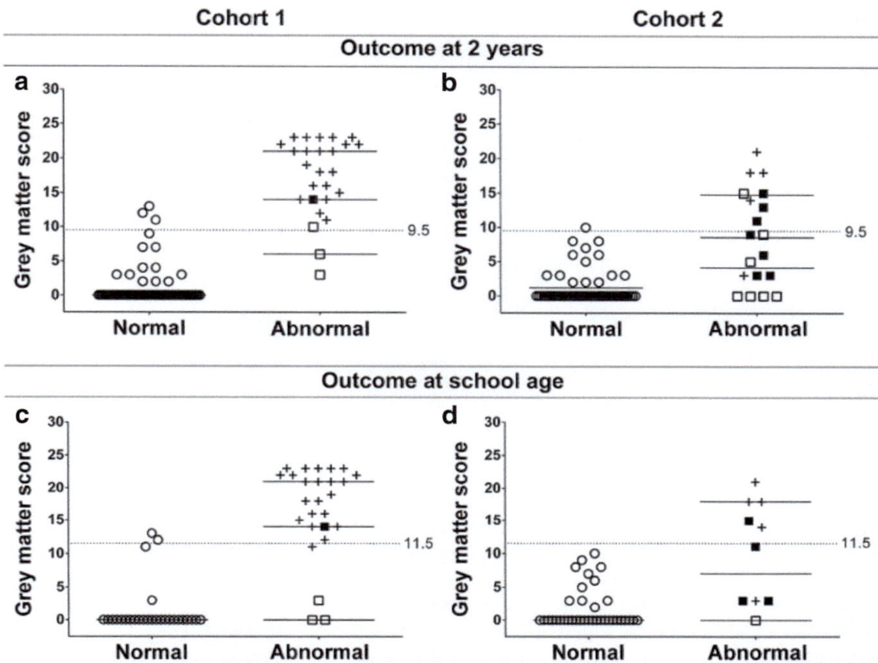

Fig. 8.15 Individual score values of the gray matter subscore of infants with normal and abnormal outcome (Weeke et al. [91])

Table 8.5 Comparison of long-term outcomes for infants with hypoxic-ischemic encephalopathy (not-cooled) with normal/mild, moderate, and severe white matter injury but without central grey matter injury

Neurodevelopmental outcomes	Normal and mild WM $n = 26$	Moderate WM $n = 34$	Severe WM $n = 22$	p
Motor outcomes				
Cerebral palsy, n (%)	0	1(3)	4(18)	0.018
Delayed walking (>18 months) n (%)	0	1(3)	5(23)	0.005
Other outcomes				
Feeding impairment, n (%)	0	3(9)	5(23)	0.026
Communication impairment, n (%)	1(4)	9(28)	14(64)	<0.001
Visual impairment, n (%)	0	1(3)	7/20(35)	<0.001
Hearing loss, n (%)	0	1(3)	1(4.5)	0.72
Behavioral problems, n (%)	1(3.5)	10(30)	13/19(68)	<0.001
Seizures (follow-up), n (%)	0	3(9)	8(36)	<0.001

(continued)

Table 8.5 (continued)

	Normal and mild WM $n = 22$	Moderate WM $n = 28$	Severe WM $n = 21$	p^a
Developmental quotient (DQ)[b]				
Total DQ ± SD	112 ± 14.1	104.3 ± 11.1	88.5 ± 20.5	<0.0001
Motor	108.4 ± 10.5	107.3 ± 15.9	92.8 ± 24.6	0.12
Social	114.3 ± 13.3	108.5 ± 12.9	96.1 ± 23.7	0.02
Hearing and language	111.7 ± 18.4	106 ± 21.2	83.2 ± 23.6	<0.001
Eye and hand coordination	109 ± 11.6	99.3 ± 11.5	83.4 ± 17.6	<0.001
Performance	115.6 ± 17.4	103.5 ± 12.4	83.6 ± 18.3	<0.001

	Normal, mild, and moderate WM $n = 52$	Severe WM $n = 20$	p
Head growth			
HC SDS at follow-up, mean ± SD	−0.05 ± 1.4	−2.1 ± 1.04	<0.001
Head growth (difference between birth HC SDS and HC SDS at follow-up, mean ± SD)	−0.37 ± 1.1	−2.02 ± 1.46	<0.001

Between mild and severe WM subgroups, significant differences were found for total DQ ($p < 0.001$), social subscale ($p < 0.05$) language, eye and hand coordination, and performance subscales ($p < 0.001$), but not for the motor subscale
Between moderate and severe subgroups, significant differences were found in total DQ ($p < 0.05$), language subscale ($p < 0.05$), and eye and hand coordination and performance subscales ($p < 0.01$), but not in motor or social subscales
Head circumference (HC) corrected for age and sex and expressed as SD from the mean for a British population
[a]Kruskal–Wallis test, Bonferroni, and Dunn multiple comparison post hoc tests: No significant differences were found between mild and moderate WM subgroups in total DQ and all subscales
[b]DQ measured using the Griffiths Mental Development Scales

References

1. Kurinczuk JJ, White-Koning M, Badawi N. Epidemiology of neonatal encephalopathy and hypoxic-ischaemic encephalopathy. Early Hum Dev. 2010;86(6):329–38.
2. Lawn J, Shibuya K, Stein C. No cry at birth: global estimates of intrapartum stillbirths and intrapartum-related neonatal deaths. Bull World Health Organ. 2005;83(6):409–17.
3. Montaldo P, Pauliah SS, Lally PJ, Olson L, Thayyil S. Cooling in a low-resource environment: lost in translation. Semin Fetal Neonatal Med. 2015;20(2):72–9.
4. Wood S, Crawford S, Hicks M, Mohammad K. Hospital-related, maternal, and fetal risk factors for neonatal asphyxia and moderate or severe hypoxic-ischemic encephalopathy: a retrospective cohort study. J Matern Fetal Neonatal Med. 2021;34(9):1448–53.
5. Aslam HM, Saleem S, Afzal R, Iqbal U, Saleem SM, Shaikh MW, Shahid N. Risk factors of birth asphyxia. Ital J Pediatr. 2014;40:94.
6. Berglund S, Grunewald C, Pettersson H, Cnattingius S. Risk factors for asphyxia associated with substandard care during labor. Acta Obstet Gynecol Scand. 2010;89(1):39–48.
7. Bouiller JP, Dreyfus M, Mortamet G, Guillois B, Benoist G. Intrapartum asphyxia: risk factors and short-term consequences. J Gynecol Obstet Biol Reprod (Paris). 2016;45(6):626–32.
8. Gardella C, Taylor M, Benedetti T, Hitti J, Critchlow C. The effect of sequential use of vacuum and forceps for assisted vaginal delivery on neonatal and maternal outcomes. Am J Obstet Gynecol. 2001;185(4):896–902.

9. Chakkarapani AA, Aly H, Benders M, Cotten CM, El-Dib M, Gressens P, Hagberg H, Sabir H, Wintermark P, Robertson NJ, Newborn Brain Society Guidelines and Publications Committee. Therapies for neonatal encephalopathy: targeting the latent, secondary and tertiary phases of evolving brain injury. Semin Fetal Neonatal Med. 2021;26(5):101256.

10. Sarnat HB, Sarnat MS. Neonatal encephalopathy following fetal distress. A clinical and electroencephalographic study. Arch Neurol. 1976;33(10):696–705.

11. Azzopardi D, Brocklehurst P, Edwards D, Halliday H, Levene M, Thoresen M, Whitelaw A, TOBY Study Group. The TOBY Study. Whole body hypothermia for the treatment of perinatal asphyxial encephalopathy: a randomised controlled trial. BMC Pediatr. 2008;8:17.

12. Jacobs SE. Selective head cooling with mild systemic hypothermia after neonatal encephalopathy: multicentre randomised trial. J Pediatr. 2005;147(1):122–3.

13. Jacobs SE, Morley CJ, Inder TE, Stewart MJ, Smith KR, McNamara PJ, Wright IM, Kirpalani HM, Darlow BA, Doyle LW, Infant Cooling Evaluation Collaboration. Whole-body hypothermia for term and near-term newborns with hypoxic-ischemic encephalopathy: a randomized controlled trial. Arch Pediatr Adolesc Med. 2011;165(8):692–700.

14. Shankaran S, Laptook AR, Ehrenkranz RA, Tyson JE, McDonald SA, Donovan EF, Fanaroff AA, Poole WK, Wright LL, Higgins RD, Finer NN, Carlo WA, Duara S, Oh W, Cotten CM, Stevenson DK, Stoll BJ, Lemons JA, Guillet R, Jobe AH, National Institute of Child Health and Human Development Neonatal Research Network. Whole-body hypothermia for neonates with hypoxic-ischemic encephalopathy. N Engl J Med. 2005;353(15):1574–84.

15. Simbruner G, Mittal RA, Rohlmann F, Muche R, neo.nEURO.network Trial Participants. Systemic hypothermia after neonatal encephalopathy: outcomes of neo.nEURO.network RCT. Pediatrics. 2010;126(4):e771–8.

16. Mendler MR, Mendler I, Hassan MA, Mayer B, Bode H, Hummler HD. Predictive value of thompson-score for long-term neurological and cognitive outcome in term newborns with perinatal asphyxia and hypoxic-ischemic encephalopathy undergoing controlled hypothermia treatment. Neonatology. 2018;114(4):341–7.

17. Thompson CM, Puterman AS, Linley LL, Hann FM, van der Elst CW, Molteno CD, Malan AF. The value of a scoring system for hypoxic ischaemic encephalopathy in predicting neurodevelopmental outcome. Acta Paediatr. 1997;86(7):757–61.

18. Thorsen P, Jansen-van der Weide MC, Groenendaal F, Onland W, van Straaten HL, Zonnenberg I, Vermeulen JR, Dijk PH, Dudink J, Rijken M, van Heijst A, Dijkman KP, Cools F, Zecic A, van Kaam AH, de Haan TR. The thompson encephalopathy score and short-term outcomes in asphyxiated newborns treated with therapeutic hypothermia. Pediatr Neurol. 2016;60:49–53.

19. Thoresen M, Hellstrom-Westas L, Liu X, de Vries LS. Effect of hypothermia on amplitude-integrated electroencephalogram in infants with asphyxia. Pediatrics. 2010;126(1):e131–9.

20. Meder U, Cseko AJ, Szakacs L, Balogh CD, Szakmar E, Andorka C, Kovacs K, Dobi M, Brandt FA, Szabo M, Szabo AJ, Jermendy A. Longitudinal analysis of amplitude-integrated electroencephalography for outcome prediction in hypoxic-ischemic encephalopathy. J Pediatr. 2022;246:19–25.e15.

21. Alharbi HM, Pinchefsky EF, Tran MA, Salazar Cerda CI, Parokaran Varghese J, Kamino D, Widjaja E, Mamak E, Ly L, Nevalainen P, Hahn CD, Tam EWY. Seizure burden and neurologic outcomes after neonatal encephalopathy. Neurology. 2023;100(19):e1976–84.

22. Kharoshankaya L, Stevenson NJ, Livingstone V, Murray DM, Murphy BP, Ahearne CE, Boylan GB. Seizure burden and neurodevelopmental outcome in neonates with hypoxic-ischemic encephalopathy. Dev Med Child Neurol. 2016;58(12):1242–8.

23. Chalak LF, Pappas A, Tan S, Das A, Sanchez PJ, Laptook AR, Van Meurs KP, Shankaran S, Bell EF, Davis AS, Heyne RJ, Pedroza C, Poindexter BB, Schibler K, Tyson JE, Ball MB, Bara R, Grisby C, Sokol GM, D'Angio CT, Hamrick SEG, Dysart KC, Cotten CM, Truog WE, Watterberg KL, Timan CJ, Garg M, Carlo WA, Higgins RD, Eunice Kennedy Shriver National Institute of Child Health and Human Development Neonatal Research Network. Association between increased seizures during rewarming after hypothermia for neonatal hypoxic ischemic encephalopathy and abnormal neurodevelopmental outcomes at 2-year follow-up: a nested multisite cohort study. JAMA Neurol. 2021;78(12):1484–93.

24. Pavel AM, Rennie JM, de Vries LS, Blennow M, Foran A, Shah DK, Pressler RM, Kapellou O, Dempsey EM, Mathieson SR, Pavlidis E, Weeke LC, Livingstone V, Murray DM, Marnane WP, Boylan GB. Neonatal seizure management: is the timing of treatment critical? J Pediatr. 2022;243:61–8.e62.

25. Bashir RA, Espinoza L, Vayalthrikkovil S, Buchhalter J, Irvine L, Bello-Espinosa L, Mohammad K. Implementation of a neurocritical care program: improved seizure detection and decreased antiseizure medication at discharge in neonates with hypoxic-ischemic encephalopathy. Pediatr Neurol. 2016;64:38–43.

26. Leijser LM, Vein AA, Liauw L, Strauss T, Veen S, Wezel-Meijler G. Prediction of short-term neurological outcome in full-term neonates with hypoxic-ischaemic encephalopathy based on combined use of electroencephalogram and neuro-imaging. Neuropediatrics. 2007;38(5):219–27.

27. Rath C, Rao S, Suryawanshi P, Desai S, Chetan C, Patil K, Patole S. Does abnormal Doppler on cranial ultrasound predict disability in infants with hypoxic-ischaemic encephalopathy? A systematic review. Dev Med Child Neurol. 2022;64(10):1202–13.

28. Epelman M, Daneman A, Kellenberger CJ, Aziz A, Konen O, Moineddin R, Whyte H, Blaser S. Neonatal encephalopathy: a prospective comparison of head US and MRI. Pediatr Radiol. 2010;40(10):1640–50.

29. Annink KV, de Vries LS, Groenendaal F, Vijlbrief DC, Weeke LC, Roehr CC, Lequin M, Reiss I, Govaert P, Benders M, Dudink J. The development and validation of a cerebral ultrasound scoring system for infants with hypoxic-ischaemic encephalopathy. Pediatr Res. 2020;87(Suppl 1):59–66.

30. Kinney HC, Volpe JJ. Hypoxic-ischemic injury in the term infant: neuropathology. In: Volpe C, editor. Volpe's neurology of the newborn, vol. 1. Elsevier; 2018. p. 484–99.

31. Vermeulen RJ, Fetter WP, Hendrikx L, Van Schie PE, van der Knaap MS, Barkhof F. Diffusion-weighted MRI in severe neonatal hypoxic ischaemia: the white cerebrum. Neuropediatrics. 2003;34(2):72–6.

32. Alderliesten T, Nikkels PG, Benders MJ, de Vries LS, Groenendaal F. Antemortem cranial MRI compared with postmortem histopathologic examination of the brain in term infants with neonatal encephalopathy following perinatal asphyxia. Arch Dis Child Fetal Neonatal Ed. 2013;98(4):F304–9.

33. Annink KV, de Vries LS, Groenendaal F, van den Heuvel MP, van Haren NEM, Swaab H, van Handel M, Jongmans MJ, Benders MJ, van der Aa NE. The long-term effect of perinatal asphyxia on hippocampal volumes. Pediatr Res. 2019;85(1):43–9.

34. Okereafor A, Allsop J, Counsell SJ, Fitzpatrick J, Azzopardi D, Rutherford MA, Cowan FM. Patterns of brain injury in neonates exposed to perinatal sentinel events. Pediatrics. 2008;121(5):906–14.

35. Shankaran S, Laptook AR, McDonald SA, Hintz SR, Barnes PD, Das A, Higgins RD, Eunice Kennedy Shriver National Institute of Child Health, and Human Development Neonatal Research Network. Acute perinatal sentinel events, neonatal brain injury pattern, and outcome of infants undergoing a trial of hypothermia for neonatal hypoxic-ischemic encephalopathy. J Pediatr. 2017;180:275–8.e272.

36. Volpe JJ. Neonatal encephalopathy: an inadequate term for hypoxic-ischemic encephalopathy. Ann Neurol. 2012;72(2):156–66.

37. Annink KV, Meerts L, van der Aa NE, Alderliesten T, Nikkels PGJ, Nijboer CHA, Groenendaal F, de Vries LS, Benders M, Hoebeek FE, Dudink J. Cerebellar injury in term neonates with hypoxic-ischemic encephalopathy is underestimated. Pediatr Res. 2021;89(5):1171–8.

38. Myers RE. Four patterns of perinatal brain damage and their conditions of occurrence in primates. Adv Neurol. 1975;10:223–34.

39. Marin-Padilla M. Developmental neuropathology and impact of perinatal brain damage. III: gray matter lesions of the neocortex. J Neuropathol Exp Neurol. 1999;58(5):407–29.

40. Li AM, Chau V, Poskitt KJ, Sargent MA, Lupton BA, Hill A, Roland E, Miller SP. White matter injury in term newborns with neonatal encephalopathy. Pediatr Res. 2009;65(1):85–9.

41. Harteman JC, Nikkels PG, Benders MJ, Kwee A, Groenendaal F, de Vries LS. Placental pathology in full-term infants with hypoxic-ischemic neonatal encephalopathy and association with magnetic resonance imaging pattern of brain injury. J Pediatr. 2013;163(4):968–95.e962.
42. Martinez-Biarge M, Bregant T, Wusthoff CJ, Chew AT, Diez-Sebastian J, Rutherford MA, Cowan FM. White matter and cortical injury in hypoxic-ischemic encephalopathy: antecedent factors and 2-year outcome. J Pediatr. 2012;161(5):799–807.
43. Hayman M, van Wezel-Meijler G, van Straaten H, Brilstra E, Groenendaal F, de Vries LS. Punctate white-matter lesions in the full-term newborn: underlying aetiology and outcome. Eur J Paediatr Neurol. 2019;23(2):280–7.
44. McAdams RM, Fleiss B, Traudt C, Schwendimann L, Snyder JM, Haynes RL, Natarajan N, Gressens P, Juul SE. Long-term neuropathological changes associated with cerebral palsy in a nonhuman primate model of hypoxic-ischemic encephalopathy. Dev Neurosci. 2017;39(1–4):124–40.
45. Hayakawa K, Tanda K, Koshino S, Nishimura A, Kizaki Z, Ohno K. Pontine and cerebellar injury in neonatal hypoxic-ischemic encephalopathy: MRI features and clinical outcomes. Acta Radiol. 2020;61(10):1398–405.
46. Steggerda SJ, de Bruine FT, Smits-Wintjens VE, Verbon P, Walther FJ, van Wezel-Meijler G. Posterior fossa abnormalities in high-risk term infants: comparison of ultrasound and MRI. Eur Radiol. 2015;25(9):2575–83.
47. Steggerda SJ, de Bruine FT, Smits-Wintjens VE, Walther FJ, van Wezel-Meijler G. Ultrasound detection of posterior fossa abnormalities in full-term neonates. Early Hum Dev. 2012;88(4):233–9.
48. Lequin MH, Steggerda SJ, Severino M, Tortora D, Parodi A, Ramenghi LA, Groenendaal F, Meys KME, Benders MJNL, de Vries LS, Vann SD. Mammillary body injury in neonatal encephalopathy: a multicentre, retrospective study. Pediatr Res. 2022;92(1):174–9. https://doi.org/10.1038/s41390-021-01436-3.
49. Annink KV, de Vries LS, Groenendaal F, Eijsermans RMJC, Mocking M, van Schooneveld MMJ, Dudink J, van Straaten HLM, Benders MJNL, Lequin M, van der Aa NE. Mammillary body atrophy and other MRI correlates of school-age outcome following neonatal hypoxic-ischemic encephalopathy. Sci Rep. 2021;11:5017. https://doi.org/10.1038/s41598-021-83982-8.
50. Spencer APC, Lequin MH, de Vries LS, Brook JCW, Jary S, Tonks J, Cowan FM, Thoresen M, Chakkarapani E. Mammillary body abnormalities and cognitive outcomes in children cooled for neonatal encephalopathy. Dev Med Child Neurol. 2023;65(6):792–802. https://doi.org/10.1111/dmcn.15453.
51. Jacobs SE, Berg M, Hunt R, Tarnow-Mordi WO, Inder TE, Davis PG. Cooling for newborns with hypoxic ischaemic encephalopathy. Cochrane Database Syst Rev. 2013;2013(1):CD003311.
52. Laptook AR, Shankaran S, Tyson JE, Munoz B, Bell EF, Goldberg RN, Parikh NA, Ambalavanan N, Pedroza C, Pappas A, Das A, Chaudhary AS, Ehrenkranz RA, Hensman AM, Van Meurs KP, Chalak LF, Khan AM, Hamrick SEG, Sokol GM, Walsh MC, Poindexter BB, Faix RG, Watterberg KL, Frantz ID 3rd, Guillet R, Devaskar U, Truog WE, Chock VY, Wyckoff MH, McGowan EC, Carlton DP, Harmon HM, Brumbaugh JE, Cotten CM, Sanchez PJ, Hibbs AM, Higgins RD, Eunice Kennedy Shriver National Institute of Child Health and Human Development Neonatal Research Network. Effect of therapeutic hypothermia initiated after 6 hours of age on death or disability among newborns with hypoxic-ischemic encephalopathy: a randomized clinical trial. JAMA. 2017;318(16):1550–60.
53. Jerez-Calero A, Salvatierra-Cuenca MT, Benitez-Feliponi A, Fernandez-Marin CE, Narbona-Lopez E, Uberos-Fernandez J, Munoz-Hoyos A. Hypothermia plus melatonin in asphyctic newborns: a randomized-controlled pilot study. Pediatr Crit Care Med. 2020;21(7):647–55.
54. Ruegger CM, Davis PG, Cheong JL. Xenon as an adjuvant to therapeutic hypothermia in near-term and term newborns with hypoxic-ischaemic encephalopathy. Cochrane Database Syst Rev. 2018;8(8):CD012753.

55. Tsuji M, Sawada M, Watabe S, Sano H, Kanai M, Tanaka E, Ohnishi S, Sato Y, Sobajima H, Hamazaki T, Mori R, Oka A, Ichiba H, Hayakawa M, Kusuda S, Tamura M, Nabetani M, Shintaku H. Autologous cord blood cell therapy for neonatal hypoxic-ischaemic encephalopathy: a pilot study for feasibility and safety. Sci Rep. 2020;10(1):4603.

56. Wu YW, Comstock BA, Gonzalez FF, Mayock DE, Goodman AM, Maitre NL, Chang T, Van Meurs KP, Lampland AL, Bendel-Stenzel E, Mathur AM, Wu TW, Riley D, Mietzsch U, Chalak L, Flibotte J, Weitkamp JH, Ahmad KA, Yanowitz TD, Baserga M, Poindexter BB, Rogers EE, Lowe JR, Kuban KCK, O'Shea TM, Wisnowski JL, McKinstry RC, Bluml S, Bonifacio S, Benninger KL, Rao R, Smyser CD, Sokol GM, Merhar S, Schreiber MD, Glass HC, Heagerty PJ, Juul SE, HEAL Consortium. Trial of erythropoietin for hypoxic-ischemic encephalopathy in newborns. N Engl J Med. 2022;387(2):148–59.

57. Ilves P, Kiisk M, Soopold T, Talvik T. Serum total magnesium and ionized calcium concentrations in asphyxiated term newborn infants with hypoxic-ischaemic encephalopathy. Acta Paediatr. 2000;89(6):680–5.

58. Ivy AS, Clark CL, Bahm SM, Meurs KP, Wusthoff CJ. Improving the identification of neonatal encephalopathy: utility of a web-based video tool. Am J Perinatol. 2017;34(5):520–2.

59. Lingappan K, Kaiser JR, Srinivasan C, Gunn AJ. Relationship between PCO_2 and unfavorable outcome in infants with moderate-to-severe hypoxic ischemic encephalopathy. Pediatr Res. 2016;80(2):204–8.

60. Mohammad K, Hicks M, Buchhalter J, Esser MJ, Irvine L, Thomas S, Scott J, Javadyan J, Kamaluddeen M. Hemodynamic instability associated with increased risk of death or brain injury in neonates with hypoxic ischemic encephalopathy. J Neonatal Perinatal Med. 2017;10(4):363–70.

61. Williams KP, Galerneau F. Intrapartum fetal heart rate patterns in the prediction of neonatal acidemia. Am J Obstet Gynecol. 2003;188(3):820–3.

62. Arriagada S, Huang H, Fletcher K, Giannone P. Prevention of excessive hypothermia in infants with hypoxic ischemic encephalopathy prior to admission to a quaternary care center: a neonatal outreach educational project. J Perinatol. 2019;39(10):1417–27.

63. Goswami I, Bello-Espinosa L, Buchhalter J, Amin H, Howlett A, Esser M, Thomas S, Metcalfe C, Lind J, Oliver N, Kozlik S, Mohammad K. Introduction of continuous video EEG monitoring into 2 different NICU models by training neonatal nurses. Adv Neonatal Care. 2018;18(4):250–9.

64. Mohammad K, Dharel D, Abou Mehrem A, Esser MJ, Paul R, Zein H, Scott JN, Fiedrich E, Murthy P, Dossani S, Kopores K, Kowal D, Montpetit J, Al Awad E, Thomas S. Impact of outreach education program on outcomes of neonates with hypoxic ischemic encephalopathy. Paediatr Child Health. 2021;26(5):e215–21.

65. Momin S, Thomas S, Zein H, Scott JN, Leijser LM, Vayalthrikovil S, Yusuf K, Paul R, Howlett A, Mohammad K. Comparing three methods of therapeutic hypothermia among transported neonates with hypoxic-ischemic encephalopathy. Ther Hypothermia Temp Manag. 2023;13(3):141–8.

66. Roychoudhury S, Esser MJ, Buchhalter J, Bello-Espinosa L, Zein H, Howlett A, Thomas S, Murthy P, Appendino JP, Scott JN, Metcalfe C, Lind J, Oliver N, Kozlik S, Mohammad K. Implementation of neonatal neurocritical care program improved short-term outcomes in neonates with moderate-to-severe hypoxic ischemic encephalopathy. Pediatr Neurol. 2019;101:64–70.

67. Cramer SC, Sur M, Dobkin BH, O'Brien C, Sanger TD, Trojanowski JQ, Rumsey JM, Hicks R, Cameron J, Chen D, Chen WG, Cohen LG, deCharms C, Duffy CJ, Eden GF, Fetz EE, Filart R, Freund M, Grant SJ, Haber S, Kalivas PW, Kolb B, Kramer AF, Lynch M, Mayberg HS, McQuillen PS, Nitkin R, Pascual-Leone A, Reuter-Lorenz P, Schiff N, Sharma A, Shekim L, Stryker M, Sullivan EV, Vinogradov S. Harnessing neuroplasticity for clinical applications. Brain. 2011;134(Pt 6):1591–609.

68. O'Brien K, Robson K, Bracht M, Cruz M, Lui K, Alvaro R, da Silva O, Monterrosa L, Narvey M, Ng E, Soraisham A, Ye XY, Mirea L, Tarnow-Mordi W, Lee SK, FICare Study Group and FICare Parent Advisory Board. Effectiveness of family integrated care in neonatal intensive care units on infant and parent outcomes: a multicentre, multinational, cluster-randomised controlled trial. Lancet Child Adolesc Health. 2018;2(4):245–54.

69. DeMaster D, Bick J, Johnson U, Montroy JJ, Landry S, Duncan AF. Nurturing the preterm infant brain: leveraging neuroplasticity to improve neurobehavioral outcomes. Pediatr Res. 2019;85(2):166–75.

70. Maguire CM, Walther FJ, Sprij AJ, Le Cessie S, Wit JM, Veen S, Leiden Developmental Care Project. Effects of individualized developmental care in a randomized trial of preterm infants <32 weeks. Pediatrics. 2009;124(4):1021–30.

71. Feldman R, Rosenthal Z, Eidelman AI. Maternal-preterm skin-to-skin contact enhances child physiologic organization and cognitive control across the first 10 years of life. Biol Psychiatry. 2014;75(1):56–64.

72. Procianoy RS, Mendes EW, Silveira RC. Massage therapy improves neurodevelopment outcome at two years corrected age for very low birth weight infants. Early Hum Dev. 2010;86(1):7–11.

73. Braid S, Bernstein J. Improved cognitive development in preterm infants with shared book reading. Neonatal Netw. 2015;34(1):10–7.

74. Chorna O, Filippa M, De Almeida JS, Lordier L, Monaci MG, Huppi P, Grandjean D, Guzzetta A. Neuroprocessing mechanisms of music during fetal and neonatal development: a role in neuroplasticity and neurodevelopment. Neural Plast. 2019;2019:3972918.

75. Shellhaas RA, Burns JW, Barks JDE, Hassan F, Chervin RD. Maternal voice and infant sleep in the neonatal intensive care unit. Pediatrics. 2019;144(3):e20190288.

76. Smith SW, Ortmann AJ, Clark WW. Noise in the neonatal intensive care unit: a new approach to examining acoustic events. Noise Health. 2018;20(95):121–30.

77. Shellhaas RA, Burns JW, Hassan F, Carlson MD, Barks JDE, Chervin RD. Neonatal sleep-wake analyses predict 18-month neurodevelopmental outcomes. Sleep. 2017;40(11):zsx144.

78. Forcada-Guex M, Pierrehumbert B, Borghini A, Moessinger A, Muller-Nix C. Early dyadic patterns of mother-infant interactions and outcomes of prematurity at 18 months. Pediatrics. 2006;118(1):e107–14.

79. Sandoval Karamian AG, Mercimek-Andrews S, Mohammad K, Molloy EJ, Chang T, Chau V, Murray DM, Wusthoff CJ, Newborn Brain Society Guidelines and Publications Committee. Neonatal encephalopathy: etiologies other than hypoxic-ischemic encephalopathy. Semin Fetal Neonatal Med. 2021;26(5):101272.

80. Dag Y, Firat AK, Karakas HM, Alkan A, Yakinci C, Erdem G. Clinical outcomes of neonatal hypoxic ischemic encephalopathy evaluated with diffusion-weighted magnetic resonance imaging. Diagn Interv Radiol. 2006;12(3):109–14.

81. Thayyil S, Pant S, Montaldo P, Shukla D, Oliveira V, Ivain P, Bassett P, Swamy R, Mendoza J, Moreno-Morales M, Lally PJ, Benakappa N, Bandiya P, Shivarudhrappa I, Somanna J, Kantharajanna UB, Rajvanshi A, Krishnappa S, Joby PK, Jayaraman K, Chandramohan R, Kamalarathnam CN, Sebastian M, Tamilselvam IA, Rajendran UD, Soundrarajan R, Kumar V, Sudarsanan H, Vadakepat P, Gopalan K, Sundaram M, Seeralar A, Vinayagam P, Sajjid M, Baburaj M, Murugan KD, Sathyanathan BP, Kumaran ES, Mondkar J, Manerkar S, Joshi AR, Dewang K, Bhisikar SM, Kalamdani P, Bichkar V, Patra S, Jiwnani K, Shahidullah M, Moni SC, Jahan I, Mannan MA, Dey SK, Nahar MN, Islam MN, Shabuj KH, Rodrigo R, Sumanasena S, Abayabandara-Herath T, Chathurangika GK, Wanigasinghe J, Sujatha R, Saraswathy S, Rahul A, Radha SJ, Sarojam MK, Krishnan V, Nair MK, Devadas S, Chandriah S, Venkateswaran H, Burgod C, Chandrasekaran M, Atreja G, Muraleedharan P, Herberg JA, Kling Chong WK, Sebire NJ, Pressler R, Ramji S, Shankaran S, HELIX Consortium. Hypothermia for moderate or severe neonatal encephalopathy in low-income and middle-income countries (HELIX): a randomised controlled trial in India, Sri Lanka, and Bangladesh. Lancet Glob Health. 2021;9(9):e1273–85.

82. Jary S, Lee-Kelland R, Tonks J, Cowan FM, Thoresen M, Chakkarapani E. Motor performance and cognitive correlates in children cooled for neonatal encephalopathy without cerebral palsy at school age. Acta Paediatr. 2019;108(10):1773–80.

83. Lee-Kelland R, Jary S, Tonks J, Cowan FM, Thoresen M, Chakkarapani E. School-age outcomes of children without cerebral palsy cooled for neonatal hypoxic-ischaemic encephalopathy in 2008-2010. Arch Dis Child Fetal Neonatal Ed. 2020;105(1):8–13.

84. Goeral K, Urlesberger B, Giordano V, Kasprian G, Wagner M, Schmidt L, Berger A, Klebermass-Schrehof K, Olischar M. Prediction of outcome in neonates with hypoxic-ischemic encephalopathy II: role of amplitude-integrated electroencephalography and cerebral oxygen saturation measured by near-infrared spectroscopy. Neonatology. 2017;112(3):193–202.
85. Lin B, Zhang P, Cheng G, Zhou W, Wang L. Meta-analysis of prognostic tests in neonates over 35-week gestational age with hypoxic-ischemic encephalopathy. Zhonghua Yi Xue Za Zhi. 2014;94(2):115–21.
86. Cainelli E, Vedovelli L, Mastretta E, Gregori D, Suppiej A, Bisiacchi PS. Long-term outcomes after neonatal hypoxic-ischemic encephalopathy in the era of therapeutic hypothermia: a longitudinal, prospective, multicenter case-control study in children without overt brain damage. Children (Basel). 2021;8(11):1076.
87. Martinez-Biarge M, Diez-Sebastian J, Wusthoff JW, Lawrence S, Aloysius A, Rutherford MA, Cowan FM. Feeding and communication impairments in infants with central grey matter lesions following perinatal hypoxic-ischaemic injury. Eur J Paediatr Neurol. 2012;16:688–96.
88. Martinez-Biarge M, Diez-Sebastian J, Kapellou O, Gindner D, Allsop JM, Rutherford MA, Cowan FM. Predicting motor outcome and death in term hypoxic-ischemic encephalopathy. Neurology. 2011;76(24):2055–61.
89. Martinez-Biarge M, Diez-Sebastian J, Rutherford MA, Cowan FM. Outcomes after central grey matter injury in term perinatal hypoxic-ischaemic encephalopathy. Early Hum Dev. 2010;86(11):675–82.
90. Trivedi SB, Vesoulis ZA, Rao R, Liao SM, Shimony JS, McKinstry RC, Mathur AM. A validated clinical MRI injury scoring system in neonatal hypoxic-ischemic encephalopathy. Pediatr Radiol. 2017;47(11):1491–9.
91. Weeke LC, Groenendaal F, Mudigonda K, Blennow M, Lequin MH, Meiners LC, van Haastert IC, Benders MJ, Hallberg B, de Vries LS. A novel magnetic resonance imaging score predicts neurodevelopmental outcome after perinatal asphyxia and therapeutic hypothermia. J Pediatr. 2018;192:33–40.e32.
92. van Steenis A, Cizmeci MN, Groenendaal F, Thoresen M, Cowan FM, de Vries LS, Steggerda S. Individualised neuroprognostication in neonates with hypoxic-ischemic encephalopathy treated with hypothermia. Neurol Clin Pract. 2025;15(1):e200370. https://doi.org/10.1212/CPJ.0000000000200370.

Focal Arterial Infarction and Lobar Hemorrhage in Term Infants

Miriam Martinez-Biarge and Frances M. Cowan

Abbreviations

Baby CIMT	Constraint-induced movement therapy for babies
CP	Cerebral palsy
CSVT	Cerebral sinus venous thrombosis
GMAs	General Movements Assessment
HINE	Hammersmith Infant Neurological Examination
HIE	Hypoxic-ischemic encephalopathy
IVH	Intraventricular hemorrhage
NAIS	Neonatal arterial ischemic stroke
MCA	Middle cerebral artery
MRI	Magnetic resonance imaging
PAIS	Perinatal arterial ischemic stroke
PLIC	Posterior limb of the internal capsule
RCT	Randomized controlled trial

M. Martinez-Biarge
Department of Paediatrics, Imperial College HealthCare NHS Trust, London, UK
e-mail: miriam.martinez-biarge@nhs.net

F. M. Cowan (✉)
Department of Paediatrics, Imperial College London, London, UK
e-mail: f.cowan@imperial.ac.uk

© The Author(s) 2024
G. Meijler, K. Mohammad (eds.), *Neonatal Brain Injury*,
https://doi.org/10.1007/978-3-031-55972-3_9

## 9.1	Focal Arterial Infarction (Stroke)

### 9.1.1	For Parents

#### 9.1.1.1	What Is a Stroke?

A stroke happens when the blood flow to an area of the brain gets interrupted. This causes brain cells not to get the oxygen and glucose they need, and they cannot survive this for more than a few minutes after the blockage. Insufficient oxygen to part of the body is known as ischemia. Usually the blood flow is interrupted by a blood clot.

#### 9.1.1.2	Aren't Strokes a Disease of Older People?

Although strokes affect older people in greater proportion, they can occur at any age, including newborn babies. In fact, babies are especially vulnerable, and stroke happens to newborns more often than older children or young adults.

#### 9.1.1.3	How Does the Clot Form?

During pregnancy (and the first few days after birth), the mother and the fetus increase the factors that produce clots in order to prevent excessive blood loss during labor. This is one reason why babies and mothers are more prone to having clots around the time of birth.

The clot that causes the stroke is usually thought to start in the placenta, and this happens more often as the placenta gets "older." If the clot loosens from the wall of a blood vessel, it can travel to the baby through the umbilical cord and reach the heart and then move to arteries going to the brain. This does not usually occur later once the cord has been cut and the baby's circulation has fully adapted to living outside the womb. However, the symptoms can occur during the first few days after birth.

#### 9.1.1.4	Why Some Babies Have Strokes, But Not Others?

We do not know yet why strokes happen in some babies. Some situations during pregnancy and labor have been related to a higher risk of having a stroke—these are called risk factors and include inflammation of the placenta, high maternal blood pressure or a long and difficult labor. However these situations are also very common in babies who do not have a stroke. We do not yet know how to prevent a stroke.

#### 9.1.1.5	How Are Strokes in Babies Diagnosed?

A stroke is suspected when a baby has seizures (fits) during the first few days after birth. Some babies do not have seizures but are sleepier than usual, irritable, do not feed well or show irregular breathing.

Seizures happen because the injured brain cells produce an abnormal electrical pattern. In babies with stroke, the most common seizures involve the arm, the leg, or both, of one side of the body. They usually last a few minutes, during which jerky and twitching movements can be seen. Babies are usually awake and calm during the episode and do not show signs of pain, although some might be a little irritable—and they are usually calm after the episode.

When a stroke is suspected, doctors will do some tests to confirm or exclude it. These tests include taking images of the brain using cranial ultrasound (can be done on the ward) and MRI (magnetic response imaging—the baby needs to be taken to the scanner), various blood tests, EEG (recording brain waves) and an echocardiogram (imaging of the heart using ultrasound).

9.1.1.6 What Is the Treatment for Strokes?

Babies with a suspected stroke are admitted to the neonatal intensive care unit. There is no specific treatment at present for the stroke itself, but it is important to keep the baby's temperature in the normal range and also the blood pressure, pulse rate, oxygen level, and blood sugar, all of which are thought to help in preventing further damage. If seizures recur, some medications will be used to stop them.

9.1.1.7 Is the Life of My Baby at Risk?

Strokes in otherwise healthy, term babies very seldom cause death. The majority of babies will recover well from the acute problems and will be able to go home approximately a week after they are diagnosed. Strokes that happen around the time of birth are not expected to recur later in life—this would be extremely rare.

If the baby has an underlying medical condition (heart problems or infection such as meningitis) or is very premature, a stroke can make the baby's general condition more severe.

9.1.1.8 What Are the Consequences of the Stroke?

A summary of problems that may occur following a stroke are shown in the illustration below (Fig. 9.1). A stroke on the left side of the infant may affect movement abilities on the right side of the body and vice versa.

Because of the stroke, one part of the baby's brain has been damaged. At present we have no means to heal this part of the brain. Depending on the size and the location of the stroke (and which brain functions are affected), the consequences for the baby's future will be different. The information below is very general, and many babies with stroke do not have all the potential issues talked about.

Small strokes near the cortex (surface) of the brain may not cause any problems. However larger strokes and strokes that involve the central part of the brain or the areas supplied by one of the major cerebral arteries (called the middle cerebral artery) often affect the main areas controlling motor (movement) and language. If this happens, it is very likely that the child will develop a condition called hemiplegia and that they will find some aspects of communication challenging. This happens in about one third of babies with stroke. Remarkably however there is usually no major problem with language.

Hemiplegia means that one side of the body is weak or stiff or a combination of both. In children with neonatal stroke, the affected side of the body is opposite to the site of the stroke, and the arm and the hand are usually more affected than the leg and the foot (see illustration). It is very uncommon that a child with hemiplegia will not be able to walk, though walking may start later than in most children.

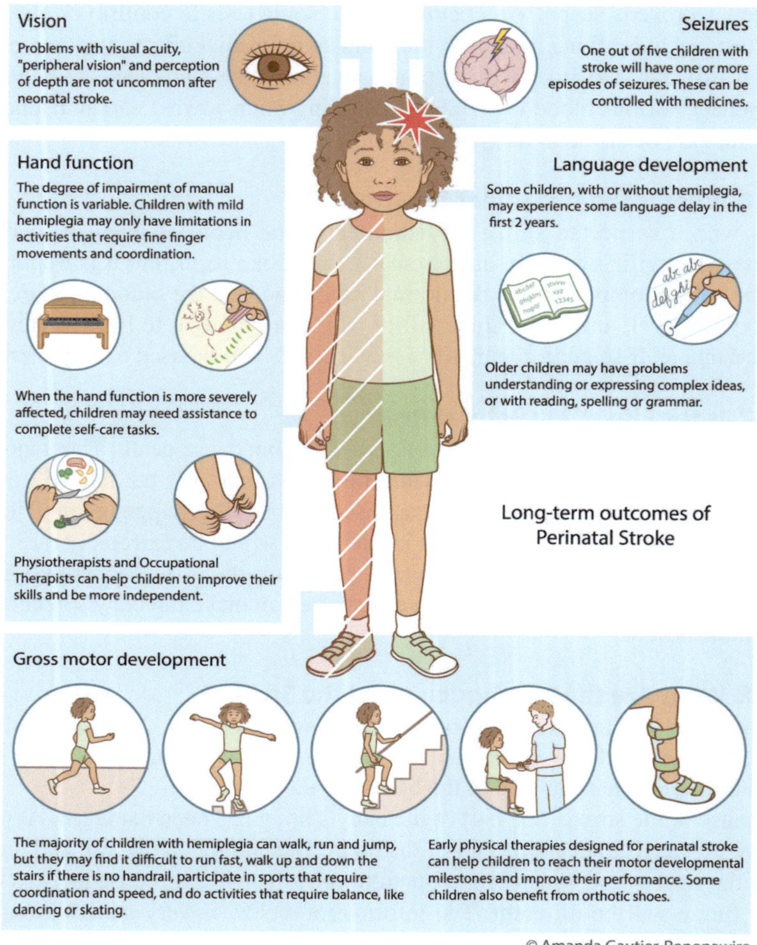

Fig. 9.1 Schematic drawing outlining possible long-term difficulties that may be faced by children with perinatal stroke. (© Amanda Gautier-Ronopawiro)

Some children may have impaired visual function. This does not mean that they cannot see, but their visual acuity or their ability to perceive distances or objects that are not in the center of where they are looking may be limited. Hearing is not expected to be affected. There is an increased risk of seizures or epilepsy in later childhood but most children do not develop this difficulty.

Although it is not possible to anticipate in detail all the problems a child may have, knowing the size and location of the stroke can predict quite accurately the risk of developing hemiplegia. The best test to obtain this information is an MRI scan.

9.1.1.9 What Happens After the Baby Is Discharged Home?

Depending on the hospital where your baby was born or admitted to, the person seeing you after your baby goes home can be a pediatrician, a neonatologist, or a pediatric neurologist. Other professionals are usually involved at different times: rehabilitation specialists, physiotherapists, occupational therapists, and speech and language therapists.

Babies at higher risk of hemiplegia will be seen more frequently during the first year, when any problems with movements usually emerge. If this happens, your baby will be referred early for physiotherapy assessment.

In some cases, a repeat MRI scan at 3 months of age will be offered; this second scan can help to define the risk of motor or visual impairment better if the first one was inconclusive.

During the first years, the developmental progress of your child will be monitored. Most children are doing well at this age, so assessments may be infrequent.

Around the time your child starts going to school, it would be useful to perform a neuropsychological assessment to see if there are any areas of development (language, attention, memory, how they process visual information, etc.) that could benefit from extra support. By doing this your child will feel more confident in school and with their peers, and their academic performance will improve.

9.1.1.10 Can Hemiplegia Be Cured?

No, but physical therapies (physiotherapy, occupational therapy), and sometimes leg support and adaptations to footwear, can improve hand and foot function, thus increasing the ability to perform everyday tasks. They can also help to correct posture and prevent pain and contractures (muscle tightening). In recent years, various rehabilitation strategies have been developed for children with hemiplegia, and others are under research. Some of them are applied intensively in summer camps for older children. This experience, as well as joining a club or group for children with hemiplegia, can be very positive and can help children to improve their skills and confidence.

In some centers one of these therapies (Baby Constraint-Induced Movement Therapy, Baby-CIMT) is now applied to babies as young as 3 months, if they are not using one hand as much or as well as the other. The long-term effects and other aspects of this early intervention are still being investigated.

9.1.1.11 Will My Child Be Able to Attend Mainstream School?

Most children with neonatal stroke can attend mainstream school. As explained before, some children may find some academic areas more difficult and may need extra help.

If the child has a hemiplegia, they may find managing a knife and fork together difficult, and getting dressed and undressed and sports challenging, and may not feel confident to participate in team sports (see illustration). Teachers and class helpers need to be aware of this and provide appropriate and discrete support.

Many parents report that their child with neonatal stroke experiences more behavioral or emotional problems than their siblings or friends. In many cases these are related to the degree of motor problems and how they are affecting your child's daily life. It is also possible that the injury to the brain itself makes the child more vulnerable to psychological problems. In any case, it is important to speak about this with your doctor and ask for help early. Some children, as they get older, perceive themselves different to other children, and this can create problems for them with peer relations.

Parents caring for a baby who so unexpectedly has very worrying symptoms often find this difficult and studies have documented that parents not uncommonly suffer from depression and other problems in the weeks and months after the birth even if the baby seem to be making good progress. If you are findings this to be the case seek help from your home doctor, visiting health professional, obstetrician or your baby's doctor.

9.1.2   For Professionals

9.1.2.1 Incidence

Perinatal stroke is the second most common cause of neonatal seizures in term-born infants after HIE and affects between 1:1600 and 1:5000 live births [1, 2], with a slight preference for males [2–4]. These different prevalence rates are likely due to differences in the populations included in studies. Perinatal stroke is the leading cause of unilateral cerebral palsy in children born at term and is also associated with other adverse outcomes in childhood: cognitive, language, and behavioral problems and an increased risk of epilepsy.

The terms perinatal arterial ischemic stroke and neonatal arterial ischemic stroke are often used interchangeably, and there is an overlap between them, but they are not exactly the same.

> **Terminology**
> **Perinatal arterial ischemic stroke (PAIS) or perinatal stroke.** Stroke that occurs at any time in the perinatal period, from 20 weeks of pregnancy to postnatal day 7.
> **Neonatal arterial ischemic stroke (NAIS) or neonatal stroke.** Stroke that occurs within the first postnatal month.
> **Arterial presumed perinatal ischemic stroke (APPIS).** Stroke that is detected after the neonatal period in infants who were not symptomatic at birth (but whose stroke, from its imaging appearances, would seem to have occurred neonatally or more likely before birth).

9.1.2.2 Pathophysiology and Risk Factors

The perinatal period is a high-risk time for cerebrovascular events. Of all arterial strokes affecting the pediatric population, 25% occur in the neonatal period [1].

Although the details are not well understood, it is accepted that in most cases a thrombo-embolus originating in the placenta crosses the patent foramen ovale to the left side of the heart and then moves onward to the aortic arch and the cerebral circulation [5] (see Fig. 9.2). Fetuses and neonates have a high hemoglobin concentration, relatively slow blood velocity and low serum activity levels of protein S and protein C, all of which contribute to create a hypercoagulable and proinflammatory state.

Some antenatal and mostly perinatal factors have been associated with a higher risk of neonatal stroke in epidemiological studies [4, 6, 7] (Fig. 9.3). None of these factors is determinant on its own, but most studies have shown that a combination of factors increases the risk.

Thrombophilic abnormalities in infants and/or their mothers were once thought to play a significant role in the pathogenesis of neonatal stroke; however results from more recent studies, along with the very low rate of recurrence of neonatal stroke,

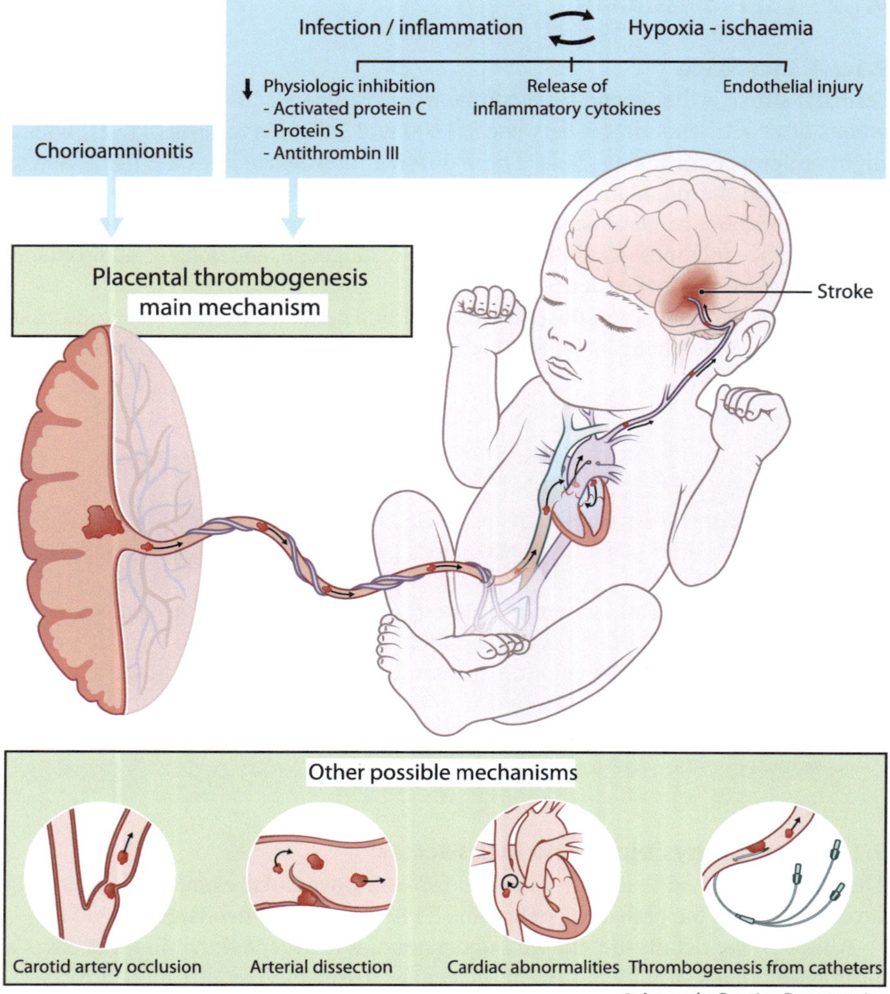

Fig. 9.2 Schematic drawing of potential mechanisms causing perinatal stroke. (© Amanda Gautier-Ronopawiro)

suggest that thrombophilia may be a predisposing factor that acts only in the specific context of the perinatal period when other risk factors are also present [8, 9]. However, if there is a strong family history, then this should be investigated in the infant.

9.1.2.3 Presentation

The typical scenario is represented in Fig. 9.4. Focal and brief seizures in a non-encephalopathic neonate who otherwise looks well are the most frequent sign; other infants may be just sleepy, not feed well or present with apneas [4]. Clinical presentation is different in neonates with congenital heart disease or in infants with sepsis

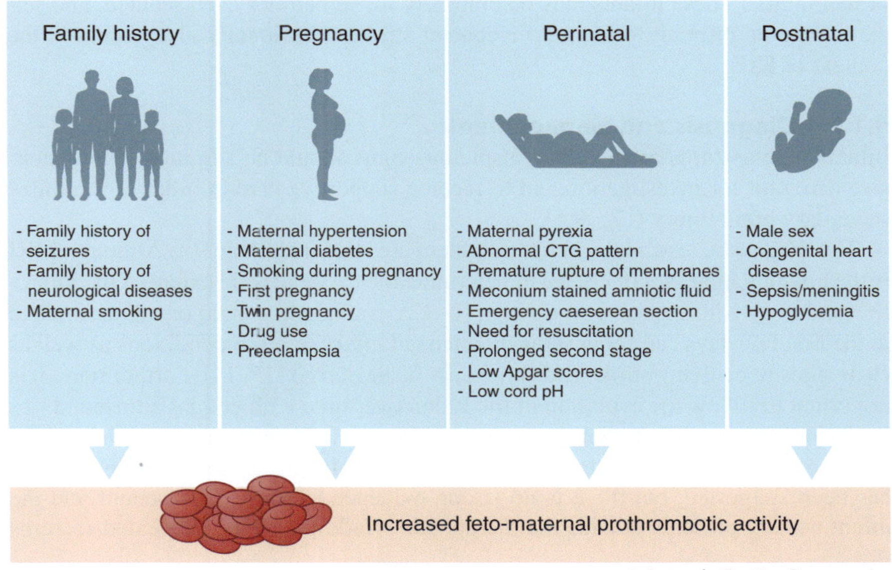

Fig. 9.3 Summary of clinical information from the family history, pregnancy, perinatally and postnatally currently thought relevant to the development of perinatal stroke. (© Amanda Gautier-Ronopawiro)

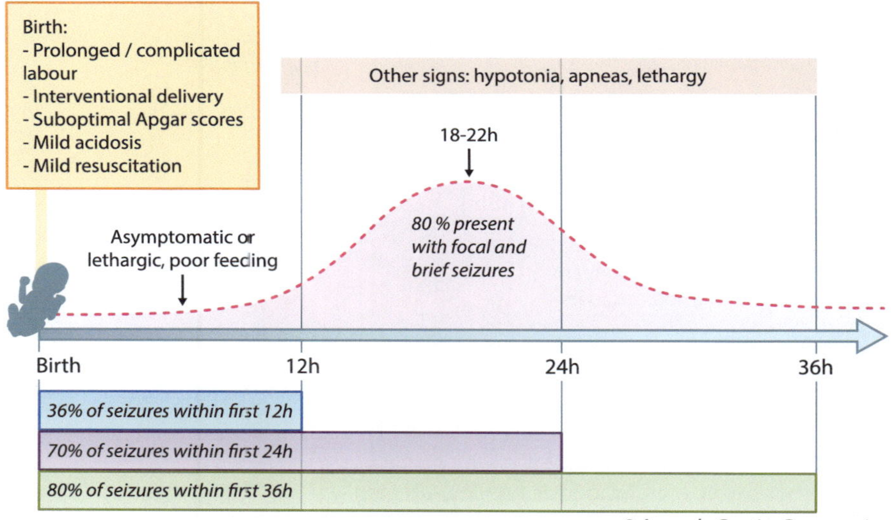

Fig. 9.4 Time course of likely presentation and symptom onset in term or near-term infants with perinatal stroke. (© Amanda Gautier-Ronopawiro)

or meningitis. These infants may be clinically ill, sometimes even sedated, and seizures may be difficult to identify. Neonatal stroke occasionally also occurs in the context of HIE.

9.1.2.4 Diagnosis and Management

Infants with seizures or any other suspicious signs should be admitted to the intensive care unit for investigation and to receive supportive care in order to minimize secondary brain injury (Fig. 9.5).

The diagnostic tests and when to use them are shown in Table 9.1. Although MRI is the imaging modality of choice to determine the existence and extent of the infarction and to give information on timing [10–12], cranial ultrasound on admission and in the first few days can show signs of antenatal injury or other conditions as well as clear signs of evolving stroke and should not be neglected [13, 14]. Furthermore, it is important to follow the evolution of the lesion over time with cranial ultrasound.

There is no specific treatment at present for neonatal stroke though trials of the early administration of erythropoietin and stems cells are underway; hypothermia has been suggested, but there is no strong evidence to support its benefit and the infant usually presents outside the therapeutic window for HIE. Repeated seizures

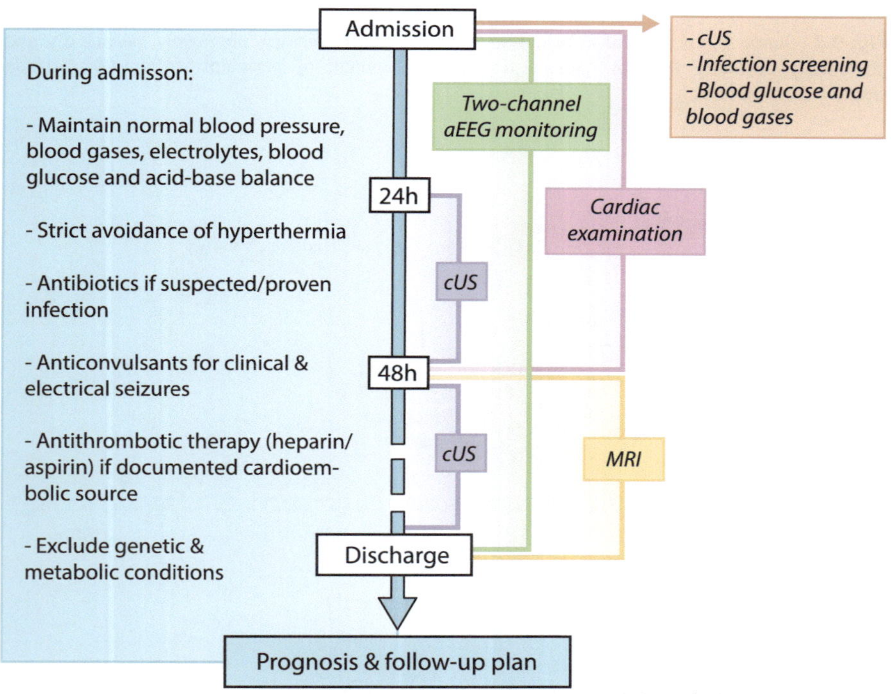

Fig. 9.5 Summary of the recommended clinical management of a newborn infant with perinatal stroke. (© Amanda Gautier-Ronopawiro)

Table 9.1 Investigations

Test	Timing	Findings
Cranial ultrasound scan	On admission	Often normal or non-specific findings if stroke onset was recent Can show signs of other conditions or prenatal injury Doppler exam of the MCA may show low/absent blood velocities on the side of stroke if the artery is still blocked
	24–48 h after admission	Asymmetries of echogenicity—can still be subtle Loss of normal echogenic interface between cortex and white matter Unilateral swelling and sometimes midline shift with larger strokes Subtle or more obvious focal echogenicity Doppler exam may show low/absent blood velocities or increased velocities from reperfusion on the side of an MCA stroke
	48–72 h after admission	More obvious focal and usually unilateral echogenicity—wedge shape if larger stroke affecting the main MCA branch
MRI	1–7 days after admission	Restricted diffusion on DWI and ADC—up to day 7 (full extent may not be seen on day 1 or 2) Changes in SI on T1-W and T2-W images (these appear later than the changes on DWI) show the size and location of the infarct and the affected structures
	3 months	DTI can show involvement of the CST and the OR if neonatal MRI was inconclusive. Atrophy can be seen with asymmetries of the PLIC, peduncles, and thalami, being less myelinated/smaller on the side of the lesion
Two-channel aEEG	From admission until normal tracing and end of seizures	Identifies seizures and monitors response to treatment - important as seizures may become sub-clinical after treatment Assessment of background activity
Full EEG	First week	Assessment of background and identifying focality of seizure activity
Cardiac/ vascular exam	First 24 h	Echocardiogram can show signs of endocarditis and thrombosis Neck ultrasound can show carotid thrombogenesis or occlusion Umbilical, abdominal, and femoral artery/vein ultrasound can show thrombosis if catheters are or were used

ADC apparent diffusion, *CST* corticospinal tract, *DTI* diffusion tensor imaging, *DWI* diffusion-weighted imaging, *MCA* middle cerebral artery, *OR* optic radiation, *PLIC* posterior limb of the internal capsule, *SI* signal intensity

should be treated urgently, usually until the (a)EEG tracing is normal and electrical seizures are no longer seen. Most infants with a stroke do not have ongoing seizure activity. Although the risk of recurrent seizures or epilepsy in infancy and childhood is increased, there is no evidence that prolonging anticonvulsant therapy after neonatal seizures has any effect in preventing later epilepsy. These drugs may have adverse neurodevelopmental effects, and prolonged use of these drugs should be avoided. Most infants do not need to be discharged home on medication [15].

9.1.2.5 Prognosis

Neonatal stroke affects many areas of development (see Table 9.2 and Figs. 9.6 and 9.7). Overall, 50–60% of children will have some developmental problems in one or

Table 9.2 Prognosis

Outcome	Prevalence	When it appears	Comorbidity	Prediction
Contralateral hemiplegia—upper limb generally more affected	30%	First signs: 2–9 months Obvious: 12–18 months Very rarely: >24 months	70–75% have ≥1 other developmental problem: Epilepsy, impaired language, cognitive deficit, visual impairment	High predictive value from neonatal MRI (see Fig. 9.5). Main predictor: location and CST involvement (PLIC and cerebral peduncles)
Language impairment	50%	Mild delay at 24 months—25% Complex maybe subtle language deficits at school age—50%	More prevalent in children with CP or epilepsy, but can be the only developmental area affected in some children	Higher risk with left-sided strokes, especially if they involve the left supramarginal gyrus (area posterior to central sulcus)
Cognitive impairment or low academic skills	20–30%	IQ is usually within the normal range, although in 20–25% IQ is between −2 and −1 SD. Specific learning difficulties/low academic performance presents at school age in up to 30% of children	More frequent in children with hemiplegia (especially with poor manual dexterity), but can occur without motor impairment. Lower academic performance in children with (active) epilepsy	Associated with larger strokes, but more difficult to predict individually
Epilepsy	20% ≥1 isolated episodes 10% active epilepsy	Variable (usually after first year)	40% if hemiplegia 10% if no hemiplegia	From neonatal MRI: higher risk with main branch MCA, large infarcts, and bilateral infarcts
Visual field defects	20–30%	First 3 years	Rare in isolation—usually co-occur with CP	From neonatal MRI: 40–60% in main branch MCA; 30–40% in PCA. Strong correlation with asymmetry of the OR at 3 months on conventional MRI and DTI

CP cerebral palsy, *CST* corticospinal tract, *DTI* diffusion tensor imaging, *MCA* middle cerebral artery, *OR* optic radiations, *PCA* posterior cerebral artery, *PLIC* posterior limb of the internal capsule

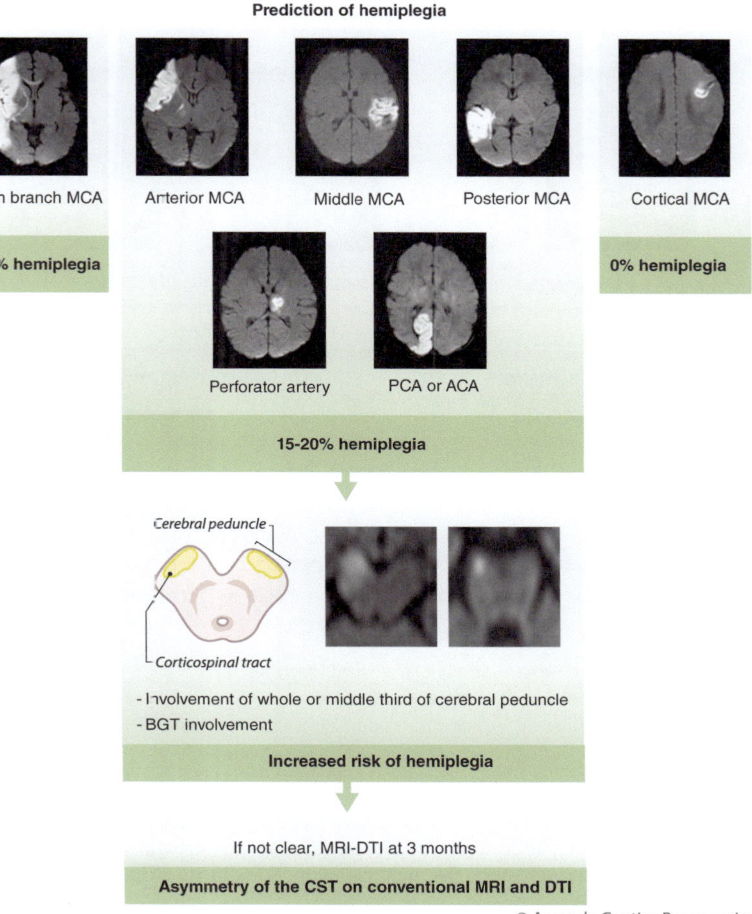

Fig. 9.6 Prediction of hemiplegia from neonatal brain imaging: the MRI scans show different sites of stroke with a range of likelihood of hemiplegia decreasing from 100% for the far left image, depending on whether the posterior limb of the internal capsule and the cerebral peduncle are also involved for the middle images, to 0% for a small cortical infarct. (From Wagenaar N et al. Pediatrics 2018 [17]. Permission to use the MR images has been from the copyright holder, AAP publications). (©AmandaGautier-Ronopawiro). *ACA* anterior cerebral artery, *MCA* Middle cerebral artery, *PCA* posterior cerebral artery, *BGT* Basal ganglia and thalamus, *CST* Cortico-spinal tract, *DTI* diffusion tensor imaging

more domains and around 25% in two or more [16]. Despite this, most children are able to attend a mainstream school.

Neonatal stroke has been traditionally associated with contralateral hemiplegia [18], but language development is the area most commonly affected—although all children with stroke are able to speak, up to half of them experience difficulties at school age, when they have to use language in more complex ways. Hemiplegia typically affects the hand function more than gross motor skills. Almost all children

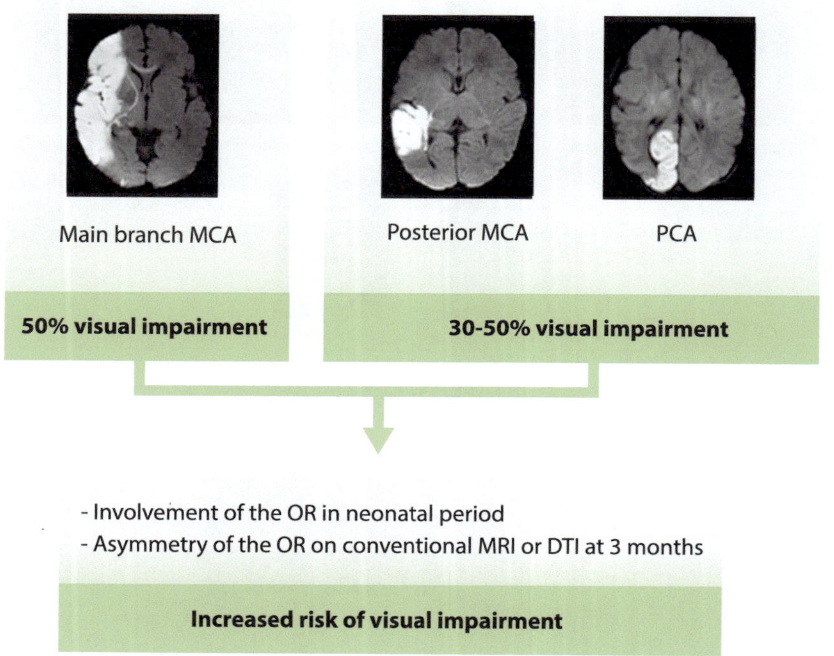

Fig. 9.7 Prediction of visual impairment from neonatal brain imaging: the MRI scans show different sites of stroke with a range of likelihood of developing some visual difficulties. (From Wagenaar N et al. Pediatrics 2018 [17]. Permission to use the MR images has been obtained from the copyright holder, AAP publications). (© Amanda Gautier-Ronopawiro). *MCA* Middle cerebral artery, *PCA* posterior cerebral artery, *OR* optic radiation, *DTI* diffusion tensor imaging

are able to walk before the age of 2 years and when the Gross Motor Function Classification System is used, most of them are classified at level I, which means that they are able to perform most daily physical activities, but with restricted speed, balance, and coordination. However children with bilateral strokes [19] may have more severe gross motor impairment and may be non-ambulant and also children with an additional underlying diagnosis.

Most children with neonatal stroke have an IQ within the normal range, but lower than their peers and lower than expected for their family background. However fewer than 10% have an IQ more than 2SD below the mean but up to 30% will experience poor academic performance and specific learning difficulties, including attention deficits and impaired executive function [20]. These problems are more frequently, but not exclusively, seen in children with hemiplegia and tend to get worse with time as academic and other demands are greater and especially in the presence of active epilepsy [21]. Epilepsy only affects 10–15% of children with neonatal stroke, although up to 25% may have isolated seizures at some point during infancy and childhood [22]. It is not clear whether the risk of febrile seizures is increased, but it seems sensible to manage high temperature early.

Recent studies have shown that children with stroke who develop hemiplegia have poorer social adjustment and participation and poorer quality of life than their peers, and this is related to the degree of manual ability, cognitive impairment and behavioral problems [23, 24]. As most children with stroke are in mainstream school, the children have to cope with peer pressure and their perception that they are different—this may be in ways that are overtly obvious such as hemiplegia or due to more subtle hidden problems relating to aspects of processing speed, vision, and language abilities and it is important that both family and schools are aware of these possibilities. As with other disabilities, parents of children with hemiplegia and other comorbidities may be psychologically affected and may need professional support themselves [25, 26].

Prognosis depends largely on the location of the infarct [17, 18] (Figs. 9.6 and 9.7); therefore it is important to look at the MRI scans yourself and/or request the following specific information from radiologists: (1) arterial territory affected; (2) involvement of the corticospinal tract (CST) at any level (motor cortex, posterior limb of the internal capsule, cerebral peduncle); (3) involvement of the basal ganglia and thalami (BGT); and (4) involvement of the optic radiation (OR). If involvement of the CST or OR is not clear from neonatal images, a repeat MRI at 3 months can help to confirm or rule out injury at these levels [27].

Middle Cerebral Artery (MCA)

Main Branch
These infarcts almost always involve the CST, and therefore they lead to contralateral hemiplegia in virtually all cases. Comorbidity is highest in this group: 85% of these children have other developmental impairments, i.e. cognitive impairment, language delay, epilepsy, behavioral problems, and visual field defects; each affects around 50% of children with main branch MCA infarct [17].

Anterior, Middle, and Posterior Branches
The overall risk of hemiplegia in these groups varies between 10 and 20%; this risk is modulated by the involvement of the BGT or the cerebral peduncle. The prevalence of other problems is in general low (10–20%), and fewer than 30% will experience adverse outcomes in more than one area [17].

Cortical Branches
Because strokes in cortical branches of the MCA do not affect the CST, hemiplegia is a very unlikely outcome in this group, unless there are other associated lesions. As these infarcts are also usually small, the risk of epilepsy and other adverse outcomes is lower than in other types (0–20%). Only 10% of the children in this group will show developmental impairment in more than one area [17].

Perforator Stroke (MCA Branches Supplying the Central Gray Matter)
The risk of hemiplegia is 15–20% and depends on involvement of the PLIC. The prevalence of other problems is low, and fewer than 10% have other developmental problems.

Posterior Cerebral Artery (PCA)

The risk of hemiplegia in this group is lower than 20% and even lower if there is no BGT or CST involvement.

Infarction in this territory is associated with an increased risk of visual impairment, specifically visual field deficits (20–30%), although lower than in children in the previous group [17, 28]. Asymmetry of the optic radiation as seen on the neonatal MRI or at 3 months is a good predictor of later visual deficit [29].

Anterior Cerebral Artery (ACA)

The rate of hemiplegia is low (10–20%) as in the previous group, but children in this group may experience higher rates of cognitive and behavioral problems [17].

9.1.2.6 Follow-Up

Follow-up and interventions in infants with neonatal stroke should be tailored to the specific risks of adverse outcomes in each patient, also taking into account the needs of the family. Children at high risk of hemiplegia should be seen more often during the first year and should be referred for physiotherapy and occupational therapy assessment soon after the first signs of motor impairment emerge. Performing General Movements Assessment (GMA) and Hand Assessment for Infants (HAI) around 3 months of age in this group is especially valuable in detecting those infants at increased risk of developing hemiplegia [30, 31].

For others, examinations in the first 2 years do not need to be so very frequent, but it is important that a full developmental assessment is done around the age of 2 years in order to detect the first signs of language delay or other problems. Additionally parents/carers need support even when the risks of neurodevelopmental problems in their child are low and they need to know how to make contact in case of concern.

All children with neonatal stroke should have a detailed neuropsychological evaluation at early school age (5–7 years) or sooner if problems are already suspected. This could anticipate future learning difficulties, and if appropriate rehabilitation based on this assessment is started, it can improve academic performance, self-esteem, and quality of life. Children who do not develop a hemiplegia may still have some signs of neuromotor impairment when examined at school age [32].

Visual assessments should be undertaken especially in those with a posterior cerebral artery or posterior branch MCA stroke. See earlier and later comments [33, 34].

Children who develop moderate or severe motor impairment or epilepsy should also be referred to a pediatric neurologist.

9.1.2.7 Communication with Parents

On Admission

In a typical scenario (term infant with or without a difficult labor/delivery who presents with focal brief seizures in the first 48 postnatal hours), tell parents the following, after excluding hypoglycemia or other electrolyte type problems:

- That the most likely cause for the seizure is an arterial stroke, but that some investigations need to be carried out before a definite diagnosis is made.

- What investigations will be done in the next hours and days and why they are important (aEEG, cranial ultrasound, infection screening, glucose and blood gases, cardiac evaluation, brain MRI).
- If the seizures recur, their infant may need anti-seizure medications, explain how they work and that they may make their baby sleepy.
- If the diagnosis is confirmed, reassure them that that arterial strokes in neonates are very seldom associated with an increased risk of mortality in the neonatal period and that the risk of recurrence is very low.

In infants with congenital heart disease or meningitis or with HIE, the short- and long-term prognosis is influenced by the underlying condition and therefore should be individualized.

Before Discharge

Discuss the prognosis, based on the MRI findings and clinical information. Some parents, but not all, prefer to look at the MRI images—it is advisable to ask them first.

Before talking to parents, investigate what is available in your hospital or community in terms of follow-up and therapeutic input. Some therapeutic programs are available, e.g. GAME initiated before 5 months which was found to be superior to equally intense standard care though this is a general developmental program and not specific for hemiplegia [35, 36]. Baby CIMT and bimanual therapy are hemiplegia specific, and even if these are not available where you work, you may be asked about them. These therapies have been shown to improve early motor outcomes [37], but there are few and only short-term studies. A large clinical trial of this therapy is underway in Australia [38]. A study is also ongoing to assess focused therapy for lower limb function in infants with hemiplegia, with encouraging early results, but the findings from the full RCT are yet to be published [39] While there are data to support early interventions, long-term effects and sustained improvements are yet to be established.

Specific Issues

- If hemiplegia is highly likely, explain what hemiplegia means and how it may affect the infant's life. If it is not quite sure whether a hemiplegia will develop, plan to assess the baby at 3–4 months, and also repeat the MRI at 3 months. If hemiplegia is unlikely, it is important to reassure parents about this.
- Describe the first signs of hemiplegia that parents may notice and when they would likely appear. Plan with the physiotherapists, a GMA assessment for fidgety movements (FMs) and HINE exam at 3–4 months post-term age. These will help in assessing the likelihood of developing cerebral palsy (CP). Infants with normal FMs are unlikely to develop a hemiplegia, though a few false-positive results have been reported [40]. Infants with absent FMs but a HINE score > 50 at 3 months are highly likely to develop a hemiplegia, while those with absent FMs and HINE scores <50 are more likely to develop bilateral CP [41].

Asymmetries in hand function can be quantified using the HAI (Hand Assessment for Infants) from 3 months post-term age [30, 31, 42].
- Explain how to provide appropriate sensory stimulation to the potentially affected limb perhaps in discussion with the physiotherapist.
- If the visual pathways seem involved in the stroke, referral for visual assessment is recommended, and advise visual stimulation to the affected side (i.e., contralateral to the side of the stroke) [28, 43].
- Explain expected outcomes in other areas (see Table 9.2), acknowledging that these are more difficult to predict in the neonatal period.
- Advise about temperature management during episodes of infection.
- Explain when you want to see their child in clinic for the first follow-up visit and when and how to seek medical assistance before then if needed. Follow-up plans should include long-term cognitive, language, and behavioral review and monitoring for later seizure occurrence as well as support for the family.
- Inform parents about national associations for children with hemiplegia. Readily accessible information and support for parents and carers is available from, for example, Hemihelp in the UK (https://contact.org.uk/help-for-families/information-advice-services/hemihelp/), and similar associations in Europe and the USA (http://chasa.org) have greatly increased both professional and public knowledge of the condition.
- Explore parental feelings regarding the cause of the stroke. Self-blame is highly prevalent among parents of infants with stroke and has been associated with persisting parental depression and poorer family functioning [25, 26, 44, 45]. It is important to stress that we do not know how to prevent perinatal stroke.

9.1.2.8 Conclusions

Perinatal arterial ischemic stroke in term-born infants is relatively common. Although significant progress has been made in understanding its pathophysiology and risk factors, we still do not know why some infants are affected and, more importantly, how to prevent it. Perinatal stroke is the main cause of congenital hemiplegia and may also lead to a complex mixture of neurodevelopmental problems, especially language and attention deficits, impaired executive function and complicated peer interactions, our understanding of which has only recently improved.

Today it is possible to predict hemiplegia with a high degree of accuracy using MRI in the neonatal period, and this examination should be offered to all infants with stroke, as early identification of motor problems may result in better function. Follow-up after perinatal stroke should be planned according to the individual risk of neurodevelopmental impairments and the needs of each family and should continue at least until school age, even in children who are doing well at 2 years.

9.2   Lobar Hemorrhage

9.2.1   For parents

9.2.1.1 What Is Lobar Hemorrhage?

Lobar hemorrhage is a bleed in one of the four lobes of the upper parts of the brain. It usually occurs around the time of birth. We generally do not know why it happens. Sometimes it may be related to a collection of blood on the surface of the brain that causes pressure and prevents the blood inside the brain from circulating normally, and this can break the blood vessels and cause bleeding inside the brain. However, small amounts of blood on the surface of the brain are common even after normal deliveries and do not cause any problems. Lobar hemorrhage can cause brain cells not to get the oxygen and glucose they need, and they can be permanently damaged.

9.2.1.2 How Are Lobar Hemorrhages Diagnosed?

A lobar hemorrhage is suspected when a baby has seizures (fits) or apneas (periods of not breathing) in the first few days after birth. The doctors will do tests including taking images of the brain using cranial ultrasound and MRI (magnetic resonance imaging), EEG (recording brain waves), and various blood tests for infection and anemia (low hemoglobin) or abnormalities of how the blood clots.

9.2.1.3 Is there Some Special Treatment?

Babies with a suspected lobar hemorrhage are admitted to the neonatal intensive care unit, and care is taken to keep baby's temperature, blood pressure, pulse rate, oxygen level, and blood sugar in the normal range. If the blood is not clotting properly, help will be given for that; if the hemoglobin is very low, blood will be given, and medication will be given to reduce the chance of further seizures. The medical team will do tests to see if there is any underlying cause for the hemorrhage, but usually this is not the case. If the hemorrhage is causing pressure effects on the brain, it may be necessary to insert a tube to drain the hemorrhage or fluid from the spaces in the brain. This would be discussed with the surgeons who specialize in this.

9.2.1.4 Is the Life of My Baby at Risk?

Most babies with lobar hemorrhages recover well and are able to go home a few days or weeks after diagnosis, depending on what other problems they have. These hemorrhages that happen around the time of birth are not expected to recur later in life; this would be extremely rare unless some underlying cause is found. However, sometimes babies with large hemorrhages are very sick and may not survive.

9.2.1.5 What Are the Consequences of a Lobar Hemorrhage?

Depending on the size and the location of the hemorrhage, consequences will be different. Small hemorrhages and even large ones that are only on one side in the front of the brain are not likely to cause difficulties with movements or vision or language, but they do increase the risk of having seizures or epilepsy later on. If the hemorrhage is near the part of the brain that carries messages about movements or in or near the visual area, then these abilities may be affected but almost never to the extent that your baby would not walk or would not see. Hearing is not expected to be affected. The best test to help in predicting the future is an MRI brain scan.

9.2.1.6 What Happens After the Baby Is Discharged Home?

Depending on the hospital where your baby was born or admitted to, the person seeing you after your baby goes home can be a pediatrician, a neonatologist, or a pediatric neurologist. Other professionals are usually involved at different times: rehabilitation specialists, physiotherapists, occupational therapists, and speech and language therapists.

Babies at higher risk of problems with movement, usually called a hemiplegia, will be seen more frequently during the first year, when any problems with movements usually emerge. If this happens, your baby will be referred early for physiotherapy assessment. For more details on this, please see the information for parents on hemiplegia earlier in this chapter (Fig 9.1).

During the first years, the developmental progress of your child will be monitored. Most children are doing well at this age, so assessments may be infrequent.

Around the time your child starts going to school, it would be useful to perform a neuropsychological assessment to see if there are any areas of your child's development (language, attention, memory, interpreting visual information) that could benefit from extra support. A proactive approach and being aware of possible difficulties is likely to help your child feel more confident in school with their peers and improve their academic performance.

9.2.2 For Professionals

9.2.2.1 Incidence

Isolated lobar parenchymal hemorrhage (or hematoma) in term neonates is uncommon, and the incidence is not well defined, but probably occurs in 1/10,000 live births with the majority of cases presenting within the first postnatal week. [46]. Lobar hemorrhage refers to supratentorial lesions affecting the neocortex, and it not generally a term used to include thalamic or cerebellar hemorrhages (see Chaps. 4 and 12). It is considerably less common than neonatal ischemic stroke, and lobar hemorrhagic lesions are not confined to an arterial territory.

Accompanying sub-arachnoid and intraventricular hemorrhage occur in about a fifth of infants with lobar hemorrhage; subdural hemorrhage is the more common. Subpial hemorrhage has now been well described and thought to be important in the development of underlying brain injury [47–50]. Associations with cerebral sinus venous thrombosis (CSVT) and with hypoxic-ischemic encephalopathy (HIE) are reported, and hemorrhagic transformation of ischemic lesions can occur, sometimes appearing as a primary hematoma.

9.2.2.2 Pathogenesis

The majority of large isolated parenchymal hematomas in full-term infants occur after an uneventful pregnancy and normal delivery. Some studies describe an increased incidence of interventional vaginal delivery, but most of these studies include sub-tentorial hemorrhage as well [51]. Lobar hemorrhages are most commonly seen in the frontal or temporal lobes but also occur in parietal and occipital regions. Mostly a clear etiology is not found, and the hemorrhage is an isolated finding and recurrence is rare. The appearances of the hemorrhage on MRI scans often suggest that there is extra-axial subpial hemorrhage extending into and widening the adjacent cerebral sulci and pressing on the underlying cortex. It is likely this causes underlying cortical and subcortical infarction from local venous compression [50]. Although earlier reports suggested that local trauma with contusion and pressure related to delivery may be causative, this association has not been upheld in later studies. Temporal hematoma is reported to be associated with thrombosis of the vein of Labbé though this also is not proven [52].

Although lobar hemorrhage in term infants is often isolated, there are some recognized associations that should be considered.

- Clotting studies should be done in all infants. Thrombocytopenia and clotting dysfunction are reported in about 25% of infants [53, 54]. These usually resolve without new hemorrhage occurring but, e.g. in the context of ECMO, reported rates of parenchymal hemorrhage range from 8.2% to 23% in ECMO survivors and in up to 52% of ECMO non-survivors [55]. Vitamin K deficiency and fetal or neonatal alloimmune thrombocytopenia also need to be considered but are uncommon associations.
- Congenital thrombophilias have been associated with venous and arterial infarctions and hemorrhage. However a recent prospective, population-based, controlled

study by Curtis et al. suggests minimal association between perinatal stroke including hemorrhagic stroke and thrombophilia [9]. Mutations in the COL4A1 and COL4A2 genes may result in hemorrhage and porencephalic cyst formation but seldom single lobar hemorrhage. However with additional hemorrhagic lesions, or a family history of adult intracranial hemorrhage, aneurysms, ocular manifestations, or nephropathy, these diagnoses should be considered. The human phenotypes are extremely variable even within families [56]. One study documented other monogenic associations with perinatal intracranial hemorrhage [57].

- Large focal hemorrhage may occur in HIE especially in infants with more severe white matter injury, multiorgan failure and derangement in the coagulation pathway, but it is uncommon [58] especially in the absence of IVH [59]. Outcomes generally relate more to the severity of the HI-related abnormality than the hemorrhage itself unless the hemorrhage damages the motor or optic pathways.
- Meningitis, HSV encephalitis, and other intracranial infections (parechoviruses (HPeVs), rotavirus, enterovirus, listeria monocytogenes, and parvovirus B19) are known associations with large intraparenchymal hemorrhage (see Chap. 13).
- Hemorrhage can occur in neonatal brain tumors. These in themselves are very rare, but up to 14–18% show spontaneous hemorrhage, attributed to the tumor's rapid growth. Prognosis depends on the tumor type and location and the general condition of the infant rather than the hemorrhage per se.
- Vascular malformations seen in the neonatal period such as vein of Galen malformation [60], developmental venous malformations [61], and hereditary hemorrhagic telangiectasia [62] may have associated hemorrhage, but rarely is hemorrhage the main presentation.

9.2.2.3 Presentation

The most common presentation of lobar hematoma in the term infant is with seizures in the first postnatal week and mostly in the first day after birth, though a proportion present with apnea, typically the temporal lesions [63]. Being hemorrhagic they are generally well seen on cranial ultrasound very soon after their occurrence [51], unless quite small or remote from the ultrasound probe. They may also be detected incidentally on cranial ultrasound done because of admission for other reasons such as HIE or systemic illness and can occur with ECMO. The frontal lesions tend to lie adjacent to the falx and superior sagittal sinus. Concurrent intraventricular hemorrhage (IVH) also may occur and thus in some infants consequent post-hemorrhagic ventriculomegaly.

9.2.2.4 Imaging

Figure 9.8 shows a large focal hemorrhage in the left temporal lobe. This was seen on the admission cranial ultrasound scan on day 2. The MRI scan was done 2 days later (see legend for further details).

Figure 9.9 shows a large focal hemorrhage in the left frontal lobe on days 3 and 9 after birth. The MRI appearances of hemorrhage in neonates change rapidly in the first days as shown in this figure (see legend for further details) and description of the time course of signal change with acute hemorrhage in neonates in Table 9.3.

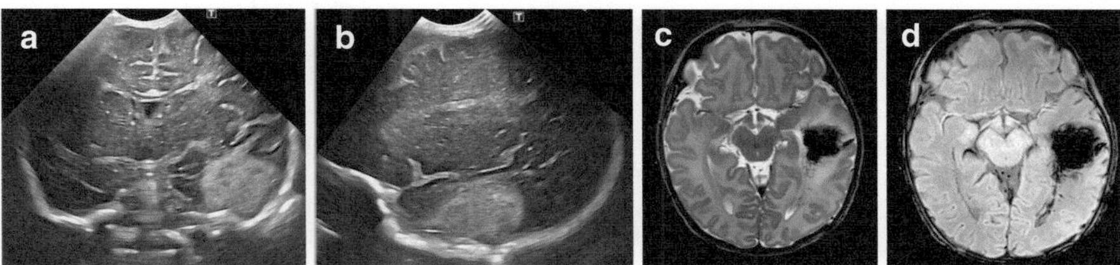

Fig. 9.8 This full-term infant, born by an uncomplicated vaginal delivery, was admitted to the neonatal unit because of apneas due to seizures seen on aEEG on day 2. Seizures ceased after two doses of phenobarbitone. Cranial ultrasound scans on admission (**a**, coronal, **b**, parasagittal) showed a large rounded echogenic lesion in the left temporal lobe. An MRI scan on day 4 (**c**, T2-W, **d**, susceptibility-weighted axial images) showed a typical lobar hemorrhage in the temporal lobe consistent with the cranial ultrasound scans. Additionally there was a small amount of hemorrhage in the left ventricle. The child had a normal neurodevelopment assessment at 1 year

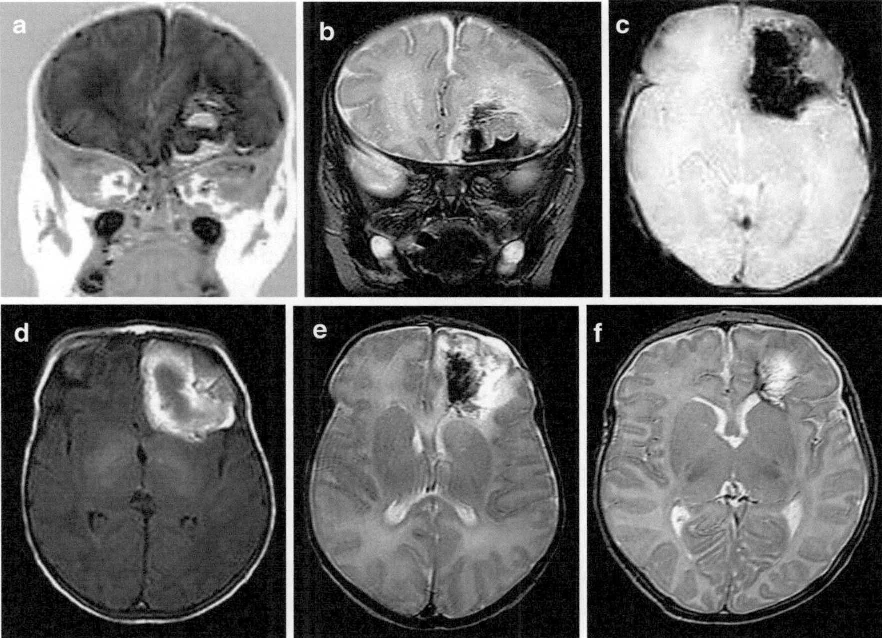

Fig. 9.9 Term-born infant presenting with seizures. The MRI done on day 3 (upper row) and day 9 (lower row) shows a large left-sided frontal subpial hemorrhage with distortion and displacement of the cortical margin. On day 3 (coronal **a** and **b**, and axial **c**), the hemorrhage is high signal intensity on the T1-W image (**a**) and low signal on the T2-W image (**b**) both within the brain and in the extracerebral space. It is also low signal on the susceptibility-weighted image (SWI) (**c**). On day 9, the hemorrhage on the T1-W image has a high signal periphery but is isointense in the center (**d**), while on the T2-W image (**e**) the hemorrhage remains of low signal in the center with a very high signal rim. Some dilated veins are also seen in **e** and better depicted in **f**

Table 9.3 Time course of signal intensity changes on MRI following acute hemorrhage

Age of hemorrhage	Parenchymal hemorrhage		Extracerebral hemorrhage	
	T1-W	T2-W	T1-W	T2-W
First 2 days	Isointense with a high SI rim	Low SI	High SI	Low SI/isointense
3 days	High SI/isointense	Low SI with high SI in the periphery	High SI	High SI
3–10 days	High SI/isointense	Low SI with high SI in the periphery	High SI	Low SI—In larger lesions, some high SI
10–21 days	High SI	High SI	High SI	Low SI—in larger lesions, some high SI
3–6 weeks	High SI	High SI with low SI in the periphery	High SI/nil	Low SI

Adapted from: Rutherford M. Hemorrhagic lesions of the newborn brain. In: MRI of the Neonatal Brain. Copyright © 2024 Dr. Mary A Rutherford. Available at: https://www.mrineonatalbrain.com/ch04-09.php

SI signal intensity

The appearances of hemorrhage on MRI often suggest that there is extra-axial subpial hemorrhage accompanying large lobar hemorrhage in newborns (Fig. 9.9) extending into and widening the adjacent cerebral sulci and pressing on the underlying cortex. It is likely this effect that causes cortical and subcortical infarction from local venous compression [47–49]. This appearance is not always seen and is not obvious in the example shown in Fig. 9.8.

9.2.2.5 Treatment

Management necessitates admission to intensive care, with the institution of supportive treatment (maintenance of normothermia, normotension, normoglycemia, normocapnia). Screening should be done for infection, and hemoglobin levels as well as platelets and clotting factors should be monitored with appropriate treatment for any derangements.

Seizures can be initially very difficult to treat but usually stop within a few days with anti-seizure medication. This should be monitored with EEG/aEEG (see Chap. 16). There is no need to continue medication after discharge.

In the first few days, serial cranial ultrasound examinations should be done to monitor whether the hemorrhage is causing a midline shift and/or significant tissue compression or ventriculomegaly. If this is seen or there are clinical signs of raised intracranial pressure, an MRI should be done urgently (or a CT if MRI is not possible, though CT not likely to be better than cranial ultrasound) to define better the pressure effects of the hemorrhage and an urgent consultation with neurosurgeons arranged. Consider doing an ultrasound-guided percutaneous needle puncture to reduce the midline shift that has been described in the management of this problem [64].

If the hemorrhage is also in the ventricles, post-hemorrhagic ventriculomegaly can develop and can be checked for using cranial ultrasound. The presence of hemorrhage in the ventricles in a term infant should also lead to a search for cerebral venous thrombosis (see Chap. 11).

9.2.2.6 Prognosis

There is a significant early mortality associated with larger or multiple cerebral hemorrhagic lesions, usually in infants who have derangements in coagulation and associated problems such as HIE or need for ECMO [51]. In general for infants with underlying conditions, it is the severity of those conditions that best informs outcomes.

For term infants not affected by additional pathologies, the outcome for supratentorial lobar hemorrhage, when it occurs as an isolated lesion in one of the hemispheres, seems to be good despite the dramatic appearances of the initial lesion. Of note, none of the studies describing outcomes contain many infants, but they are in agreement with each other regarding relatively good outcomes; there is little long-term outcome data in the literature[51, 53, 63, 65, 66].

The principles for predicting outcomes for these focal hemorrhagic lesions are similar to those used for arterial territory stroke. If the lesion affects the parietal lobe and the motor pathway is involved, a hemiplegia would be expected. However this is not so common with these large lobar lesions. There is an increased risk for later seizures although the rates are not well defined. If the hemorrhage affects the optic radiations or visual cortex, monitoring for squint and testing of the visual fields and visual processing are recommended.

References

1. DeVeber GA, MacGregor D, Curtis R, et al. Neurologic outcome in survivors of childhood arterial ischemic stroke and sinovenous thrombosis. J Child Neurol. 2000;15:316–24.
2. Grunt S, Mazenauer L, Buerki SE, et al. Incidence and outcomes of symptomatic neonatal arterial ischemic stroke. Pediatrics. 2015;135(5):e1220–8.
3. Darmency-Stamboul V, Chantegret C, Ferdynus C, et al. Antenatal factors associated with perinatal arterial ischemic stroke. Stroke. 2012;43:2307–12.
4. Martinez-Biarge M, Cheong JL, Diez-Sebastian J, et al. Risk factors for neonatal arterial ischemic stroke: the importance of the intrapartum period. J Pediatr. 2016;173:62–8.
5. Chabrier S, Husson B, Dinomais M, et al. New insights (and new interrogations) in perinatal arterial ischemic stroke. Thromb Res. 2011;127(1):13–22.
6. Harteman JC, Groenendaal F, Kwee A, et al. Risk factors for perinatal arterial ischaemic stroke in full-term infants: a case-control study. Arch Dis Child Fetal Neonatal Ed. 2012;97:F411–6.
7. Srivastava R, Dunbar M, Shevell M, Oskoui M, Basu A, Rivkin MJ, Shany E, de Vries LS, Dewey D, Letourneau N, Hill MD, Kirton A. Developmental and validation of a prediction model for perinatal arterial ischemic stroke in term neonates. JAMA Network Open. 2022;5(6):e2219203. https://doi.org/10.1001/jamanetworkopen.2022.19203.
8. Arnaez J, Arca G, Martín-Ancel A, et al. Coagulation factor V G1691A, factor II G20210A and methylenetetrahydrofolate reductase C677T gene mutations do not play a major role in symptomatic neonatal arterial ischaemic stroke. Br J Haematol. 2018;180(2):290–2.
9. Curtis C, Mineyko A, Massicotte P, Leakerr M, Jiang XY, Kirton A. Thrombophilia risk is not increased in children after perinatal stroke. Blood. 2017;129(20):2793–800. https://doi.org/10.1182/blood-2016-11-750893.
10. Dudink J, Mercuri E, Al-Nakib L, et al. Evolution of unilateral perinatal arterial ischemic stroke on conventional and diffusion-weighted MR imaging. Am J Neuroradiol. 2009;30:998–1004.
11. van der Aa NE, Benders MJ, Vincken KL, et al. The course of apparent diffusion coefficient values following perinatal arterial ischemic stroke. PLoS One. 2013;8(2):e56784.
12. Wagenaar N, van der Aa NE, Groenendaal F, et al. MR imaging for accurate prediction of outcome after perinatal arterial ischemic stroke: sooner not necessarily better. Eur J Paediatr Neurol. 2017;21(4):666–70.

13. Cowan F, Mercuri E, Groenendaal F, Bassi L, Ricci D, Rutherford M, de Vries L. Does cranial ultrasound imaging identify arterial cerebral infarction in term neonates? Arch Dis Child Fetal Neonatal Ed. 2005;90(3):F252–6.
14. Olivé G, Agut T, Echeverría-Palacio CM, Arca G, García-Alix A. Usefulness of cranial ultrasound for detecting neonatal middle cerebral artery stroke. Ultrasound Med Biol. 2019;45(3):885–90. https://doi.org/10.1016/j.ultrasmedbio.2018.11.004.
15. Glass HC, Soul JS, Chang T, Wusthoff CJ, Chu CJ, Massey SL, Abend NS, Lemmon M, Thomas C, Numis AL, Guillet R, Sturza J, McNamara NA, Rogers EE, Franck LS, McCulloch CE, Shellhaas RA. Safety of early discontinuation of antiseizure medication after acute symptomatic neonatal seizures. JAMA Neurol. 2021;78(7):817–25. https://doi.org/10.1001/jamaneurol.2021.1437. Erratum in: JAMA Neurol. 2021 Jul 1;78(7):882.
16. Chabrier S, Peyric E, Drutel L, et al. Multimodal outcome at 7 years of age after neonatal arterial ischemic stroke. J Pediatr. 2016;172:156–61.e3.
17. Wagenaar N, Martinez-Biarge M, van der Aa NE, van Haastert IC, Groenendaal F, Benders MJNL, Cowan FM, de Vries LS. Neurodevelopment after perinatal arterial ischemic stroke. Pediatrics. 2018;142(3):e20174164. https://doi.org/10.1542/peds.2017-4164.
18. Mercuri E, Rutherford M, Cowan F, et al. Early prognostic indicators of outcome in infants with neonatal cerebral infarction: a clinical, electro- encephalogram, and magnetic resonance imaging study. Pediatrics. 1999;103:39–46.
19. Mineyko A, Kirton A. Long-term outcome after bilateral perinatal arterial ischemic stroke. Pediatr Neurol Dec. 2019;101:39–42. https://doi.org/10.1016/j.pediatrneurol.2019.07.013.
20. Bosenbark DD, Krivitzky L, Ichord R, Vossough A, Bhatia A, Jastrzab LE, Billinghurst L. Clinical predictors of attention and executive functioning outcomes in children after perinatal arterial ischemic stroke. Pediatr Neurol. 2017;69:79–86. https://doi.org/10.1016/j.pediatrneurol.2017.01.014.
21. Westmacott R, Macgregor D, Askalan R, et al. Late emergence of cognitive deficits after unilateral neonatal stroke. Stroke. 2009;40(6):2012–9.
22. Wusthoff CJ, Kessler SK, Vossough A, Ichord R, Zelonis S, Halperin A, Gordon D, Vargas G, Licht DJ, Smith SE. Risk of later seizure after perinatal arterial ischemic stroke: a prospective cohort study. Pediatrics. 2011;127(6):e1550–7.
23. Caspar-Teuscher M, Studer M, Regényi M, Steinlin M, Grunt S, Swiss Neuropediatric Stroke Registry Group. Health related quality of life and manual ability 5 years after neonatal ischemic stroke. Eur J Paediatr Neurol. 2019;23(5):716–22. https://doi.org/10.1016/j.ejpn.2019.08.002.
24. Kirton A, deVeber G. Life after perinatal stroke. Stroke. 2013;44:3265–71.
25. Bemister TB, Brooks BL, Dyck RH, Kirton A. Predictors of caregiver depression and family functioning after perinatal stroke. BMC Pediatr. 2015;15:75. https://doi.org/10.1186/s12887-015-0397-5.
26. Khan U, Watson R, Pearse JE, Irwin L, Rapley T, Basu AP. Grappling with uncertainty—experiences of parents of infants following perinatal stroke. Res Dev Disabil. 2022;124:104201. https://doi.org/10.1016/j.ridd.2022.104201.
27. van der Aa N, Leemans A, Northington FJ, et al. Does diffusion tensor imaging-based tractography at 3 months of age contribute to the prediction of motor outcome after perinatal arterial ischemic stroke? Stroke. 2011;42(12):3410–4.
28. Mercuri E, Spano M, Bruccini G, et al. Visual outcome in children with congenital hemiplegia: correlation with MRI findings. Neuropediatrics. 1996;27:184–8.
29. van der Aa NE, Dudink J, Benders MJ, Govaert P, van Straaten HL, Porro GL, Groenendaal F, de Vries LS. Neonatal posterior cerebral artery stroke: clinical presentation, MRI findings, and outcome. Dev Med Child Neurol. 2013;55(3):283–90. https://doi.org/10.1111/dmcn.12055.
30. Pascal A, Govaert P, Ortibus E, Naulaers G, Lars A, Fjørtoft T, Oostra A, Zecic A, Cools F, Cloet E, Casaer A, Cornette L, Laroche S, Samijn B, Van den Broeck C. Motor outcome after perinatal stroke and early prediction of unilateral spastic cerebral palsy. Eur J Paediatr Neurol. 2020;29:54–61. https://doi.org/10.1016/j.ejpn.2020.09.002.
31. Ryll UC, Krumlinde-Sundholm L, Verhage CH, Sicola E, Sgandurra G, Bastiaenen CH, Eliasson AC. Predictive validity of the hand assessment for infants in infants at risk of unilateral cerebral palsy. Dev Med Child Neurol. 2021;63(4):436–43. https://doi.org/10.1111/dmcn.14739.

32. Mercuri E, Barnett A, Rutherford M, et al. Neonatal cerebral infarction and neuromotor outcome at school age. Pediatrics. 2004;113:95–100.
33. Guzzetta A, Fazzi B, Mercuri E, et al. Visual function in children with hemiplegia in the first years of life. Dev Med Child Neurol. 2001;43:321–9.
34. Mercuri E, Anker S, Guzzetta A, et al. Neonatal cerebral infarction and visual function at school age. Arch Dis Child Fetal Neonatal Ed. 2003;88:F487–91.
35. Morgan C, Novak I, Badawi N. Enriched environments and motor outcomes in cerebral palsy: systematic review and meta-analysis. Pediatrics. 2013;132:e735–46.
36. Morgan C, Badawi N, Novak I. "A Different Ride": a qualitative interview study of parents' experience with early diagnosis and goals, activity, motor enrichment (GAME) intervention for infants with cerebral palsy. J Clin Med. 2023;12(2):583. https://doi.org/10.3390/jcm12020583.
37. Eliasson AC, Nordstrand L, Ek L, Lennartsson F, Sjöstrand L, Tedroff K, Krumline-Sundholm L. The effectiveness of Baby-CIMT in infants younger than 12 months with clinical signs of unilateral-cerebral palsy; an explorative study with randomized design. Res Dev Disabil. 2018;72:191–201.
38. Boyd RN, Ziviani J, Sakzewski L, et al. REACH: study protocol of a randomised trial of rehabilitation very early in congenital hemiplegia. BMJ Open. 2017;7(9):e017204.
39. Hurd C, Livingstone D, Brunton K, et al. Early intensive lower extremity rehabilitation show preliminary efficacy after perinatal stroke; results of a pilot randomised controlled trial. Neurorehabil Neural Repair. 2022;36(6):360–70.
40. Guzzetta A, Mercuri E, Rapisardi G, et al. General movements detect early signs of hemiplegia in term infants with neonatal cerebral infarction. Neuropediatrics. 2003;34:61–6.
41. Romeo DMM, Cioni M, Scoto M, Mazzone L, Palermo F, Romeo MG. Neuromotor development in infants with cerebral palsy investigated by the Hammersmith Infant Neurological Examination during the first year of age. Eur J Paediatr Neurol. 2008;12:24–31. https://doi.org/10.1016/j.ejpn.2007.05.006.
42. Guzzetta A, Pizzardi A, Belmonti V, et al. Hand movements at 3 months predict later hemiplegia in term infants with neonatal cerebral infarction. Dev Med Child Neurol. 2010;52(8):767–72.
43. Fazzi E, Micheletti S, Calza S, Merabet L, Rossi A, Galli J, Early Visual Intervention Study Group. Early visual training and environmental adaptation for infants with visual impairment. Dev Med Child Neurol. 2021;63(10):1180–93.
44. Bemister TB, Brooks BL, Dyck RH, Kirton A. Parent and family impact of raising a child with perinatal stroke. BMC Pediatr. 2014;14:182. https://doi.org/10.1186/1471-2431-14-182.
45. Peterson RK, Williams T, Dlamini N, Westmacott R. Parent experiences and developmental outcomes following neonatal stroke. Clinic Neuropsychol. 2021;l35(5):973–87.
46. Rooks VJ, Eaton JP, Ruess L, Petermann GW, Keck-Wherley J, Pedersen RC. Prevalence and evolution of intracranial hemorrhage in asymptomatic term infants. AJNR Am J Neuroradiol. 2008;29(6):1082–9. https://doi.org/10.3174/ajnr.A1004.
47. Assis Z, Kirton A, Pauranik A, Sherriff M, Wei X-C. Idiopathic neonatal subpial hemorrhage with underlying cerebral infarct: imaging features and clinical outocme. AJNR Am J Neuroradiol. 2021;42(1):185–93.
48. Barreto ARF, Carrasco M, Dabrowski AK, Sun LR, Tekes A. Subpial hemorrhage in neonates: what radiologists need to know. AJR Am J Roentgenol. 2021;216:1–10.
49. Cain DW, Dingman AL, Armstrong J, Stence NV, Jensen AM, Mirsky DM. Subpial hemorrhage of the neonate. Stroke. 2020;51(1):315–8. https://doi.org/10.1161/STROKEAHA.119:025987.
50. Dabrowski AK, Carrasco M, Gatti JR, Barreto ARF, Parkinson C, Robinson S, Tekes A, Sun LR. Neonatal subpial hemorrhage: clinical factors, neuroimaging and outcomes in a quaternary care children's center. Pediatr Neurol. 2021;120:52–8.
51. Brouwer AJ, Groenendaal F, Koopman C, Nievelstein RJA, Han SK, De Vries LS. Intracranial hemorrhage in full-term newborns: a hospital-based cohort study. Neuroradiology. 2010;52(6):567–76. https://doi.org/10.1007/s00234-010-0698-1.
52. Kalpatthi R, Coley BD, Rusin JA, Blanchong CA. Neonatal temporal lobar hemorrhage secondary to thrombosis of the vein of Labbé. J Perinatol. 2005;25(9):605–7.
53. Cole L, Dewey D, Letourneau N, et al. Clinical characteristics, risk factors, and outcomes associated with neonatal hemorrhagic stroke. JAMA Pediatr. 2017;171(3):230. https://doi.org/10.1001/jamapediatrics.2016.4151.

54. Jhawar BS, Ranger A, Steven D, Del Maestro RF. Risk factors for intracranial hemorrhage among full-term infants: a case-control study. Neurosurgery. 2003;52(3):581–90; discussion 588–90.
55. Wien MA, Whitehead MT, Bulas M, Melbourne L, Oldenburg G, Short BL, Massaro AN. Petterns of brain injury in newborns treated with extracorporeal membrane oxygenation. AJNR Am J Neuroradiol. 2017;38:820–6. https://doi.org/10.3174/ajnr.A5092.
56. Meuwissen MEC, Halley DJJ, Smit LS, Lequin MH, Cobben JM, de Coo R, van Harssel J, Sallevelt S, Woldringh G, van der Knaap MS, de Vries LS, Mancini GMS. The expanding phenotype of COL4A1 and COL4A2 mutations: clinical data on 13 newly identified families and a review of the literature. Genet Med. 2015;17(11):843–53. https://doi.org/10.1038/gim.2014.210.
57. Hausman-Kedem M, Malinger G, Modai S, Kushner SA, Shiran SI, Ben-Sira L, Roth J, Constantini A, Fattal-Valevski A, Ben-Shachar S. Monogenic causes of apparently idiopathic perinatal intracranial hemorrhage. Ann Neurol. 2021;89(4):813–22.
58. Wisnowski JL, Wintermark P, Bonifacio SL, Smyser CD, Barkovich AJ, Edwards AD, de Vries LS, Inder TE, Chau V, Newborn Brain Society Guidelines and Publications Committee. Neuroimaging in the term newborn with neonatal encephalopathy. Semin Fetal Neonatal Med. 2021;26(5):101304.
59. Al Yazidi G, Boudes E, Tan X, Saint-Martin C, Shevell M, Wintermark P. Intraventricular hemorrhage in asphyxiated newborns treated with hypothermia: a look into incidence, timing and risk factors. BMC Pediatr. 2015;15:106–14.
60. Meyers PM, Hallback VV, Phatouros CP, Dowd CF, Malek AM, Lempert TE, Lefler JE, Higashida RT. Hemorrhagic complications in vein of Galen malformation. Ann Neurol. 2000;47:748–55.
61. Horsch S, Govaert P, Cowan FM, Benders MJNL, Groenendaal F, Lequin M, Saliou G, de Vries LS. Developmental venous anomaly in the newborn brain. Neuroradiology. 2014;56(7):579–88. https://doi.org/10.1007/s00234-014-1367-6.
62. Delaney HM, Rooks VJ, Wolfe SQ, Sawyer TL. Term neonate with intracranial hemorrhage and hereditary hemorrhagic telangiectasia: a case report and review of the literature. J Perinatol. 2012;32:642–4.
63. Slaughter L, Egelhoff J, Balmakund T. Neurologic outcome in neonatal temporal lobe hemorrhagic venous infarcts. J Child Neurol. 2009;24(10):1236–42. https://doi.org/10.1177/0883073809333529.
64. Cizmeci MN, Thewissen L, Zecic A, Woerdeman PA, de Boer B, Baert E, Govaert P, Dudink J, Groenendaal F, Lequin M, de Vries LS. Bedside ultrasound-guided percutaneous needle aspiration of intra- and extra-axial intracranial hemorrhage in neonates. Neuropediatrics. 2018;49(4):238–45. https://doi.org/10.1055/s-0038-1641568.
65. Hanigan WC, Powell FC, Palagallo G, Miller TC. Lobar hemorrhages in full-term neonates. Childs Nerv Syst. 1995;11:276–80.
66. Jhawar BS, Ranger A, Steven DA, Del Maestro RF. A follow-up study of infants with intracranial hemorrhage at full-term. Can J Neurol Sci. 2005;32(3):332–9.

Birth-Related Mechanical Head Injuries

10

Khorshid Mohammad (iD), Gerda Meijler (iD),
and Linda S. de Vries (iD)

Abbreviations

AIFM1	Apoptosis-inducing factor mitochondria associated 1
AVM	Arteriovenous malformation
COL4A1 and A2	Collagen type IV alpha 1 and alpha 2
CSVT	Cerebral sinovenous thrombosis
HIE	Hypoxic-ischemic encephalopathy
HR	Heart rate
IVH	Intraventricular hemorrhage
MRI	Magnetic resonance imaging

K. Mohammad (✉)
Section of Newborn Critical Care, Department of Pediatrics, Alberta Children's Hospital and
University of Calgary, Calgary, AB, Canada
e-mail: mkhorshi@ucalgary.ca; khorshid.mohammad@albertahealthservices.ca

G. Meijler
Department of Neonatology, Isala Women and Children's Hospital, Zwolle, The Netherlands
e-mail: gmeijler@gmail.com

L. S. de Vries
Department of Neonatology, University Medical Center Utrecht (UMCU),
Utrecht, The Netherlands

Department of Pediatrics, Division of Neonatology, Willem-Alexander Children's Hospital,
Leiden University Medical Center (LUMC), Leiden, The Netherlands

© The Author(s) 2024
G. Meijler, K. Mohammad (eds.), *Neonatal Brain Injury*,
https://doi.org/10.1007/978-3-031-55972-3_10

10.1 For Parents

Birth is a life event and can be stressful for both the mother and her newborn infant. The newborn head is large in proportion to the rest of the body, yet must pass through a narrow canal at the time of birth. Fortunately, both mother and baby are well adapted to get through this without complications. However, some trauma to the head may occur and may even cause brain injury due to the delivery itself and/or to interventions to assist the birth when the baby's head has difficulties passing through the birth channel or when the baby's or mother's condition necessitates intervention.

10.1.1 What Is Traumatic Brain Injury?

Traumatic brain injury during delivery can be divided into three categories from the surface of the head to the brain tissue. Of note, these injuries can co-exist:

1. Injuries outside the skull.
2. Injuries inside the skull and outside the brain.
3. Injuries to or inside the brain.

10.1.2 Head Injuries outside the Skull

- Caput succedaneum (edema of the scalp): this is a superficial swelling of the scalp over the presenting part (the part of the head that comes first) (Fig. 10.2). The maximum size of the lesion is at the time of birth and it subsides thereafter. This type of lesion is benign and very common.
- Cephalohematoma (bleed of the scalp): this is a collection of blood between the skull bone and its cover (the periosteum) (Fig. 10.2). Unlike the previous lesion, this increases in size in the first days of birth and then eventually disappears by 6–7 weeks of birth. Cephalohematoma does not cross the sutures of the skull. It can cause jaundice due to the blood that needs to breakdown during the first few days after birth.
- Subgaleal hemorrhage: this type of lesion is the most serious among the three and requires close attention as it can lead to significant blood loss if not diagnosed early (Fig. 10.2). It is a blood collection underneath the membrane that separates the skin from the bone. It crosses the sutures of the skull and can cause a large fluctuating swelling on the scalp, forward displacement of the ears, and swelling extending to the neck and around the eyes. The bleed can become larger shortly after birth.

10.1.3 Injuries inside the Skull and outside the Brain

- Epidural bleed: Is a collection of blood between the outer layers covering the brain and the skull (Fig. 10.2). This rare condition can be "silent" (thus not cause any symptoms) or may cause increased pressure inside the skull and/or seizures.

- Subdural bleed: Is a collection of blood underneath the previous layer (dura mater) and above the layer immediately covering the brain (Fig. 10.2). It can be without symptoms or cause similar problems like the epidural bleed.
- Subarachnoid bleed: Is the deepest hemorrhage outside the brain below the innermost layer that covers the brain immediately (Fig. 10.2). This is the most common among the three; it is usually without symptoms and underdiagnosed but can cause apnea (periods of breath cessation) or seizures during the first few days of birth.

10.1.4 Injuries to or inside the Brain

- Intraparenchymal (inside brain tissue) bleed: This type of injury is very rare. In full-term infants, it often presents with seizures, but can also go undiagnosed [1]. Large lesions can cause seizures and apneas (periods of breath cessation) and can have long-term consequences.
- Intraventricular bleed: This is a bleed into the fluid-filled structures in the brain called the lateral ventricles. This lesion is far more common in preterm infants and rare in full-term infants. Intraventricular bleed can be without symptoms, but infants sometimes present with apneas and/or seizures, and the intraventricular bleed can cause blockage of fluid, leading to hydrocephalus (distended ventricles that may lead to abnormal head growth). Depending on the degree of the ventricular enlargement, the treatment can range from just observation to surgical intervention.

10.1.5 How Will I Know if My Baby Has Traumatic Brain Injury?

A medical team will be examining your baby closely, especially the head for any signs of injury such as swelling; they may run some blood tests and may do imaging of the brain to make sure your baby is not affected by the traumatic delivery. You will be informed if your baby requires treatment or admission to the neonatal intensive care unit.

10.1.6 Why Did My Baby Develop Traumatic Brain Injury?

It is hard to know the exact cause. However, your baby may have had instrumental help to assist the birth when the head had difficulties passing through the birth channel or when the baby's or mother's condition necessitated immediate intervention. This necessary intervention may increase the risk of traumatic brain injury.

10.1.7 What Is the Treatment for Traumatic Brain Injury?

Most of the injuries to the head during the delivery are benign and don't require any treatment. In a small number of cases, your baby may need admission for monitoring and/or requires blood transfusion, treatment for blood pressure, or seizures. In rare cases neurosurgery intervention may be required. Your medical team will keep you updated about your baby's condition and progress.

10.1.8 What Will Happen to My Baby (Prognosis)?

Most of the injuries to the head during the delivery are benign and don't cause any long-term complications. However, depending on the severity of the symptoms and findings on imaging, there may be a risk of long-term impact. Your physician will communicate the blood tests and imaging (cranial ultrasound, CT scan, or MRI) results with you and explain possible prognosis.

10.2 For Professionals

10.2.1 Incidence and Risk Factors

Birth (even when spontaneous) is a traumatic event and can lead to different types of head injury. The incidence of birth-related head injuries is underreported and estimated to be between 0.82 and 9.5 per 1000 live births with cephalohematoma being the most common injury [2–4]. A recent study, looking at yearly trends between 2006 and 2014, showed a significant decrease from 0.37 to 0.35/1000 discharge records [2]. Risk factors for mechanical birth injuries include large for gestational age, male sex, vaginal delivery, primiparity, forceps delivery, vacuum delivery, and maternal distress [3].

10.2.2 Anatomy

It is important to get familiar with the anatomy of the scalp and meninges layers to understand different types of mechanical brain injuries in the newborn. Figure 10.1 illustrates the scalp layers from the surface to the brain, while Fig. 10.2 shows different types of bleeds to the head (within different layers of meninges and scalp).

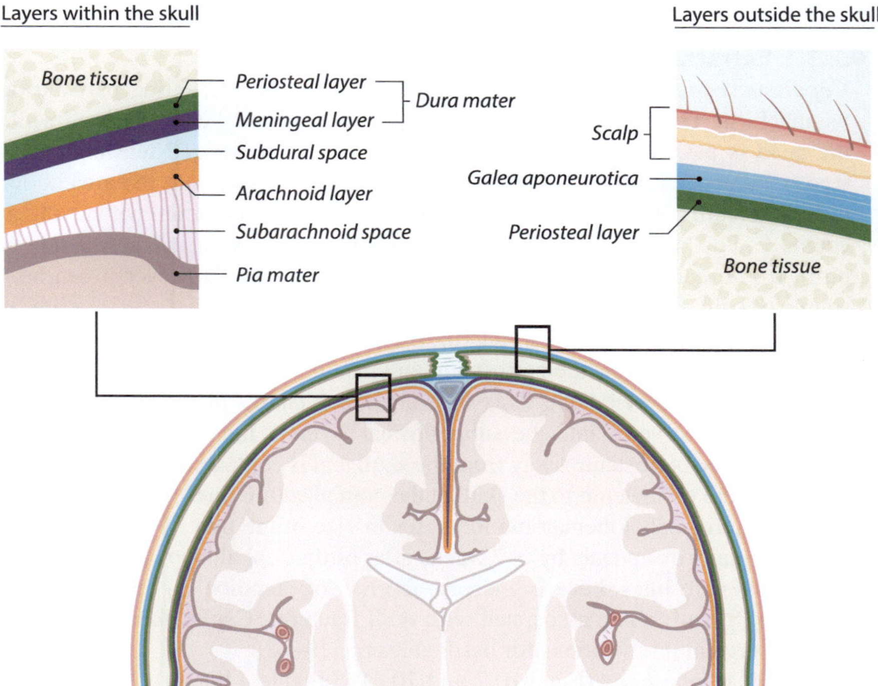

Fig. 10.1 Illustration demonstrating the layers of scalp, skull, meninges, and brain on a coronal section. (© Amanda Gautier-Ronopawiro)

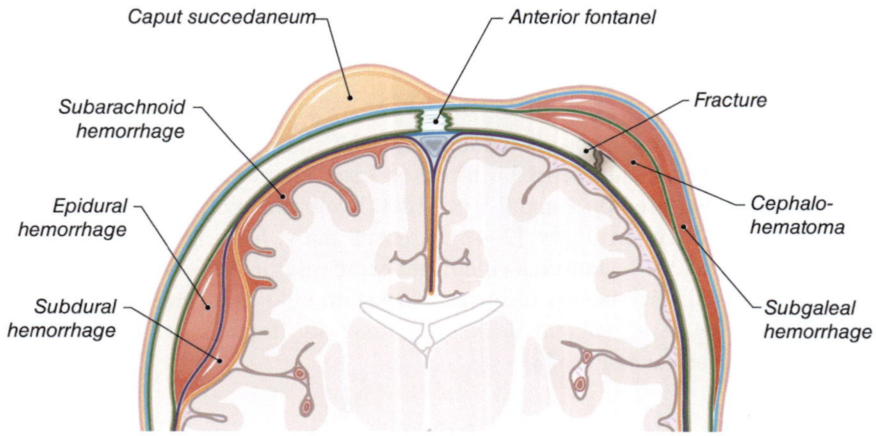

Fig. 10.2 Illustration depicting hemorrhages by location within the different layers of the meninges and scalp. (© Amanda Gautier-Ronopawiro)

10.2.3 Diagnosis and Treatment

Mechanical birth-related brain injury can be divided into extracranial and intracranial injuries:

10.2.3.1 Extracranial Injuries

- *Caput succedaneum* (Fig. 10.2): Is an edema over the presenting part during vaginal birth. The edema forms due to the pressure against the vaginal wall while the head is passing through the narrow canal. This prolonged tension causes serosanguineous fluid to leak from the subcutaneous tissue into the area above the periosteum between the scalp and the lining of the periosteum with resultant edema and/or bruising [5]. The lesion is visible and has its maximum size at birth. It is usually asymptomatic and subsides over time. However it can be a source of pain, irritation, and alopecia in extreme cases [6].
- *Cephalohematoma* (Figs. 10.2 and 10.3): This is a collection of bloody or serosanguinous fluids below the periosteum and results from the compression of the skull against the pelvic bone. This shearing action causes bleeding of the emissary and diploic veins into the subperiosteal layer of the skull. The bleeding slowly lifts the periosteum away from the skull and is contained by the ligaments that attach the periosteum to the skull at the cranial suture lines [5]. Unlike caput succedaneum, cephalohematoma increases in size in the first days of birth and then eventually disappears by 6–7 weeks after birth. Cephalohematoma does not cross the suture lines, but can increase the risk of jaundice [7] and secondary infection [8] and can be associated with skull fractures. Cephalohematoma may require surgical interventions for ossified lesions [9–12].
- *Subgaleal hemorrhage* (Figs. 10.2 and 10.4): Subgaleal hemorrhage can be a life-threatening emergency commonly associated with perinatal asphyxia. It

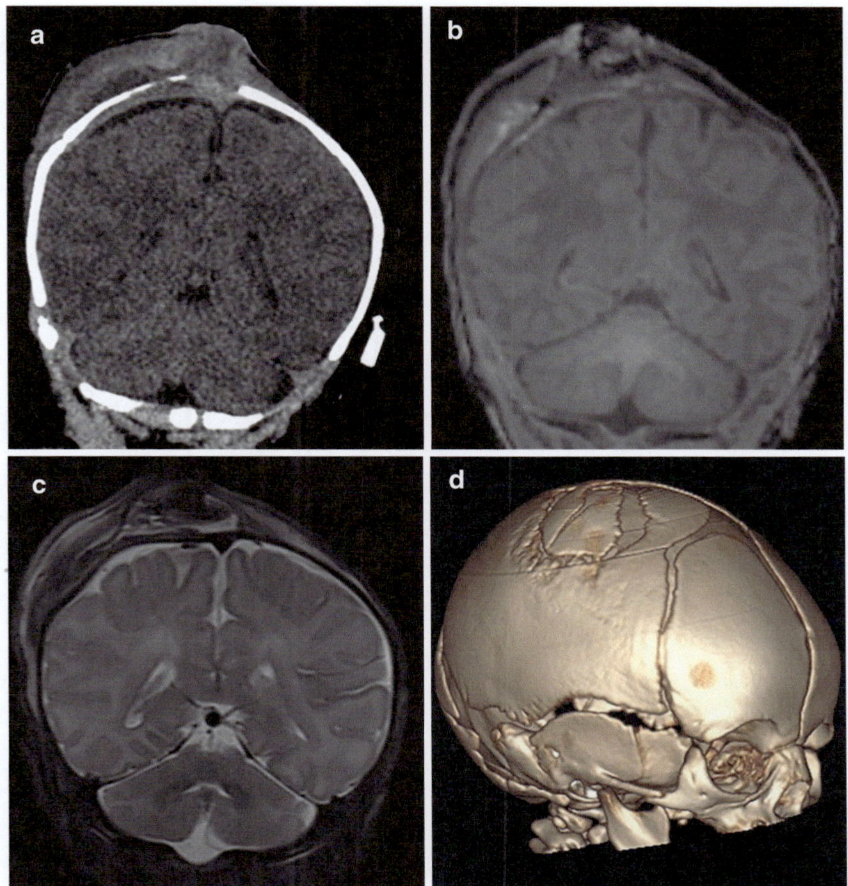

Fig. 10.3 2-week-old term male with history of forceps delivery presenting with right parietal soft tissue swelling. Neuroimaging demonstrated right-side cephalohematoma on coronal CT scan (**a**) and coronal T1- (**b**) and T2- (**c**) weighted brain MRI images. CT reconstruction of the skull (**d**) demonstrated complex fracture beneath the cephalohematoma

may require immediate intervention with fluid resuscitation and blood products. Infants with a history of traumatic birth or vacuum/forceps-assisted delivery should be checked and monitored closely for the presence and/or progression of subgaleal hemorrhage. Subgaleal hemorrhage can present with diffuse fluctuating scalp swelling, the scalp feels like "leather pouch filled with water," displaced earlobes, puffy eyelids, head circumference increase by ½ cm or more, pallor, poor perfusion, lethargy, poor feeding, tachypnea, increased work of breathing, tachycardia (HR > 160 bpm), apneas, and/or seizures. Infants with suspected subgaleal hemorrhages should be assessed following a strict protocol:

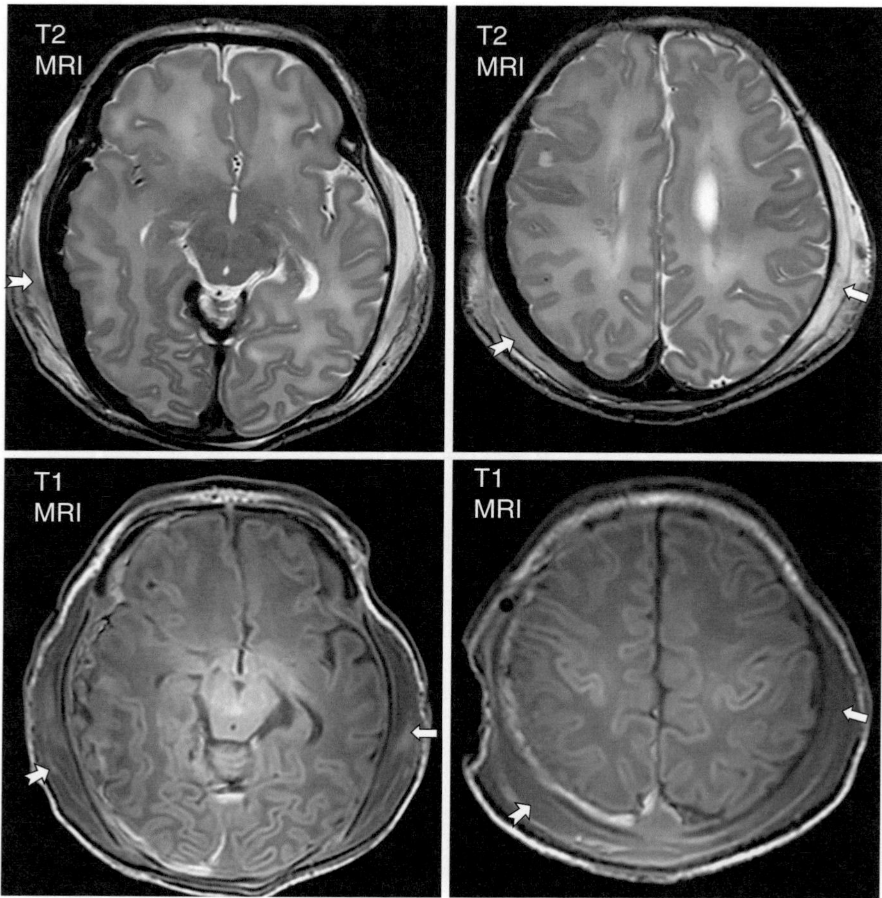

Fig. 10.4 Brain MRI in a full-term baby after traumatic delivery showing bilateral subgaleal hemorrhage on T2- and T1-weighted sequences (arrows) and subdural hemorrhage as decreased signal intensity on T2 and increased signal intensity on T1

- Frequent head circumference measurement (every 2 h in the first few hours after birth).
- Frequent physical examination.
- Continuous cardiorespiratory monitoring for at least 24 h.
- Complete blood count, coagulation profile, and cross-matched erythrocytes should be ordered.
- Close follow-up after discharge especially for hyperbilirubinemia.

- *Epidural hematoma* (Fig. 10.2): Is rare in neonates possibly due to underdeveloped meningeal arteries [13]. Risk factors for epidural hematoma include instrumental delivery, nulliparity, or fall after birth [4]. Epidural hematoma can be asymptomatic or may cause increased pressure inside the skull and/or seizures. Large and symptomatic epidural hemorrhages may require surgical intervention [14].

- *Subdural hemorrhage* (Figs. 10.4 and 10.5): Is a common intracranial hemorrhage in term infants and can be an incidental finding on brain MRI. Risk factors are similar to other mechanical birth injuries such as instrumental delivery, nulliparous, and fetal distress. Subdural hemorrhage is usually small and asymptomatic, especially infratentorially, but, when large, can present with seizures and/or apneas [15]. Subdural hemorrhages usually require no intervention. But if large and symptomatic and/or causing a midline shift or imminent herniation of the cerebellar tonsils, emergency neurosurgical drainage may be necessary. It is also possible to perform an ultrasound-guided needle aspiration [16]. Subdural hemorrhage can be associated with poor outcome especially with associated perinatal asphyxia [15].

- *Subarachnoid hemorrhage* (Fig. 10.2): Is another common injury in the newborn which can be an incidental finding on brain MRI [15]. Subarachnoid hemorrhage can be small. Larger subarachnoid hemorrhages can be associated with seizures and/or apneas and bradycardia. Prognosis is usually favorable unless comorbidities such as hypoxic ischemic encephalopathy (HIE) and hydrocephalus exist [17]. Treatment is usually supportive and symptomatic.

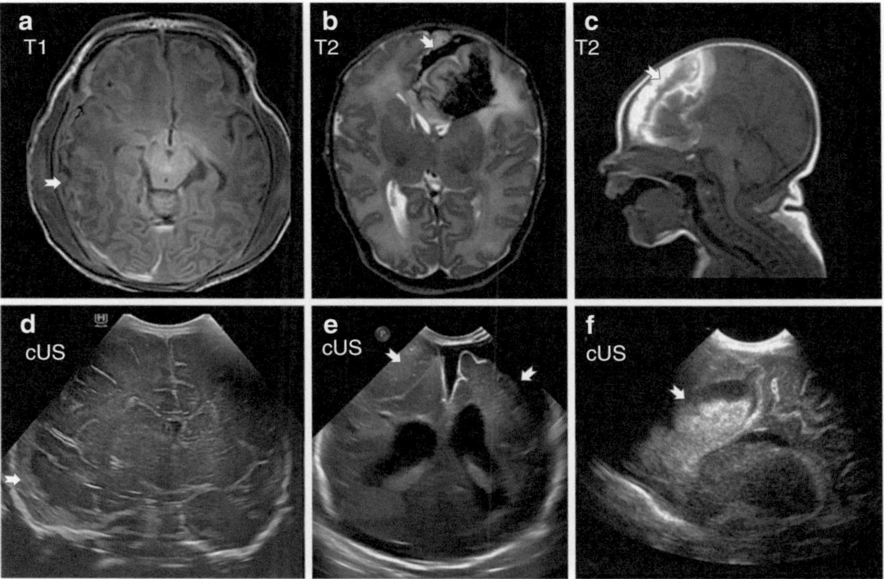

Fig. 10.5 MRI (axial T1 and T2, and sagittal T1) top row, and cUS (coronal and sagittal plane) bottom row. (**a** and **c**) Showing subdural hemorrhage (blue arrows) on T1-weighted MRI sequence (increased signal intensity), (**b**) T2-weighted MRI sequence (decreased signal intensity), and cUS (**d–f**) (bright for subacute and dark for acute hemorrhage). Also note the large frontal lobe hematoma (white arrows) (**b, c, f**)

10.2.3.2 Intracranial Hemorrhages (Fig. 10.6)

Intraparenchymal and intraventricular hemorrhages may be the result of traumatic birth or trauma after birth. In full-term infants, most intraparenchymal and intraventricular hemorrhages are secondary to other conditions. Cerebral sinus venous thrombosis (CSVT) leading to hemorrhagic infarction and/or intraventricular hemorrhage (IVH) is the most common cause (see Chap. 11 "CSVT"). Lobar hematoma especially in the temporal lobe may also occur in the context of thrombocytopenia and of specific genetic mutations (apoptosis-inducing factor mitochondria-associated 1 (AIFM1), Collagen Type IV Alpha 1 and 2 Chain (COL 4A1 or COL4A2)) or vascular malformations such as a vein of Galen malformation [18], AVM in infants with Rendu-Osler-Weber [19, 20], or pial arteriovenous fistulae [21]. Some congenital syndromes such as Sturge-Weber may present with

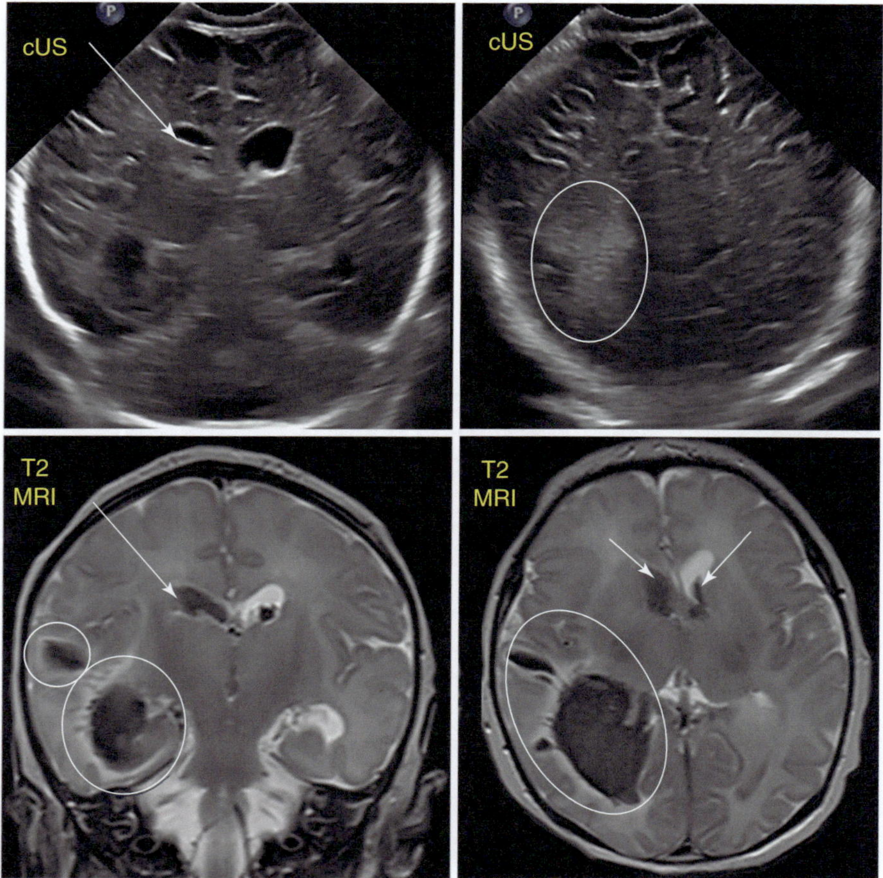

Fig. 10.6 Term newborn born by emergency Caesarean section due to failure to progress. cUS and brain MRI show intraventricular hemorrhage (arrows) and intraparenchymal hemorrhage (circles) on T2 MR sequence (decreased signal intensity) and cUS (increased echogenicity)

encephalopathy, intracranial hemorrhages, or refractory seizures, and imaging indicates the etiology in these cases.

10.2.4 Prognosis

Mechanical birth-related head injuries usually carry a favorable outcome if asymptomatic or identified and treated early, especially in the case of subgaleal hemorrhage. However, the prognosis worsens when comorbidities such as HIE, progressive hydrocephalus, or seizures exist [15, 22]. Prognosis is also more guarded in large injuries such as large intraparenchymal and intraventricular hemorrhages, depending on the site and extent of the injury. Outcome tends to be favorable for infants with an isolated large frontal lobe hemorrhage (as shown in Fig. 10.5). Some possible long-term implications are hydrocephalus secondary to IVH, sometimes needing ventriculo-peritoneal-shunt, epilepsy secondary to neonatal seizures and intraparenchymal hemorrhage [23], and language and/or motor impairment secondary to large intracranial hemorrhage or HIE [24]. Careful case-by-case consideration is recommended when counseling parents. Early identification and intervention programs are crucial.

References

1. Carney O, Hughes E, Tusor N, Dimitrova R, Arulkumaran S, Baruteau KP, Collado AE, Cordero-Grande L, Chew A, Falconer S, Allsop JM, Rueckert D, Hajnal J, Edwards AD, Rutherford M. Incidental findings on brain MR imaging of asymptomatic term neonates in the developing human connectome project. EClinicalMedicine. 2021;38:100984.
2. Gupta R, Cabacungan ET. Neonatal birth trauma: analysis of yearly trends, risk factors, and outcomes. J Pediatr. 2021;238(174–180):e173.
3. Hughes CA, Harley EH, Milmoe G, Bala R, Martorella A. Birth trauma in the head and neck. Arch Otolaryngol Head Neck Surg. 1999;125(2):193–9.
4. Rabelo NN, Matushita H, Cardeal DD. Traumatic brain lesions in newborns. Arq Neuropsiquiatr. 2017;75(3):180–8.
5. Nicholson L. Caput succedaneum and cephalohematoma: the cs that leave bumps on the head. Neonatal Netw. 2007;26(5):277–81.
6. Volpe JJ. Neurology of the newborn. New York: W.B. Saunders; 2001.
7. Tan KL, Lim GC. Phototherapy for neonatal jaundice in infants with cephalohematomas. Clin Pediatr (Phila). 1995;34(1):7–11.
8. Chang HY, Chiu NC, Huang FY, Kao HA, Hsu CH, Hung HY. Infected cephalohematoma of newborns: experience in a medical center in Taiwan. Pediatr Int. 2005;47(3):274–7.
9. Chung HY, Chung JY, Lee DG, Yang JD, Baik BS, Hwang SG, Cho BC. Surgical treatment of ossified cephalohematoma. J Craniofac Surg. 2004;15(5):774–9.
10. Fan HC, Hua YM, Juan CJ, Fang YM, Cheng SN, Wang CC. Infected cephalohematoma associated with sepsis and scalp cellulitis: a case report. J Microbiol Immunol Infect. 2002;35(2):125–8.
11. Kendall N, Woloshin H. Cephalohematoma associated with fracture of the skull. J Pediatr. 1952;41(2):125–32.
12. Menkes JH. Perinatal central nervous system asphyxia and trauma. In: Schaffer & Avery's diseases of the newborn. 6th ed. Philadelphia: W.B. Saunder; 1991. p. 406–8.

13. Monson SA, Henry E, Lambert DK, Schmutz N, Christensen RD. In-hospital falls of newborn infants: data from a multihospital health care system. Pediatrics. 2008;122(2):e277–80.
14. Vachharajani A, Mathur A. Ultrasound-guided needle aspiration of cranial epidural hematoma in a neonate: treating a rare complication of vacuum extraction. Am J Perinatol. 2002;19(8):401–4.
15. Hong HS, Lee JY. Intracranial hemorrhage in term neonates. Childs Nerv Syst. 2018;34(6):1135–43.
16. Cizmeci MN, Thewissen L, Zecic A, Woerdeman PA, Boer B, Baert E, Govaert P, Dudink J, Groenendaal F, Lequin M, de Vries LS. Bedside ultrasound-guided percutaneous needle aspiration of intra- and extra-axial intracranial hemorrhage in neonates. Neuropediatrics. 2018;49(4):238–45.
17. Palmer TW, Donn SM. Symptomatic subarachnoid hemorrhage in the term newborn. J Perinatol. 1991;11(2):112–6.
18. Meyers PM, Halbach VV, Phatouros CP, Dowd CF, Malek AM, Lempert TE, Lefler JE, Higashida RT. Hemorrhagic complications in vein of Galen malformations. Ann Neurol. 2000;47(6):748–55.
19. Delaney HM, Rooks VJ, Wolfe SQ, Sawyer TL. Term neonate with intracranial hemorrhage and hereditary hemorrhagic telangiectasia: a case report and review of the literature. J Perinatol. 2012;32(8):642–4.
20. Hausman-Kedem M, Malinger G, Modai S, Kushner SA, Shiran SI, Ben-Sira L, Roth J, Constantini S, Fattal-Valevski A, Ben-Shachar S. Monogenic causes of apparently idiopathic perinatal intracranial hemorrhage. Ann Neurol. 2021;89(4):813–22.
21. Barreto ARF, Carrasco M, Dabrowski AK, Sun LR, Tekes A. Subpial hemorrhage in neonates: what radiologists need to know. AJR Am J Roentgenol. 2021;216(4):1056–65.
22. Brouwer AJ, Groenendaal F, Koopman C, Nievelstein RJ, Han SK, de Vries LS. Intracranial hemorrhage in full-term newborns: a hospital-based cohort study. Neuroradiology. 2010;52(6):567–76.
23. Soul JS. Acute symptomatic seizures in term neonates: etiologies and treatments. Semin Fetal Neonatal Med. 2018;23(3):183–90.
24. Halpin S, McCusker C, Fogarty L, White J, Cavaliere E, Boylan G, Murray D. Long-term neuropsychological and behavioral outcome of mild and moderate hypoxic ischemic encephalopathy. Early Hum Dev. 2022;165:105541.

Sinovenous Thrombosis

11

Linda S. de Vries and Sylke J. Steggerda

Abbreviations

ACT	Anticoagulation therapy
AF	Anterior fontanel
CSVT	Cerebral sinovenous thrombosis
cUS	Cranial ultrasound
ESES	Electrical status epilepticus in sleep
IVH	Intraventricular hemorrhage
MRI	Magnetic resonance imaging
SSS	Superior sagittal sinus
SWAS	Spike wake activation during sleep
SWI	Susceptibility-weighted imaging

L. S. de Vries (✉)
Department of Pediatrics, Division of Neonatology, Willem-Alexander Children's Hospital, Leiden University Medical Center (LUMC), Leiden, The Netherlands

Department of Neonatology, University Medical Center Utrecht (UMCU), Utrecht, The Netherlands
e-mail: l.s.de_vries@lumc.nl

S. J. Steggerda
Department of Pediatrics, Division of Neonatology, Willem-Alexander Children's Hospital, Leiden University Medical Center (LUMC), Leiden, The Netherlands
e-mail: S.J.Steggerda@lumc.nl

© The Author(s) 2024
G. Meijler, K. Mohammad (eds.), *Neonatal Brain Injury*,
https://doi.org/10.1007/978-3-031-55972-3_11

11.1   For Parents

There are several large blood vessels located over the surface of the brain that carry blood from the brain back to the heart. These blood vessels are called "sinuses" (Fig. 11.1). It is not common to develop a blood clot that blocks one or several of these sinuses, but it does occur in both full-term and preterm infants. Such a clot is called a thrombosis. A thrombosis in one of these sinuses occurs in fewer than 1 in 1000 live births. Brain imaging using high-quality cranial ultrasound (cUS) and especially MRI has led to better recognition of this problem.

11.1.1 How Will I Know if My Baby Has Symptoms of a Sinus Thrombosis?

Most full-term infants will be at home when they develop a thrombosis. The parents may find it more difficult to feed the baby, may not find the baby very alert, or may see jerky movements of the limbs. The baby may also have blue lips at times, because breathing may become irregular. When the infant is admitted to the hospital and an EEG recording (a test that measures electrical activity in the brain) is performed, the jerky movements are often found to be caused by seizures. The baby may also be a bit dehydrated because of the feeding difficulties. Sometimes when a baby is in the hospital for other reasons including being born preterm, a thrombosis

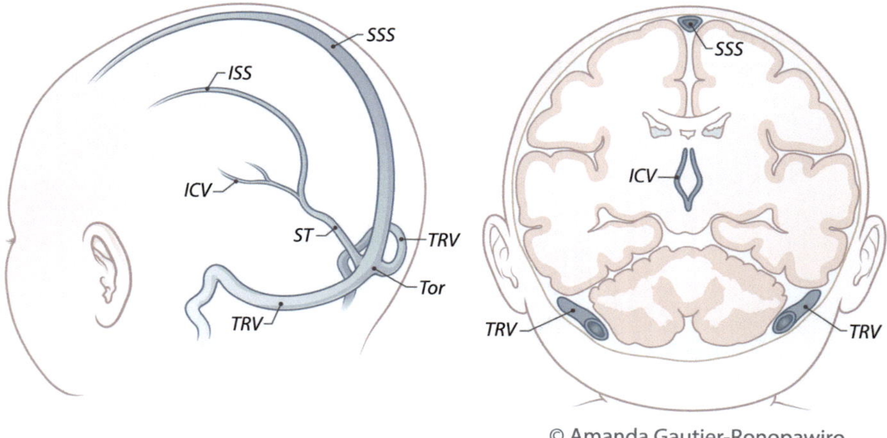

Fig. 11.1 The sinuses are shown in blue; the larger ones are situated on the surface of the brain. The main ones are the SSS, superior sagittal sinus; the TRV, transverse sinus, ISS, inferior sagittal sinus, ICV, internal cerebral vein, Tor, torcular herophili (from [1]; this is an open-access article distributed under the terms of the Creative Commons CC-BY license, which permits unrestricted use, distribution, and reproduction in any medium, provided the original work is properly cited) (© Amanda Gautier-Ronopawiro)

in a sinus may be a chance finding on a cUS or MRI or be associated with a change in behavior, like irritability.

11.1.2 Why Did My Baby Develop a Sinus Thrombosis?

The cause of a thrombosis in a sinus is often not well understood. Known risk factors are dehydration, infection, and especially meningitis. It is more common in babies who have had surgery, e.g., for a congenital heart defect. Very often however it is not clear why the thrombosis occurred.

11.1.3 What Is the Treatment if My Baby Is Diagnosed with a Sinus Thrombosis?

A thrombus in a sinus can become larger over time, and this happens in around 25% of cases. As a larger thrombus creates a higher risk for injury developing in brain tissue, thrombosis is nowadays more often treated with heparin, an anticoagulant, than in the past. This helps to prevent the thrombus from growing. In one study it was shown that after 3 months of treatment, the sinus was open again in 85% of infants. Treatment is usually started in the hospital, but can be continued at home. The medication is administered using a very thin needle, inserted just under the skin either by a health professional or by parents. Several studies have now shown that this treatment is safe and reduces the risk of developing a larger thrombus and also developing brain injury.

11.1.4 What Will Happen to My Baby (Prognosis)?

Fortunately, most babies will survive, but some will have considerable long-term problems, especially when the MRI shows injury in the brain tissue. The child without associated brain injury will usually have a favorable outcome. However, when associated brain injury is seen, then the longer-term effects depend on its size and especially where it is located in the brain. One type of injury that can be seen is hemorrhage in a central part of the brain called the thalamus. Damage in this area often leads to a special type of epilepsy starting when the child is a bit older (usually more than 3 years of age), and this form of epilepsy is typically present during sleep. Now that we are aware of this association, we suggest that a child with this type of injury to the thalamus has an EEG during sleep once a year from 3 to about 7 years, to help with early recognition and treatment of this type of epilepsy. We also recommend longer-term follow-up well into school age to ensure the child is doing well with learning and memory and is also normally developing social skills.

11.2 For Professionals

11.2.1 Incidence

The incidence of neonatal sinovenous thrombosis (CSVT) varies widely in the literature from 1/1000 to 6.6/100.000 live births. This variation is probably due to the different thresholds of performing neuroimaging in different centers [2–6]. Looking at the entire childhood period, CSVT is most commonly seen in the neonatal period [7].

Although often no causation is found, there are many risk factors for CSVT; the most important ones are listed below:

- Maternal health related: gestational hypertension, pre-eclampsia, gestational diabetes, or chorioamnionitis.
- Newborn related: male sex, asphyxia, hypoxia, preterm birth, dehydration, sepsis, meningitis, surgery for congenital heart disease.
- Delivery related: assisted delivery.

11.2.2 Clinical Signs

The clinical presentation of neonatal CSVT has been described in cohorts of predominantly full-term infants. In one study however 29% of the affected infants were born preterm [4–6]. Presentation of CSVT tends to be a bit later than for perinatal arterial stroke (PAIS) [4–6], and the diagnosis was made with a median of 10 days (IQR 4–14) in CSVT compared to 3 days (IQR 1–5) for PAIS. In two studies, the mean postnatal age at presentation was found to be slightly later in preterm infants as compared to full-term infants (9 and 5 days, respectively) [6, 8]. The main presenting symptoms consist of generalized or focal seizures and/or apnea, especially in infants with associated brain lesions. Other symptoms include encephalopathy, lethargy, irritability, feeding problems, and hyper- or hypotonia [2, 8–10]. In the study by *Berfelo et al.* CSVT was a chance finding in 13% of the cases. CSVT is not uncommon in preterm infants; of the 51 infants reported recently, 14 were born preterm [5]. No major differences in symptoms were noted for full-term or preterm infants.

11.2.3 Diagnosis

Both cranial ultrasound (cUS) and MRI can be used for the diagnosis of neonatal CSVT and are considered complementary as each has its own specific advantages. Serial imaging can be best performed with cUS as this technique is especially useful to assess the evolution of the thrombus (clot propagation, thrombus recanalization) and shows most of the associated lesions (Figs. 11.2, 11.3, and 11.4). MRI is best to show residual damage (gliosis) and possible effects on myelination and volume loss, especially reduced thalamic volume following a thalamic hemorrhage [11] (Fig. 11.5). Several studies reported the sinus(es) involved in CSVT in both full-term and preterm infants. The superior sagittal sinus (SSS), transverse sinus, and straight sinus are most often affected in the full-term infant and the transverse sinus in the preterm infant (Table 11.1). In many infants, multiple sinuses are affected.

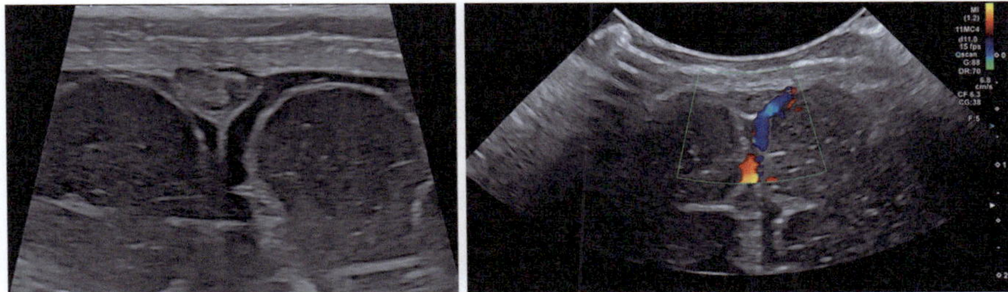

Fig. 11.2 Preterm infant born at 33 weeks gestation. Uncomplicated delivery and good Apgar scores, irritable on day 3. cUS recognized the echogenic area in the SSS, and absent flow was confirmed with color Doppler ultrasound

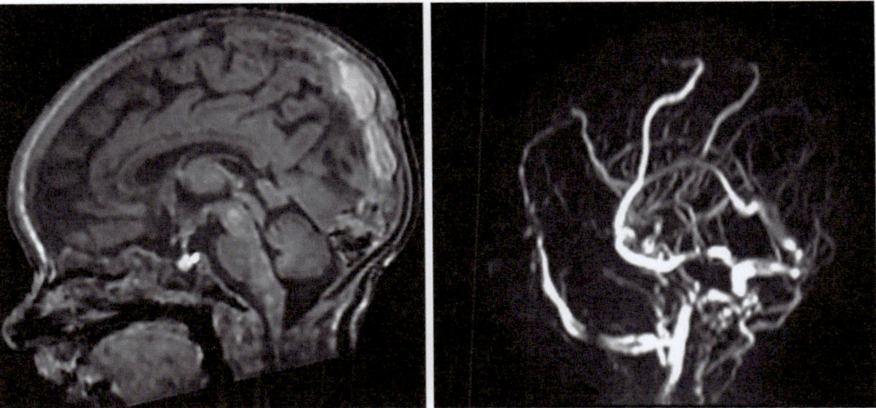

Fig. 11.3 An MRI was performed with the T1 sequence showing the thrombus and the MRV showing absence of flow in the entire SSS

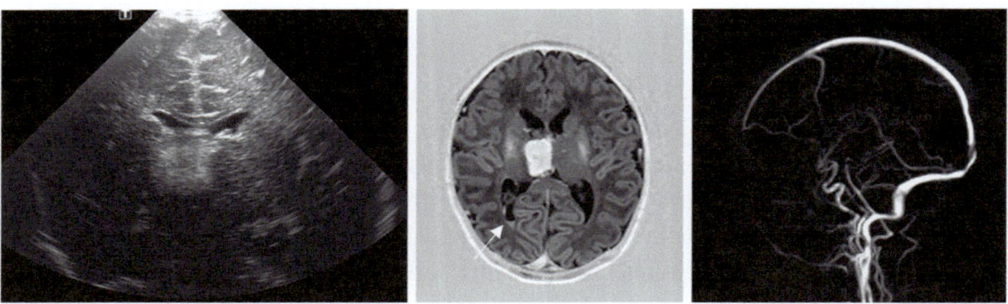

Fig. 11.4 Full-term infant, with a square-shaped echogenicity reaching to the midline in the right thalamus, highly suggestive of hemorrhage, seen on cUS. Hemorrhage of the same shape is clearly seen on the T1W transverse MRI, and some blood is also seen in the right occipital horn (arrow). The MRV does not show any flow across the straight sinus

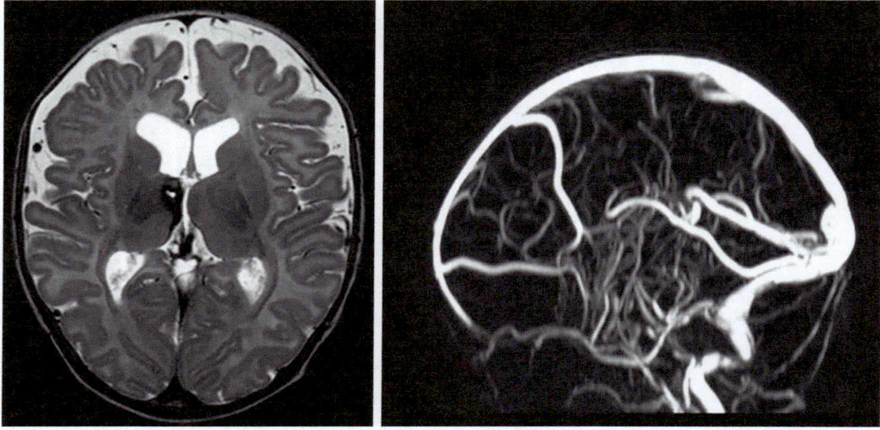

Fig. 11.5 The infant was treated with low-molecular-weight heparin for 3 months, and the MRI then showed remnants of the thalamic hemorrhage with a slightly reduced thalamic volume. Myelination of the posterior limb of the internal capsule is seen bilaterally, but there is increased extracerebral space and widening of the interhemispheric fissure, indicating white matter volume loss. The MRV shows recanalization of the straight sinus

Table 11.1 Pooled data from references by [8–10, 12, 13] (term infants), and [14] (preterm infants)

Sinus	Full-term infants ($n = 88$)	Preterm infants ($n = 32$)
Superior sagittal sinus	**56 (64)**	14 (44)
Transverse sinus	43 (49)	**22 (69)**
Straight sinus	40 (45)	10 (31)
Torcula	8 (9)	5 (16)
Jugular sinus	10 (11)	2 (6)
Sigmoid sinus	11 (12)	6 (19)
Deep venous system	17 (19)	4 (12)

11.2.4 Cranial Ultrasound

When a full-term infant presents with seizures and cUS shows an intraventricular hemorrhage (IVH) with/without a thalamic hemorrhage or unexplained white matter injury CSVT should be suspected. Color Doppler ultrasound should be performed to assess the patency of the venous sinuses and has a high specificity to rule out neonatal CSVT [1, 15]. Using the anterior fontanel (AF) as an acoustic window, the superior sagittal sinus, internal cerebral veins, and transverse sinuses can be visualized; in the AF midsagittal plane, the anterior-middle and posterior parts of the superior sagittal sinus, the inferior sagittal sinus, internal cerebral veins, and straight sinus can be seen [1, 16]. Color Doppler cUS can demonstrate partial or a total absence of flow in combination with a partial or complete occlusion of the affected sinus(es). Furthermore, cUS can identify associated brain lesions such as (late onset) IVH, thalamic hemorrhage, and white matter injury. Although it is feasible to screen the venous system in neonates, retrospective studies have reported only a moderate sensitivity of cUS for the detection of CSVT. In the study by Berfelo et al. [2], 37% of cases were diagnosed with cUS and 63% solely on MRI, and in another study approximately half of CSVT were detected with cUS [17]. Nevertheless, the use of targeted cUS screening, including color Doppler, high-frequency linear transducers, and additional mastoid fontanel views, has the potential to increase the diagnostic accuracy of cUS for the detection of CSVT [18]. Performing mastoid window ultrasound will improve recognition of a CSVT of the transverse sinus and will also allow differentiating between low flow and a true thrombosis which may be difficult with MRV (see case).

11.2.5 MRI

Even though color Doppler cUS may be very suggestive of a CSVT, we recommend obtaining an MRI, including MR venography (MRV), to confirm the diagnosis and to help in deciding whether to start anticoagulation therapy (ACT). MRI will provide more detailed information on associated brain injury. In the full-term infant, an IVH with a thalamic hemorrhage is common when there is a thrombosis of the straight sinus and deep internal venous system [19] (Fig. 11.2). In the preterm infant, associated white matter injury is more often seen [8, 9]. Diffusion weighted imaging (DWI) and Susceptibility weighted imaging (SWI) will help to distinguish between hemorrhagic and ischemic brain injury. The MRV can be acquired by both time-of-flight and phase contrast techniques. The MRI appearance of the thrombus depends on the stage (acute, subacute, or chronic) and is best seen with the T1 sequence (Fig. 11.3). A potential pitfall of MRV is that there tends to be one dominant transverse sinus, and the other may suggest absence of flow/thrombosis. The T1 sequence will be helpful to visualize the thrombosed sinus, and Doppler cUS with very low flow velocity settings can be helpful to demonstrate flow and exclude CSVT [1, 15].

11.2.6 Treatment

There is no consensus on whether or not to use ACT for CSVT. There are guidelines that recommend repeating an MRI 5 days after the first MRI to look for propagation (extension) of the thrombus which is seen in around 25% of cases [20–22]. Unfortunately, associated brain injury can occur during this 5-day time window. A comparison between international centers showed less use of ACT in the United States compared to Europe [23]. An RCT was considered but has not yet been performed, and there no longer appears to be equipoise to do such a trial, as most centers now prefer to treat, even in the presence of an IVH and/or parenchymal hemorrhage and as the use of ACT does not seem to worsen the IVH [24].

11.2.7 Prognosis

Neurodevelopmental outcome is moderate to severely abnormal in 40–50% of infants with CSVT [2, 22] (Table 11.2). In the study of Moharir, there was a 6% mortality. As expected, the outcome will be more favorable in the absence of associated parenchymal injury [10]. No or only partial recanalization and propagation of the clot were also identified as predictors of an unfavorable outcome [22]. In preterm infants with associated white matter injury that mimics cystic PVL, cerebral palsy is likely to develop. In the full-term infant with IVH and associated thalamic hemorrhage, cerebral palsy is not common, but there is a high risk of developing spike wake activation during sleep (SWAS) previously referred to as electrical status epilepticus in sleep (ESES) [25, 26]. In a prospectively studied cohort of 23 infants, as many as 83% developed SWAS [11]. By measuring thalamic volume on the 3-month MRI, it was found that a smaller thalamic volume predicted poorer cognitive outcome. Among the 13 infants who were tested before and after SWAS

Table 11.2 Prognosis [2, 11, 22]

cUS finding (maximum extent)	Conjunctive MRI finding at TEA	Prognosis
Absent flow in SSS/SS or TS without parenchymal injury	No parenchymal injury	Favorable at 18–24 months (corrected) age
Absent flow in SSS and inhomogeneous echogenicity in the white matter	Associated WMI (medullary vein distribution)	Low risk of CP, mildly increased risk of cognitive problems
Absent flow in SS/internal cerebral vein and thalamic hemorrhage	Thalamic hemorrhage	Low risk of CP, significant risk (60–80%) to develop spike wave activation during sleep (SWAS) with associated cognitive problems
Multi-sinus thrombosis and inhomogeneous echogenicity in the white matter with/ without hemorrhage	Associated WMI/ hemorrhage	Increased risk of mortality and high risk of severely abnormal outcome

TEA term-equivalent age, *WMI* white matter injury, *CP* cerebral palsy, *SSS* superior sagittal sinus, *SS* straight sinus, *TS* transverse sinus

onset (average time interval 43 months), a significant decrease in IQ score was noted (89–82; $p = 0.046$). As seizures are present during sleep, the diagnosis of SWAS will often be delayed and only made following the cognitive decline. By performing serial sleep EEGs once a year between 3 and 7 years, the diagnosis can be made early and treatment considered, especially when a cognitive decline is noted.

11.3 Case

A male infant was born at 31 weeks gestation with a birth weight of 1500 g. His mother became ill a week before delivery, after a hitherto uneventful pregnancy, and developed fever due to a bacterial pneumonia. She was treated with intravenous antibiotics.

A caesarean section was performed because of fetal distress. The infant's Apgar scores were 4, 7, 8 at 1, 5, and 10 min, respectively. He had an umbilical cord pH of 6.99 and a lactate of 11 mmol/L which normalized within the first 12 hours after birth.

He was admitted to the neonatal intensive care unit. Because of respiratory distress syndrome, he was supported with CPAP and received caffeine and a single dose of surfactant via a minimally invasive procedure. He was stable from a circulatory point of view. He was started on intravenous antibiotics; his blood culture remained sterile.

The first glucose level on admission was unmeasurable, but this normalized after the start of enteral and parenteral feeding.

On day 2 he was thrombocytopenic (platelets $97* 10^9/L$) which worsened to a lowest value of $39*10^9/L$ on day 4. Without any signs of bleeding, this was managed expectantly.

His cUS on day 1 scan showed a germinal matrix hemorrhage (IVH grade I) on the left which remained stable over the following days. On day 4 he became restless and irritable and the cUS scan was repeated. This showed an absence of flow in the right transverse sinus. Based on the clinical symptoms and the cUS image, a CSVT was suspected, and this was confirmed on an MRI scan (Figs. 11.6 and 11.7). He was treated with low-molecular-weight heparin for 3 months without any additional complications. Follow-up cUS scans showed no propagation of the clot and no additional brain abnormalities; a repeat MRI at 3 months showed full recanalization, and there were no brain lesions except for single punctate white matter lesion.

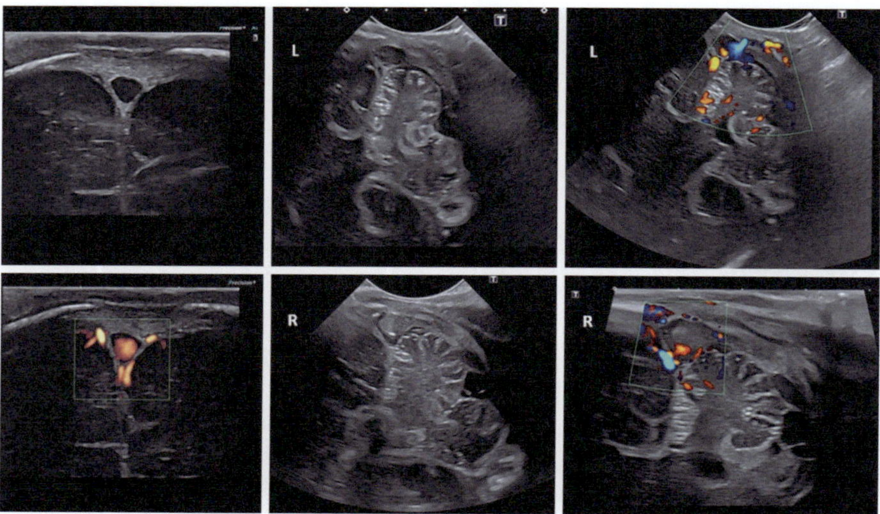

Fig. 11.6 The superior sagittal sinus is open and shows flow in the coronal view through the anterior fontanel (left). Using the mastoid window, a clot and absence of flow are shown in the right transverse sinus

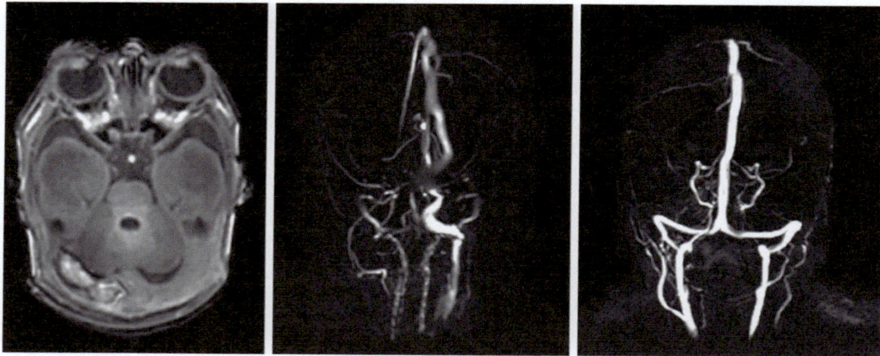

Fig. 11.7 An MRI was performed to confirm the diagnosis, and indeed a thrombus was seen on the transverse T1-weighted sequence (left). The MRV (middle) showed lack of flow in the right transverse sinus. A repeat MRI after 3 months of low-molecular-weight heparin showed full recanalization (right)

References

1. Steggerda SJ, de Vries LS. Neonatal stroke in premature neonates. Semin Perinatol. 2021;45(7):151471.
2. Berfelo FJ, Kersbergen KJ, van Ommen CH, Govaert P, van Straaten HL, Poll-The BT, et al. Neonatal cerebral sinovenous thrombosis from symptom to outcome. Stroke. 2010;41(7):1382–8.

3. Dunbar M, Mineyko A, Hill M, Hodge J, Floer A, Kirton A. Population based birth prevalence of disease-specific perinatal stroke. Pediatrics. 2020;146:e2020013201.

4. Sorg AL, von Kries R, Klemme M, Gerstl L, Felderhoff-Müser U, Dzietko M. Incidence estimates of perinatal arterial ischemic stroke in preterm- and term-born infants: a national capture-recapture calculation corrected surveillance study. Neonatology. 2021a;118(6):727–33.

5. Sorg AL, Von Kries R, Klemme M, Gerstl L, Beyerlein A, Lack N, Felderhoff-Müser U, Dzietko M. Incidence and risk factors of cerebral sinovenous thrombosis in infants. Dev Med Child Neurol. 2021b;63(6):697–704.

6. Sorg AL, Klemme M, von Kries R, Felderhoff-Müser U, Flemmer AW, Gerstl L, Dzietko M. Clinical diversity of cerebral sinovenous thrombosis and arterial ischaemic stroke in the neonate: a surveillance study. Neonatology. 2021c;118(5):530–6.

7. Deveber G, Andrew M, Adams C, Bjornson B, Booth F, Buckley DJ, Camfield CS, David M, Humphreys P, Langevin P, MacDonald E, Gillett J, Meaney B, Shevell M, Sinclair DB, Yager J. Cerebral sinovenous thrombosis in children. N Engl J Med. 2001;345:417–23.

8. Kersbergen KJ, Groenendaal F, Benders MJ, van Straaten HL, Niwa T, Nievelstein RA, de Vries LS. The spectrum of associated brain lesions in cerebral sinovenous thrombosis: relation to gestational age and outcome. Arch Dis Child Fetal Neonatal Ed. 2011a;96(6):F404–F9.

9. Kersbergen KJ, Groenendaal F, Benders MJ, de Vries LS. Neonatal cerebral sinovenous thrombosis: neuroimaging and long-term follow-up. J Child Neurol. 2011b;26(9):1111–20.

10. Fitzgerald KC, Williams LS, Garg BP, Carvalho KS, Golomb MR. Cerebral sinovenous thrombosis in the neonate. Arch Neurol. 2006;63(3):405–9.

11. van den Munckhof B, Zwart AF, Weeke LC, Claessens NHP, Plate JDJ, Leemans A, Kuijf HJ, van Teeseling HC, Leijten FSS, Benders MJN, Braun KPJ, de Vries LS, Jansen FE. Perinatal thalamic injury: MRI predictors of electrical status epilepticus in sleep and long-term neurodevelopment. Neuroimage Clin. 2020;26:102227.

12. Filip C, Zonda GI, Vasilache I-A, Scripcariu IS, Vicoveanu P, Dima V, Socolov D, Paduraru L. Neonatal cerebral sinovenous thrombosis and the main perinatal risk factors-a retrospective unicentric study. Children (Basel). 2022;9(8):1182. https://doi.org/10.3390/children9081182.

13. Pergami P, Abraham L. Impact of anticoagulation on the short-term outcome in a population of neonatal infants with cerebral sinovenous thrombosis: a retrospective study. J Child Neurol. 2011;26:844–50.

14. Christensen R, Krishnan P, deVeber G, Dlamini N, MacGregor D, Pulcine E, Moharir M. Cerebral venous sinus thrombosis in preterm infants. Stroke. 2022;53(7):2241–8.

15. Miller E, Daneman A, Doria AS, Blaser S, Traubici J, Jarrin J, et al. Color Doppler US of normal cerebral venous sinuses in neonates: a comparison with MR venography. Pediatr Radiol. 2012;42(9):1070–9.

16. Meijler, Steggerda. Cranial ultrasonography. Springer; 2019.

17. Grunt S, Wingeier K, Wehrli E, Boltshauser E, Capone A, Fluss J, et al. Swiss Neuropaediatric Stroke Registry. Cerebral sinus venous thrombosis in Swiss children. Dev Med Child Neurol. 2010;52(12):1145–50.

18. Raets MM, Sol JJ, Govaert P, Lequin MH, Reiss IK, Kroon AA, et al. Serial cranial US for detection of cerebral sinovenous thrombosis in preterm infants. Radiology. 2013;269(3):879–86.

19. Wu YW, Hamrick SE, Miller SP, Haward MF, Lai MC, Callen PW, Barkovich AJ, Ferriero DM. Intraventricular hemorrhage in term neonates caused by sinovenous thrombosis. Ann Neurol. 2003;54(1):123–6.

20. Monagle P, Chan AKC, Goldenberg NA, et al. Antithrombotic therapy in neonates and children: antithrombotic therapy and prevention of thrombosis, 9th ed: American College of Chest Physicians Evidence-Based Clinical Practice Guidelines. Chest. 2012;141(Suppl. 2):e737S–801S.

21. Rossor T, Arichi T, Bhate S, Hart AR, Singh RR. Anticoagulation in the management of neonatal cerebral sinovenous thrombosis: a systematic review and meta-analysis. Dev Med Child Neurol. 2018;60:884–91.

22. Moharir MD, Shroff M, Stephens D, et al. Anticoagulants in pediatric cerebral sinovenous thrombosis: a safety and outcome study. Ann Neurol. 2010;67:590–9.4.

23. Jordan LC, Rafay MF, Smith SE, Askalan R, Zamel KM, deVeber G, Ashwal S, International Pediatric Stroke Study Group. Antithrombotic treatment in neonatal cerebral sinovenous thrombosis: results of the International Pediatric Stroke Study. J Pediatr. 2010;156(5):704–10. 710.e1–710.e2

24. Kersbergen KJ, de Vries LS, van Straaten HLM, Benders MJNL, Nievelstein RAJ, Groenendaal F. Anticoagulation therapy and imaging in neonates with a unilateral thalamic hemorrhage due to cerebral sinovenous thrombosis. Stroke. 2009;40(8):2754–60.

25. Kersbergen KJ, de Vries LS, Leijten FS, Braun KP, Nievelstein RA, Groenendaal F, Benders MJ, Jansen FE. Neonatal thalamic hemorrhage is strongly associated with electrical status epilepticus in slow wave sleep. Epilepsia. 2013;54(4):733–40.

26. Specchio N, Wirrell EC, Scheffer IE, et al. International league against epilepsy classification and definition of epilepsy syndromes with onset in childhood: position paper by the ILAE Task Force on Nosology and Definitions. Epilepsia. 2022;63(6):1398–442.

## Part IV

Neonatal Brain Infections

Viral Infections

12

Linda S. de Vries and Sylke J. Steggerda

Abbreviations

CMV	Cytomegalovirus infection
cUS	Cranial ultrasound
HIV	Human immunodeficiency virus
HSV	Herpes simplex virus
PCR	Polymerase chain reaction
SEM	Skin eye mouth

L. S. de Vries (✉)
Department of Pediatrics, Division of Neonatology, Willem-Alexander Children's Hospital, Leiden University Medical Center (LUMC), Leiden, The Netherlands

Department of Neonatology, University Medical Center Utrecht (UMCU), Utrecht, The Netherlands
e-mail: l.s.de_vries@lumc.nl

S. J. Steggerda
Department of Pediatrics, Division of Neonatology, Willem-Alexander Children's Hospital, Leiden University Medical Center (LUMC), Leiden, The Netherlands
e-mail: S.J.Steggerda@lumc.nl

© The Author(s) 2024
G. Meijler, K. Mohammad (eds.), *Neonatal Brain Injury*,
https://doi.org/10.1007/978-3-031-55972-3_12

12.1 For Parents

12.1.1 Viral Infections Acquired During Pregnancy

During pregnancy the mother may have a mild cold or other mild symptoms that she may not even remember—many of these are due to viruses, e.g., influenza which is not problematic for the baby. Some viruses, although they may hardly cause symptoms in the mother, may cross through the placenta and infect the baby. One of the most common of these is cytomegalovirus (CMV). In most cases, it does not lead to severe brain injury, but when the infection happens early in pregnancy, it may interfere with normal brain development, and the superficial layer of the brain (the cortex) may not develop normal folding. The virus may cause polymicrogyria, meaning that there are too many and too shallow infoldings or it may lead to a lack of folding which is called lissencephaly, or incomplete development of the cerebellum. In less severely affected infants, small fluid-filled spaces (cysts) may be present next to the lateral ventricles (the normal fluid-filled spaces in the brain), or the white matter may look too bright on an MRI scan. In other infants, the lining of some of the smaller vessels in the brain may show calcification, which can be seen on ultrasound but not on MRI. Finally, CMV infection may cause damage to the nerve cells of the inner ear. This may result in hearing loss, and the infant may need hearing aids or a cochlear implant in infancy. Depending on where you live, screening for CMV is performed during pregnancy, and the diagnosis can be confirmed, by performing a test on the amniotic fluid (the fluid around the baby in the womb). Without this screening, a diagnosis before birth is only made in more severely affected fetuses, when a small head, poor growth of the baby, and/or larger ventricles are seen on routine ultrasound examinations. Such findings are suggestive of CMV infection, so additional tests will then be performed. Besides antenatal ultrasound, an antenatal MRI is nowadays often performed as well. In very severely affected fetuses, termination of the pregnancy may be considered.

After birth, it is important to assess the brain with ultrasound and MRI and to perform a hearing test. Early intervention for hearing loss is very important to achieve (near) normal speech development.

Other viruses that may affect the baby's brain are rubella, varicella, HIV, herpes simplex, and ZIKA. Rubella is now very rare due to vaccination in infancy. As most mothers have had varicella before becoming pregnant, this is also not commonly seen. HIV is more common in low- and middle-income countries, and the outcome is now much better due to treatment of the mother during pregnancy. Herpes simplex infection may occur during pregnancy, but more often the infant may acquire the infection during a vaginal delivery when there are genital lesions at the time of delivery and also after birth from a caregiver with cold sores. During the ZIKA epidemic, many fetuses were affected and developed severe brain lesions, showing a small head size at birth.

Another type of infection, caused by a parasite that is also important to be aware of, is toxoplasmosis. Mothers are generally advised during pregnancy not to eat raw meat and to be careful when looking after cats at home. An affected fetus may develop severely enlarged lateral ventricles leading to a condition called hydrocephalus, before birth.

12.1.1.1 How Will I Know if My Baby Has Symptoms of a Congenital Viral Infection?

With CMV and toxoplasmosis, the diagnosis is often already made during pregnancy. Babies with CMV may be small, have a small head, and have blue spots on the skin due to bleeding because of low platelet levels. They can also be jaundiced and may have an enlarged liver or spleen. But importantly they may also not have any of these symptoms. Tests will be done after birth to confirm the diagnosis.

Babies with toxoplasmosis may have a large head due to hydrocephalus, and babies with rubella may have cataracts.

When an infection with herpes simplex is acquired during or shortly after delivery, symptoms may first develop after the end of the second week. Sometimes there are blisters on the skin, but more often the infant will not have these but will be drowsy, not feeding well and present with seizures.

12.1.1.2 Why Did My Baby Develop a Viral or Toxoplasmosis Infection?

This happens because the mother developed an infection during pregnancy and the virus crossed the placenta and infected the fetus (CMV, toxoplasmosis) or the infection was acquired during or shortly after the delivery (herpes simplex). For CMV, it is quite common that the infected infant is the second child in the family. Young children are often infected with CMV at the nursery, and the mother can get the infection when changing the nappies, kissing the child on the mouth, or sharing a spoon when feeding. This is because an infected child will secrete the virus in the urine and saliva for many months.

For toxoplasmosis it is possible that the mother was eating raw or undercooked meat or was exposed to the stools (feces) of an infected cat at home.

12.1.1.3 What Is the Treatment if My Baby Is Diagnosed with a Viral or Toxoplasmosis Infection?

Treatment is usually not given during pregnancy for these antenatally acquired infections except for toxoplasmosis. For CMV there have been some recent trials giving antiviral therapy during the first trimester of pregnancy. To be able to possibly benefit from this treatment, screening early in pregnancy is required. Once the diagnosis is made after birth in an infant presenting with symptoms, or when imaging of the brain shows abnormalities, antiviral medication can be given. For CMV, treatment with oral medication can be started immediately and continued for

6 months and has been shown to prevent further hearing loss and according to some studies may even improve hearing. When a hearing test shows severe hearing loss, it is very important to get hearing aids very early and preferably within 3 months after birth, in order to preserve speech development. Careful follow-up is required as hearing loss due to CMV can get worse over time or even first develop up till 6 years of age. Infants with abnormal development of the cortex are at risk of developing epilepsy that needs to be treated with antiseizure medication.

For toxoplasmosis and herpes simplex infections, medication is also available. As herpes simplex infection is usually acquired during delivery but the infant will only develop symptoms several days after birth, it is very important to make the diagnosis as soon as possible to prevent further brain injury or severe illness. Therefore, when a baby gets ill after birth, pediatricians often start a treatment against herpes just in case the baby has this infection.

If there is already established brain injury, like abnormal development of the cortex (CMV) or hydrocephalus (toxoplasmosis), a cure is no longer possible. Infants with toxoplasmosis are at risk of developing eye problems at a later age and should be seen on a regular basis by an ophthalmologist.

12.1.1.4 What Will Happen to My Baby (Prognosis)?

The prognosis very much depends on the brain lesions seen on brain imaging. These can be absent or very mild in CMV and the outcome can be normal. However, when the development of the cortex is abnormal, then the risk of motor (movement), epilepsy, and learning problems is high. In infants who developed hydrocephalus following toxoplasmosis infection, the enlarged ventricles may need to be drained, using a tube (shunt), led under the skin from the lateral ventricle to the peritoneal cavity (the fluid-filled space surrounding the bowels). The shunt will allow fluid to flow from the lateral ventricles if the pressure in the lateral ventricles becomes too high. The severity of brain lesions in herpes simplex infection can vary and determines the child's outcome. Some babies may develop motor and learning problems and/or epilepsy.

12.1.2 Infections Acquired After Birth

It is also possible for the baby to get a viral infection within the first weeks after birth. The infection can be acquired through somebody at home or in the hospital. There are many viral infections that can occur, but there are only a few that affect the brain. The most common ones are enterovirus, parechovirus, and rotavirus.

Herpes infection is most often acquired during delivery but can also be acquired after birth from a caregiver. Depending on where you live, chikungunya infection (the virus that causes dengue) can also affect the brain.

12.1.2.1 How Will I Know if My Baby Has Symptoms of a Postnatal Viral Infection?

The infection usually occurs at the end of the first week or during the second week after birth. There may be a skin rash, fever, diarrhea, and difficulties feeding, and the baby may be drowsy. It is also possible that the baby presents with seizures. After admission to the hospital, an ultrasound scan will be performed, and if the baby develops seizures, the clinician will also perform an MRI scan as this will give more detailed information. The white matter of the brain may show some changes that still can disappear after some time. But in rare cases, it will result in loss of brain tissue and cysts can develop.

12.1.2.2 Why Did My Baby Develop a Viral Infection?

It is likely that another member of the family or a visitor carried the virus and infected the baby. If the baby was in the hospital, this can also be somebody visiting or looking after your baby.

12.1.2.3 What Is the Treatment if My Baby Is Diagnosed with a Viral Infection?

For viral infections that occur after birth, there is no treatment, except for herpes (see above). The doctors and nurses will support the baby and treat the seizures. Usually, these viruses have a mild course and only give symptoms for a couple of days. Rarely enterovirus may affect the heart and this can be a serious complication.

12.1.2.4 What Will Happen to My Baby (Prognosis)?

Most infants will recover and will not develop any problems when they are seen in the clinic. In those with abnormalities on MRI and especially when cysts develop, the prognosis is a bit more guarded. Cerebral palsy is uncommon, but learning disabilities may become apparent after the first couple of years.

12.2 For Professionals

12.2.1 Congenital Infections

12.2.1.1 Incidence

Cytomegalovirus (*CMV*) is the most common cause of a congenital infection. The birth prevalence is threefold greater in low- and middle-income countries (LMIC) than in high-income countries (1.48% versus 0.48%) [1]. Transplacental passage of the virus occurs during pregnancy, and intrauterine transmission increases from 5% during the preconception period to 21% during the first trimester, 36.8% during the second trimester, and 66.2% in the third trimester, respectively [2]. However, severe sequelae mainly occur following an infection during the pre-conceptional period or the first trimester, when the brain is developing rapidly.

The second most common cause of congenital infection is *toxoplasmosis gondii*, an infection that occurs following transplacental transmission of the parasite. The incidence varies across different parts of the world. A recently reported incidence in the United States was 0.23 cases per 10.000 live births [3]. The fetus is more likely to become infected later in pregnancy, and 15% of infants will become infected after maternal seroconversion at 13 weeks, 44% at 26 weeks, and 71% at 37 weeks [4]. Similar to CMV, the fetus is more likely to be severely infected when infection takes place during the first trimester.

Due to the widespread use of *rubella* vaccination, the incidence of congenital rubella infection is very low, being one per million live births in high-income countries. However, in LMICs the incidence was still reported to be as high as 12 per 10,000 live births [5]. Infection that carries a high risk of sequelae usually takes place between the first and second month of gestation.

Varicella zoster infection is uncommon, and the so-called congenital varicella syndrome can follow maternal-fetal infection in the first 20 weeks of pregnancy. The estimated risk of developing the congenital varicella syndrome is estimated to be 0.5% following a maternal infection before 13 weeks gestation and 2% for infections between 13 and 20 weeks [6, 7]. Perinatally occurring varicella infection can also be seen and is due to a maternal-fetal infection within 21 days of delivery, but this is rarely associated with brain injury. When the mother develops a varicella infection beyond 36 weeks gestation, there is a risk of 25% of perinatal varicella infection.

Neonatal *herpes* simplex virus (HSV) infection develops most often following passage through an infected birth canal. Less often it can develop due to an ascending infection near the time of birth. It is even less common to develop a HSV infection following transplacental passage of the virus or due to postnatal acquisition of the virus from infected adults. The incidence of neonatal HSV infection varies from 6 to 60 per 100,000 live births [8]. Both HSV-1 and HSV-2 infections are seen, with HSV-1 being more common nowadays.

Parvovirus, HIV and COVID infections may also affect the brain, but are beyond the scope of this review.

12.2.1.2 CMV

Diagnosis As few as 10–15% of infected infants with congenital CMV will be symptomatic at birth. They often are growth retarded and have hepatosplenomegaly and thrombocytopenia. They can be microcephalic as well. When the diagnosis is suspected, neuroimaging needs to be performed to look for brain lesions. In some infants the diagnosis will be made during pregnancy (PCR in the amniotic fluid). After birth the PCR in the urine within 21 days after birth is the gold standard. A PCR can also be performed in saliva. When the diagnosis is suspected later in infancy, for instance, when the hearing test is abnormal, a PCR can be performed on a stored Guthrie test. Besides a hearing test, the ophthalmologist should check for the presence of chorioretinitis.

Neuroimaging Cranial ultrasound (cUS) is useful and will detect calcifications usually near the ventricular margins or lenticulostriate vasculopathy (LSV), ventriculomegaly, germinolytic cysts, occipital and temporal horn cysts or adhesions, and less often cysts in the periventricular white matter. cUS is not good in detecting cortical malformation (polymicrogyria, lissencephaly) and cerebellar hypoplasia, unless the mastoid view is used and the transcerebellar distance is actually measured. An MRI is therefore recommended in any infant who shows, even mild, cUS abnormalities (Figs. 12.1 and 12.2). To better appreciate the severity of the brain lesions, several scoring systems can be used, both before and after birth. The prenatal scoring system by Cannie et al. [9] is based on MRI, while the postnatal one by Alarcon et al. [10] uses cUS and MRI.

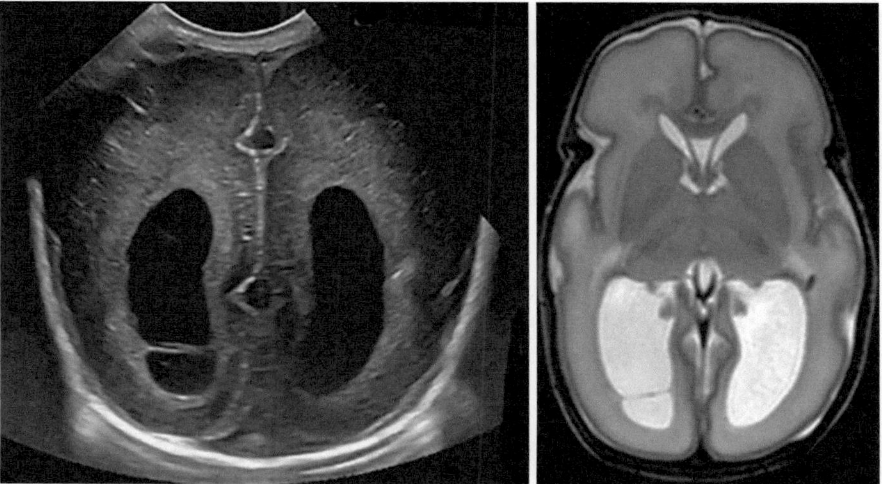

Fig. 12.1 Very preterm infant with congenital CMV infection. Cranial ultrasound, coronal view showing an occipital adhesion on the right side, confirmed with an MRI, T2-weighted sequence, axial plane, at 30 weeks' gestation

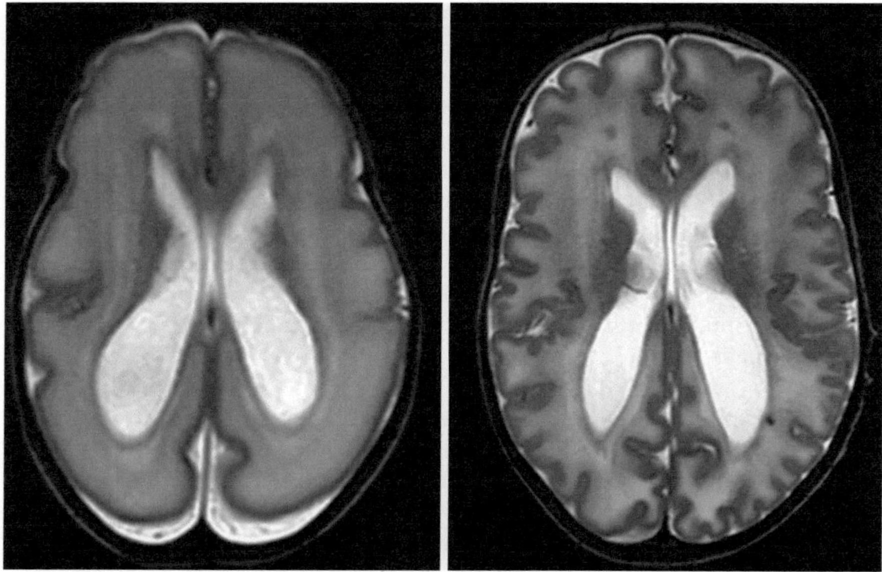

Fig. 12.2 Same infant, mid axial plane, at 30 and 40 weeks' gestation. Perisylvian polymicrogyria was suspected on the first MRI and confirmed on the TEA MRI. Also note mild ventriculomegaly and the increased signal intensity in the white matter, with a few punctate lesions (low signal intensity), best seen on the TEA MRI

12.2.1.3 Toxoplasmosis

Diagnosis Due to the increased use of antenatal treatment, the risk of a severe fetal infection has reduced considerably, and the majority of infants with a congenital infection are asymptomatic (74%). The most common finding is chorioretinitis, which was noted in 28/112 (26%) infants with a fetal infection. In this study, only one infant had severe neurological sequelae [11]. Sometimes a "systemic syndrome" can be seen with hepatosplenomegaly, hyperbilirubinemia, and anemia. These infants do not have overt neurological symptoms, but when an LP is performed, pleocytosis is seen in 85% confirming the presence of additional meningoencephalitis [12].

The diagnosis can be made just using PCR on the amniotic fluid and after birth on the CSF, but as the PCR in the CSF was only positive in 46% of those without and 70% of those with hydrocephalus, a combination of PCR and IgM and IgA antibodies is recommended [13].

Neuroimaging cUS will identify calcifications that are usually more peripheral to the ventricles than in CMV. Ventriculomegaly that can be severe and hyperechogenic nodules are also reported [14]. As these noduli can be located in the subcortical white matter, they can be missed with cUS, and MRI is recommended as well, especially to look at the cortex that may be abnormal overlying the noduli (Fig. 12.3).

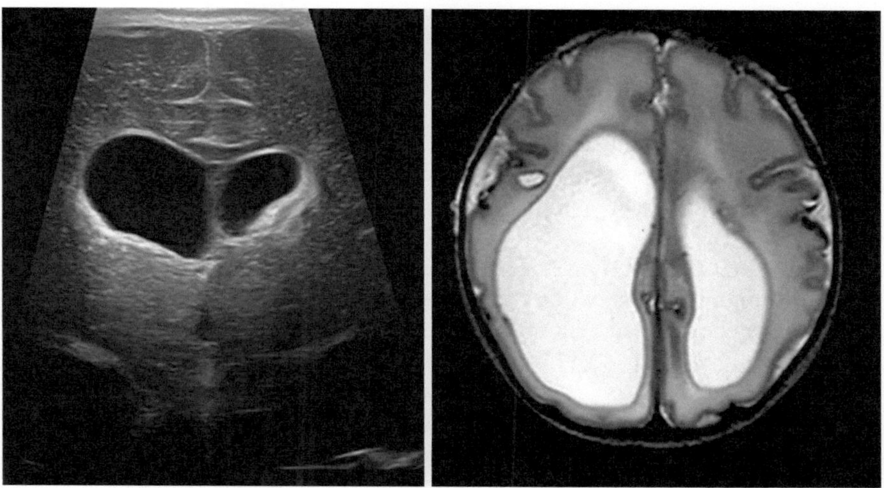

Fig. 12.3 Fetal diagnosis of toxoplasmosis infection. Postnatal cUS shows severe ventricular dilatation. The MRI, axial plane, T2-weighted sequence, additionally shows cysts in the subcortical white matter with abnormal overlying cortex

12.2.1.4 Rubella

Diagnosis Two thirds of infants with congenital rubella are asymptomatic at birth, but most will become symptomatic. Similar to CMV they may be growth retarded and have hepatosplenomegaly and thrombocytopenia. When the diagnosis is suspected, a cardiac echo should be performed as the infant often has a peripheral pulmonary stenosis and patent ductus arteriosus. The metaphyses of the long bones may show radiolucency. From the neurological perspective, the infant may have a full fontanel (25–50%) and is often irritable. Central cataracts can be seen on clinical assessment, and ophthalmoscopy will show chorioretinitis and the typical "salt and pepper" spotty hyperpigmentation of the retina. Microphthalmia may also be present. The diagnosis can be made by testing for IgM antibodies in blood from the umbilical cord or serum. IgM antibodies persist for 6–12 months [15].

Neuroimaging There is hardly any data reported in the literature. Temporal lobe cysts as well as LSV and subependymal cysts can be seen with cUS, while MRI will provide more detail about ischemic white matter lesions and delayed myelination [16].

12.2.1.5 Varicella

Diagnosis With congenital varicella syndrome, cutaneous scars can be seen in a segmental distribution, with a zigzag appearance. In severe cases hypoplastic limbs and muscles have been reported. Infants with perinatal varicella will have a vesicular rash, and there usually is a history of maternal infection. If the infant is born within 5 days of a maternal varicella infection, there will not have been time for transfer of maternal antibodies, and in case of a severe neonatal illness, the mortality rate is as high as 30% [17].

The diagnosis is usually considered based on maternal illness. Viral DNA in CSF using PCR has been reported and varicella-specific IgM in about half of the cases, as well as varicella-zoster antibodies.

Neuroimaging Brain lesions have not been reported, but ocular abnormalities are almost invariably present and vary from chorioretinitis to optic atrophy or cataracts. Outcome may be affected by limb hypoplasia.

12.2.1.6 HSV

Diagnosis Infants with HSV may present with localized or disseminated disease. The localized disease may be either restricted to the CNS or to the skin, eye, or mouth (SEM). SEM is most common (45%), followed by localized CNS disease (30%) and disseminated disease (25%). Disseminated disease presents at day 10–12 with lethargy and poor feeding, followed by stupor and seizures, with progression to coma and opisthotonic posturing. Multiple organs are affected, and in spite of antiviral therapy, mortality is still around 29% and long-term morbidity is seen in 17% [8, 18]. Symptoms in infants with CNS disease present day 16–19, and many infants (35%) do not have any skin lesions. CSF will show pleocytosis and elevated protein, and a PCR will confirm the diagnosis. Outcome is much better since the introduction of antiviral therapy, with a mortality of 4% but still a high rate of neurologic sequelae of 40% [8, 18]. Infants with SEM disease usually present day 10–12. If left untreated, progression to CNS or disseminated disease occurs in 75%. Following the introduction of antiviral therapy, the outcome is almost invariably favorable. Prompt *diagnosis* is of great importance, as timely treatment may prevent death and severe morbidity.

Diagnosis can be made using PCR in scrapings from a vesicular lesion in SEM disease and in CSF for those with disseminated or CNS disease.

Neuroimaging MRI is the preferred imaging technique, and especially DWI will help to identify ischemic lesions at an early stage. Three patterns of injury were reported: involvement of the inferior frontal/temporal lobe area, watershed areas, and corticospinal tracts [19] (Figs. 12.4 and 12.5).

12.2.1.7 Treatment

Antiviral medication is used in infants with *CMV* who are symptomatic and/or have CNS involvement. The medication, oral valganciclovir, used for 6 months, has been reported to prevent hearing loss, and in some studies even some improvement of hearing deficits occurred [20]. While medication is still mostly used after birth, there have been recent trials showing a positive effect of antenatal valaciclovir, but this is not yet standard of care [21].

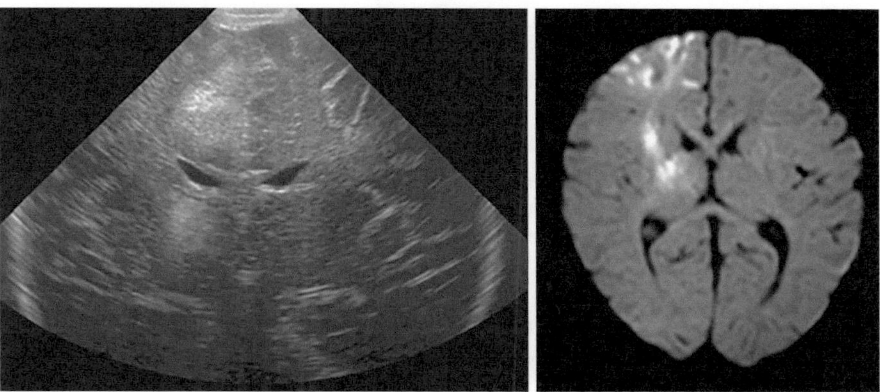

Fig. 12.4 Male term infant with herpes infection, echogenicity seen in the right frontal lobe and right thalamus, confirmed with DWI, with PLIC involvement

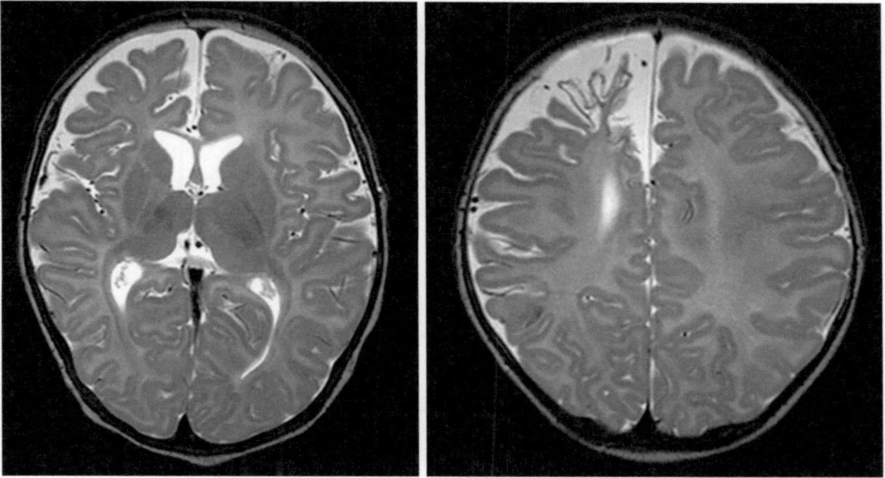

Fig. 12.5 A repeat MRI (T2-weighted sequence) shows atrophy and cystic evolution of the right frontal lobe, and asymmetry of myelination of the PLIC

In infections due to *toxoplasmosis* gondii, treatment of the maternal infection and affected fetus is important. After birth the infant will be treated as well. Spiramycin should be given within 3 weeks of seroconversion, for 1 week, followed by a combination of pyrimethamine plus sulfadiazine and folinic acid continued till the end of pregnancy. Following delivery, the infant should be treated during the first year [3].

If the infant is delivered less than 5 days after the onset of a maternal *varicella* infection, varicella zoster immune globulin should be given. If the infant shows signs of varicella infection and is severely affected, the infants should be isolated, and a course of iv acyclovir should be started. Treatment is not given to infants who acquired the infection during early pregnancy.

Antiviral therapy should be started in any infant where the diagnosis of *herpes* infection is suspected and before the diagnosis is confirmed. High-dose intravenous acyclovir is recommended. This high dose has reduced mortality and has also led to an improved outcome. After 21 days of iv therapy, oral medication is now continued till the infant reaches the age of 6 months. This has further improved neurodevelopmental outcome and reduced a relapse in those with SEM disease [22].

12.2.1.8 Prognosis

The prognosis of congenital *CMV* very much depends on time of onset of the infection and presence of brain lesions on neuro-imaging. Recent data suggest, that only an infection acquired during the first trimester will result in neurological sequelae [23]. Permanent sequelae are reported in 40–58% of those with symptomatic CMV, consisting of cognitive impairment, cerebral palsy, epilepsy, and sensorineural hearing loss. Performing cUS and MRI allows better prediction, and using a dedicated scoring system is recommended [10]. The presence of increased signal intensity on the T2-weighted sequence in the temporal lobe, the presence of cerebellar hypoplasia, and especially the presence of polymicrogyria are predictive of more severe sequelae. Of those who are asymptomatic at birth, 10–15% will develop sequelae, and this will mostly be sensorineural hearing loss [24].

The outcome varies widely following *toxoplasmosis* infection, and similar to CMV the outcome is related to the presence of neuroimaging abnormalities as well as neonatal symptoms. Infants who present with neurological symptoms or abnormal neuro-imaging findings (calcification, hydrocephalus) often have a poor outcome (50–90%), with cognitive impairment, cerebral palsy, and epilepsy [25, 26]. Most of these infants also have chorioretinitis, and this will result in severe visual impairment in 70%. In those presenting with systemic symptoms, only 10–50% will do poorly.

Data on the prognosis of congenital *varicella* infection are scarce. Following a varicella in the first 20 weeks of pregnancy, hydrocephalus, meningocele, and club-feet may be seen [6, 7].

Outcome following *herpes simplex* infection has improved with the use of early high-dose acyclovir therapy. An infection affecting the CNS carries a 4–6% mortality risk and a 55–80% risk to develop adverse sequelae, including cognitive impairment, cerebral palsy, and epilepsy. Disseminated herpes disease has a higher mortality rate (25–40%) but a better chance of a normal outcome (20–40% of survivors) [27]. Similar to the other viral infections, outcome is associated with neuroimaging findings.

12.2.2 Postnatally Acquired Infections

12.2.2.1 Incidence

The incidence reported for enterovirus and parechovirus encephalitis is 0.77/1000 and 0.04/1000 live births, respectively [28]. No population-based data have been reported for rotavirus encephalitis.

12.2.2.2 Diagnosis

The diagnosis should be suspected in an infant who develops symptoms at the end of the first week. There is often a family member with a mild illness, and the infant may present with feeding problems, rash, fever, diarrhea, and/or seizures. Rotavirus infection is often only considered in the presence of diarrhea, but this is present in only 20% of the cases. The infants tend to present on day 4–6 with seizures which have in the past been referred to as "fifth day fits." The diagnosis will be made by performing a PCR in the CSF for enterovirus and parechovirus infection. In rotavirus infection, despite the neurologic symptoms, the CSF-PCR is typically negative, and the stools should be sent for culture.

Neuroimaging cUS can detect increased white matter echogenicity, usually present on admission, in infants presenting with seizures. MRI, especially when using DWI within a week of presentation, will better delineate white matter abnormalities. Serial cUS and/or a repeat MRI will show whether these abnormalities evolve into cystic lesions, which is more common in the (late) preterm infant than in the full-term infant. The volume of white matter abnormalities, as seen with DWI, was significantly correlated to white matter volume loss on the second MRI performed at 3–4 months in a study of infants with a rotavirus infection (Fig. 12.6) [29, 30].

Treatment is supportive, with aEEG monitoring and controlling the seizures with antiseizure medication. Most infants are not very ill, but infants with an enterovirus infection may rarely develop a myocarditis, a severe complication, not uncommonly resulting in death or long-term cardiac morbidity [31].

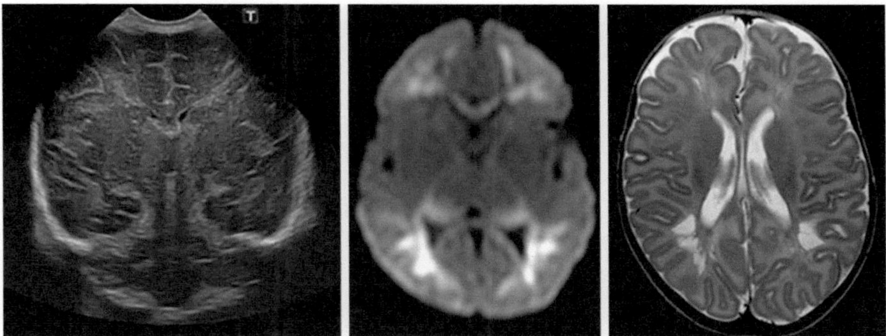

Fig. 12.6 Female infant, born at 35 weeks and admitted with seizures on day 16 and diagnosed with rotavirus encephalitis. cUS shows increased echogenicity of the white matter and thalami. The MRI-DWI shows restricted diffusion in the periventricular white matter as well as the pulvinar. A repeat MRI 6 weeks later shows cystic evolution. The child did not develop cerebral palsy, but has cognitive impairment

12.2.2.3 Prognosis

The prognosis for the postnatally acquired viral infections is considerably better compared to the congenitally acquired infections. Once again, outcome depends on involvement of the CNS, and this will most often consist of white matter damage that is clearly seen with DWI. As is to be expected, outcome is better for those without cystic evolution of the (early) white matter abnormalities. Long-term data are emerging, especially for parechovirus and rotavirus infection, and show once more that children should be followed into school age, as cognitive problems only become apparent by then [29, 30, 32].

12.3 Case

This infant was born at 36 weeks' gestation and admitted for observation of blood sugar levels and feeding and discharged home after 4 days. At day 16 the infant became ill, had feeding problems and a subfebrile temperature, and was readmitted with a suspected sepsis. Treatment with broad-spectrum antibiotics and acyclovir was started.

Blood count, glucose, sodium, calcium, and magnesium levels and liver function were all normal.

The day after readmission, the infant developed clinical seizures and was transferred to the neonatal intensive care unit for aEEG monitoring and treatment. The seizures were confirmed electrographically, and a total of three doses of phenobarbital were needed to achieve seizure control.

A lumbar puncture was performed which showed a normal cell count and glucose level. All bacterial cultures (blood, CSF, and urine) remained sterile but the PCR on plasma and CSF were positive for enterovirus (human echovirus 16).

Cranial ultrasound was performed on admission and showed increased periventricular echogenicity, most pronounced in the frontal areas, and mild echogenicity of the thalami (Fig. 12.7).

The child was followed in the outpatient clinic until the age of 7 years and has a normal motor and cognitive development and good verbal skills but shows some difficulties in attention and concentration, problem solving and working memory. He is now almost 9 years old and is attending regular education.

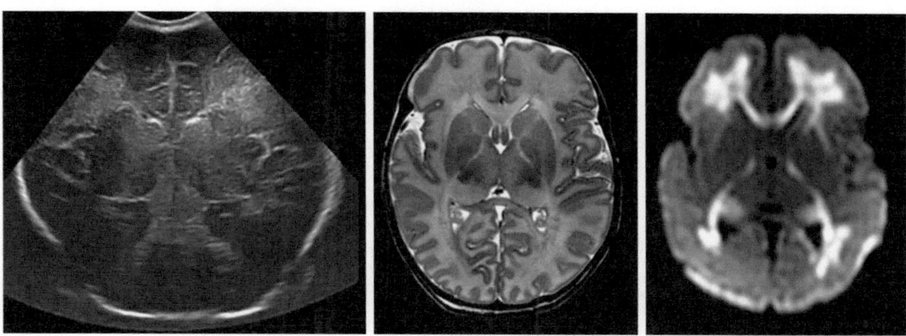

Fig. 12.7 Cranial ultrasound (left) performed on admission, shows increased echogenicity in the periventricular white matter. The MRI, performed 4 days later, shows increased signal intensity in the white matter, corpus callosum, and pulvinar on the T2-weighted sequence (middle). Diffusion weighted MRI showed restricted diffusion in the periventricular white matter, corpus callosum, optic radiations, posterior limb of internal capsule, and posterior part of the thalami (pulvinar) (right)

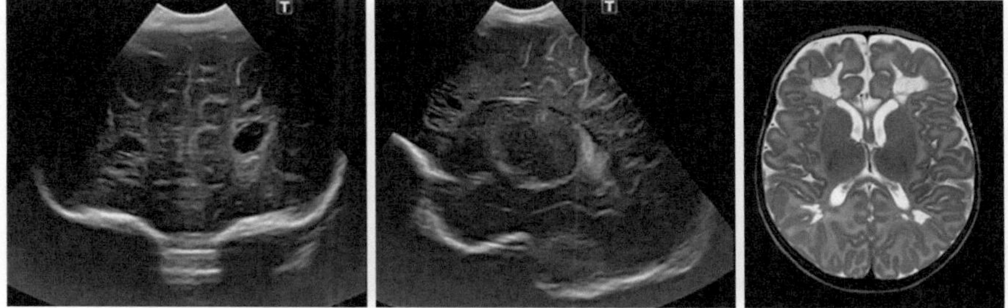

Fig. 12.8 The follow-up cranial ultrasound (left, middle) 1 month later showed cystic evolution, again most prominent in the frontal white matter. This was confirmed on MRI, axial T2 sequence (right) after 1 month which additionally showed also cyst formation in the occipital white matter (Fig. 12.8)

References

1. Ssentongo P, Hehnly C, Birungi P, et al. Congenital cytomegalovirus infection burden and epidemiologic risk factors in countries with universal screening: a systematic review and meta-analysis. JAMA Netw Open. 2021;4:e2120736.
2. Chatzakis C, Ville Y, Makrydimas G, et al. Timing of primary maternal cytomegalovirus infection and rates of vertical transmission and fetal consequences. Am J Obstet Gynecol. 2020;223:870–83.e11
3. Khalil A, Sotiriadis A, Chaoui R, et al. ISUOG Practice Guidelines: role of ultrasound in congenital infection. Ultrasound Obstet Gynecol. 2020;56:128–51.
4. Dunn D, Wallon M, Peyron F, et al. Mother-to-child transmission of toxoplasmosis: risk estimates for clinical counselling. Lancet. 1999;353:1829–33.
5. Bloom S, Rguig A, Berraho A, et al. Congenital rubella syndrome burden in Morocco: a rapid retrospective assessment. Lancet. 2005;365:135–41.
6. Pastuszak AL, Levy M, Schick B, et al. Outcome after maternal varicella infection in the first 20 weeks of pregnancy. N Engl J Med. 1994;330(13):901–5.
7. Trotta M, Borchi B, Niccolai A, et al. Epidemiology, management and outcome of varicella in pregnancy: a 20-year experience at the Tuscany Reference Centre for Infectious Diseases in Pregnancy. Infection. 2018;46(5):693–9.
8. Corey L, Wald A. Maternal and neonatal herpes simplex virus infections. N Engl J Med. 2009;361:1376–85.
9. Cannie MM, Devlieger R, Leyder M, et al. Congenital cytomegalovirus infection: contribution and best timing of prenatal MR imaging. Eur Radiol. 2016;26(10):3760–9.
10. Alarcon A, Martinez-Biarge M, Cabanas F, et al. A prognostic neonatal neuroimaging scale for symptomatic congenital cytomegalovirus infection. Neonatology. 2016;110:277–85.
11. Xu F, Markowitz LE, Gottlieb SL, Berman SM. Seroprevalence of herpes simplex virus types 1 and 2 in pregnant women in the United States. Am J Obstet Gynecol. 2007;196:43.e1-6.
12. MacDonald MG, Seshia MMK. Avery's neonatology: pathophysiology and management of the newborn. 7th ed. Philadelphia: Wolters Kluwer; 2016.
13. Olariu TR, Remington JS, Montoya JG. Polymerase chain reaction in cerebrospinal fluid for the diagnosis of congenital toxoplasmosis. Pediatr Infect Dis J. 2014;33:566–70.
14. Dhombres F, Friszer S, Maurice P, et al. Prognosis of fetal parenchymal cerebral lesions without ventriculomegaly in congenital toxoplasmosis infection. Fetal Diagn Ther. 2017;41:8–14.
15. McLean HQ, Redd S, Abernathy E, et al. Congenital rubella syndrome. In: Roush SW, Baldy LM, editors. Manual for the surveillance of vaccine-preventable diseases. Atlanta GA: Centers for Disease Control and Prevention; 2014.
16. Sawlani V, Shankar JJ, White C. Magnetic resonance imaging findings in a case of congenital rubella encephalitis. Can J Infect Dis Med Microbiol. 2013;24(4):e122–e3.
17. Mandelbrot L. Fetal varicella—diagnosis, management, and outcome. Prenat Diagn. 2012;32:511–8.
18. Kimberlin DW. Herpes simplex virus infections in neonates and early childhood. Semin Pediatr Infect Dis. 2005;16:271–81.
19. Kidokoro H, Neil JJ, Inder TE. New MR imaging assessment tool to define brain abnormalities in very preterm infants at term. AJNR Am J Neuroradiol. 2013;34(11):2208–14.
20. Jones CE, Bailey H, Bamford A, Calvert A, Dorey RB, Drysdale SB, Khalil A, Heath PT, Lyall H, Ralph KMI, Sapuan S, Vandrevala T, Walter S, Whittaker E, Wood S, UK Congenital CMV Infection Collaboration (UKCCIC). Managing challenges in congenital CMV: current thinking. Arch Dis Child. 2022.:archdischild-2022-323809; https://doi.org/10.1136/archdischild-2022-323809.
21. Shahar-Nissan K, Pardo J, Peled O, et al. Valaciclovir to prevent vertical transmission of cytomegalovirus after maternal primary infection during pregnancy: a randomised, double-blind, placebo-controlled trial. Lancet. 2020;396:779–85.

22. Kimberlin DW, Whitley RJ, Wan W, et al. Oral acyclovir suppression and neurodevelopment after neonatal herpes. N Engl J Med. 2011;365:1284–92.
23. Leruez-Ville M, Foulon I, Pass R, Ville Y. Cytomegalovirus infection during pregnancy: state of the science. Am J Obstet Gynecol. 2020;223:330–49.
24. Dollard SC, Grosse SD, Ross DS. New estimates of the prevalence of neurological and sensory sequelae and mortality associated with congenital cytomegalovirus infection. Rev Med Virol. 2007;17:355–63.
25. Berrebi A, Assouline C, Bessieres MH, et al. Long-term outcome of children with congenital toxoplasmosis. Am J Obstet Gynecol. 2010;203(552):e1–6.
26. Auriti C, Bucci S, Umberto De Rose D, et al. Maternal-fetal infections (cytomegalovirus, *toxoplasma*, syphilis): short-term and long-term neurodevelopmental outcomes in children infected and uninfected at birth. Pathogens. 2022;11(11):1278.
27. Melvin AJ, Mohan KM, Vora SB, et al. Neonatal herpes simplex virus infection: epidemiology and outcomes in the modern era. J Pediatric Infect Dis Soc. 2022;11(3):94–101.
28. Kadambari S, Okike I, Ribeiro S, et al. Seven-fold increase in viral meningo-encephalitis reports in England and Wales during 2004–2013. J Infect. 2014;69:326–32.
29. Lee KY, Weon YC, Choi SH, Oh KW, Park H. Neurodevelopmental outcomes in newborns with neonatal seizures caused by rotavirus-associated leukoencephalopathy. Seizure. 2018a;56:14–8.
30. Lee KY, Weon YC, Choi SH, et al. Neurodevelopmental outcomes in newborns with neonatal seizures caused by rotavirus-associated leukoencephalopathy. Seizure. 2018b;56:14–9.
31. Cortina G, Best D, Deisenberg M, et al. Extracorporeal membrane oxygenation for neonatal collapse caused by enterovirus myocarditis. Arch Dis Child Fetal Neonatal Ed. 2018;103:F370–6.
32. van Hinsbergh TMT, Elbers RG, Hans Ket JCF, et al. Neurological and neurodevelopmental outcomes after human parechovirus CNS infection in neonates and young children: a systematic review and meta-analysis. Lancet Child Adolesc Health. 2020;4:592–605.

Bacterial and Fungal Infections

13

Sylke J. Steggerda and Linda S. de Vries

Abbreviations

CNS   Central nervous system
CSF   Cerebrospinal fluid
cUS   Cranial ultrasound
E. coli   *Escherichia coli*
GBS   Group B streptococcus
LP   Lumbar puncture

S. J. Steggerda (✉)
Department of Pediatrics, Division of Neonatology, Willem-Alexander Children's Hospital,
Leiden University Medical Center (LUMC), Leiden, The Netherlands
e-mail: S.J.Steggerda@lumc.nl

L. S. de Vries
Department of Pediatrics, Division of Neonatology, Willem-Alexander Children's Hospital,
Leiden University Medical Center (LUMC), Leiden, The Netherlands

Department of Neonatology, University Medical Center Utrecht (UMCU), Utrecht,
The Netherlands

© The Author(s) 2024
G. Meijler, K. Mohammad (eds.), *Neonatal Brain Injury*,
https://doi.org/10.1007/978-3-031-55972-3_13

13.1   For Parents

13.1.1 Introduction

Infections in and around the brain (often called the central nervous system (CNS)) in newborn babies are serious and potentially life-threatening. Here we discuss infections caused by bacteria and fungi. Babies are particularly vulnerable to CNS infections because their immune system (the system in the body that helps to prevent and fight infections) is not fully mature. Usually the infection affects the membranes (meninges) covering the brain surface, and this is called meningitis. However, bacteria and fungi can spread throughout the fluid passages of the brain causing hydrocephalus (dilated fluid compartments within the brain) and also enter the brain tissue either from this fluid or the blood coming to the brain, causing damage from abscesses (localized areas of infection) or affecting the blood flow to the brain tissue. It is important that infections in and around the brain are recognized and treated early as they may lead to rapid worsening of illness, permanent brain damage, and even death.

13.1.2 Why Did My Baby Develop a Bacterial or Fungal Infection?

CNS infections can be caused by several bacteria or fungi. The commonest bacteria are *group B streptococcus (GBS)* and *Escherichia coli (E. coli)*. The baby is usually infected during delivery or shortly after birth. Often the bacteria first enter the baby's bloodstream, causing infection (called septicemia or sepsis), and from there spread to the brain. When this happens within the first 3 days after birth, this is called an early-onset sepsis/meningitis.

Some babies only become ill later, although the bacteria were already transmitted to the baby at birth. Or they acquire the infection later, through contact with caregivers or visitors, or because they have other risk factors making them susceptible to developing an infection. This is called late-onset sepsis/meningitis. Preterm and sick newborn babies who need treatment in a neonatal intensive care unit have an increased risk of developing late-onset infections.

A severe fungal infection (meaning a fungal infection of the blood, brain, or urinary tract) is rare in newborn babies, but extremely preterm and/or low-birth-weight infants are especially vulnerable to this type of infection. This is due to a combination of risk factors including their immature immune system and impaired barriers to infection, e.g., thin and vulnerable skin, and other factors that are present when these babies are in the neonatal intensive care unit.

13.1.3 How Will I Know if My Baby Has Symptoms of a CNS Infection?

Bacterial and fungal CNS infections can present with various symptoms including an unstable temperature (either low temperature or fever), lethargy (the baby is very sleepy and/or does not wake up for feeding), or irritability and crying a lot. Other signs are a full fontanel (when the soft spot on the top of the head feels rounded rather than mostly flat), pale color, breathing problems, and seizures. It is important to realize that not all of these symptoms may occur and that these symptoms can also be seen in other conditions, so CNS infections can be suspected when they are not actually present. But if a CNS infection is present, the symptoms can become rapidly worse. Therefore, in a sick newborn baby with, for example, temperature instability, lethargy, or breathing problems, it is important to consult a children's healthcare professional for a prompt examination.

13.1.4 Diagnosis

The diagnosis of a CNS infection involves a combination of clinical examination, laboratory tests, and imaging of the brain. The blood will be examined for signs of infection, and additional blood will be taken, and a lumbar puncture (spinal tap) will be done to see if any infection can be grown in the laboratory from the blood or spinal fluid (cerebrospinal fluid (CSF)) around the brain. With a spinal tap, a small amount of CSF is obtained through a thin needle that is gently inserted into the lower back of the baby. Examining the CSF is important as it can help to exclude or confirm a CNS infection, and when bacteria are found, it can help to choose the best antibiotics.

As explained earlier, CNS infections can lead to further complications and brain damage; therefore, most babies will also have imaging of the brain. The first and most commonly used way to do this is with cranial ultrasound (cUS). This is performed at the bedside and is very helpful in detecting abnormalities already present; it is then repeated to detect any later occurring problems and complications. If abnormalities are seen on the cUS scan or when the baby is very ill or has neurologic symptoms like seizures, an MRI scan can be performed as well though this involves moving the baby to the scanner. An MRI scan is more sensitive for detecting smaller lesions and abnormalities in areas of the brain that are difficult to examine with cUS. Also, the MRI scan can provide more detailed information about the severity and specific location of abnormalities, and this helps to determine the prognosis (likely future problems).

Babies with a CNS infection are at risk for developing seizures, especially in the acute period of infection. Therefore, when seizures are suspected, or when the baby is very ill, additional monitoring of brain activity with (a)EEG should be performed.

13.1.5 What Is the Treatment if My Baby Is Diagnosed with a CNS Infection?

Early recognition and adequate treatment are crucial in newborns with CNS infection as explained earlier. Therefore, when an infection is suspected and as soon as the appropriate tests are done, intravenous antibiotics will be started, rather than waiting for the results. If the cultures show particular bacteria, this can help to determine which antibiotics would be best to use, and thereafter the initial treatments may be changed. Getting results from the culture usually takes 24–48 h. The length of treatment depends on the type of bacteria found but will be at least 14–21 days. If a severe fungal infection is suspected, intravenous antifungal treatment will be started. As the babies can be very ill, they may require additional care such as help with breathing and nutrition and also medicines to control fluid balance, blood pressure, and seizures.

13.1.6 What Are the Complications and What Will Happen to My Baby (Prognosis)?

Different bacteria can cause different types of brain injury. In some cases, CNS infections can impede the normal flow of CSF and lead to hydrocephalus (dilated fluid compartments within the brain). When this is progressive, an additional treatment to decrease the pressure on the brain may be necessary. When babies are at risk for developing this complication, they should be closely monitored with follow-up cUS examinations.

In other cases, a brain abscess may develop. This is rare, but when it occurs it is more difficult to treat and may require drainage and longer antibiotic therapy. In the rare event of a severe fungal infection, the fungus may spread through the brain tissue to form tiny abscesses. This also requires long treatment with antifungal medication.

Both bacterial and fungal CNS infections can lead to brain injury and, depending on the severity, this may lead to difficulties with development in the future. This includes learning difficulties, motor (movement) problems, behavioral problems, visual impairments, and epilepsy (later seizures) depending on the site and extent of injury. Bacterial CNS infection can also cause hearing loss. Not all babies with a CNS infection will develop these problems; however, when they do early recognition and adequate intervention are important to support the child's further development. Therefore, newborn babies with proven CNS infection need to be included in follow-up programs with regular investigation of developmental milestones and hearing tests and access to early interventions such as physiotherapy, occupational therapy, and speech therapy.

13.2   For Professionals

13.2.1 Incidence

CNS infections in the newborn infant are of major clinical importance as they carry a high risk of mortality and long-term morbidities. Several types of organisms can be involved, including bacteria, viruses, and fungi (see also Chap. 12; viral infection). Bacterial CNS infection occurs in approximately 0.3/1000 newborns (<1 month old) [1]. This age group is more vulnerable to this type of infection than older infants, even in the era of GBS prophylaxis. Preterm infants are especially at risk.

Group B streptococcus (GBS; *Streptococcus agalactiae*) is the most commonly isolated organism in newborns with early onset infection. It is mostly seen in term infants and accounts for approximately 30–50% of all the cases of neonatal sepsis and meningitis, followed by ***Escherichia coli*** (*E. coli*) which accounts for approximately 25–35% of cases and has a higher prevalence in preterm infants and cases with late-onset infection [1–7]. Other gram-negative Enterobacteriaceae, including ***Enterobacter species, Pseudomonas aeruginosa***, ***Klebsiella***, ***Proteus***, and ***Serratia species***, can also cause neonatal meningitis; together they account for approximately 10–20% of cases. Finally, gram-positive rods such as ***Listeria monocytogenes*** and ***Bacillus cereus*** are rare but also important causative microorganisms as they carry a high risk of mortality and severe long-term impairments.

In bacterial meningitis the microorganism usually first enters the bloodstream, causing bacteremia, and then spreads to the brain and infiltrates the arachnoid membrane and space and the meninges covering the brain surface, thereby causing arachnoiditis and meningitis. However, not all cases with meningitis have a positive blood culture. In one series of 9461 very low-birth-weight infants, one third of those with meningitis did not have a positive blood culture [8]. In meningitis, bacteria can further spread throughout the cerebrospinal fluid (CSF) compartments of the brain, and this may lead to choroid plexitis, ventriculitis, intraventricular adhesions, subdural effusion, empyema, and hydrocephalus. Bacteria can also invade the brain tissue and cause vasculitis, leading to ischemic brain lesions (most commonly in GBS infection), liquefaction necrosis, and brain abscesses (most commonly gram-negative microorganisms and ***Staphylococcus aureus***) [9]. A neonatal brain abscess usually occurs as a complication of bacterial meningitis; however several cases of brain abscesses without meningitis have also been reported. In these cases the organism was cultured only by direct puncture of the abscess [10–12].

Most of the invasive fungal infections in newborns are caused by ***Candida albicans*** but also other Candida species like ***Candida parapsilosis***, ***Candida glabrata***, and ***Candida krusei*** may be involved. Disseminated fungal infection can affect the urinary tract but also the brain where it leads to meningitis, often in combination with micro abscesses. Invasive fungal infections are less common than bacterial infections and mainly occur in extremely preterm and/or low-birth-weight infants, due to a combination of an immature immune system and risk factors that impair their natural barrier. The incidence varies considerably between neonatal units and patient populations, from 0.5% to 20%. Recent studies show a decrease in incidences, likely due to the use of fluconazole or nystatin prophylaxis and decreased use of broad-spectrum antibiotics and indwelling venous catheters [13–16].

13.2.2 Presentation

As in neonatal sepsis, meningitis can be distinguished into two types of presentation based on the postnatal age at onset of illness: early onset infection (occurring within the first 72 hours after birth) and late-onset infection.

In the majority of cases with an **early-onset infection**, the newborn is exposed to the bacteria, most commonly GBS or *E. coli*, around the time of delivery (vertical transmission). Risk factors include prolonged rupture of membranes and/or signs of maternal peripartum infection, for example chorioamnionitis or infection of the urinary tract. However, asymptomatic women may also be colonized with GBS in their urinary or genital tract and subsequently colonize the newborn during delivery. In a single-center historical cohort study in the USA, investigating more than 60,000 deliveries between 2003 and 2015, 21.6% of the population was GBS colonized, and this led to invasive GBS disease in 0.1% of their offspring [17].

Typically, newborns with early-onset infection, regardless of the bacterial agent, have signs of systemic illness with temperature instability, respiratory distress, apnea, and feeding problems and can deteriorate rapidly into septic shock with respiratory and circulatory failure. Neurological symptoms are usually less prominent.

An exception is early onset infection with *Listeria monocytogenes* where infection can be the result of transplacental passage days to weeks before delivery. In these cases the infection can be caused by maternal ingestion of contaminated food products such as raw cheese, undercooked meat, and smoked seafood. The mother can experience some flu-like or gastro-intestinal symptoms but is usually not very ill. However, when the infection is transmitted to the fetus or newborn, this can result in a severe infection leading to fetal loss in approximately 25% of cases, preterm birth, and a fulminating infection in the newborn called neonatal listeriosis. Due to the infection, the newborn can develop necrotizing miliary granuloma in many organs including the brain. Treatment of the mother early in the course of her infection can prevent infection and sequelae in the fetus and newborn [18–20].

Late-onset infection in the neonate usually occurs after the first postnatal week. These infections may still be due to colonization around the time of birth (due to the same organisms that are involved in early onset infection), but more often other factors play a role, including transmission from caregivers (horizontal transmission) and hospital-acquired infection, for example, through indwelling catheters and other devices. So where maternal factors primarily influence the risk of early-onset infection, late-onset infections are often mediated by neonatal risk factors such as prematurity, low birth weight, and other neonatal complications requiring intensive care treatment, including central venous catheters and/or other invasive procedures [21]. In these cases other microorganisms can play a role, mainly gram-positive bacteria such as coagulase-negative staphylococci and *Staphylococcus aureus*, but also *E. coli*, *Klebsiella*, other gram-negative Enterobacteriaceae, and *Bacillus cereus* can be involved [22]. In newborns with late-onset meningitis, neurological symptoms are much more common than in early-onset infection and include irritability, impaired consciousness, a bulging fontanel, and either focal or generalized seizures.

Most of the invasive fungal infections in preterm infants are also of late-onset and occur between 2 and 6 weeks after birth; an exception is congenital candidiasis which is extremely rare. It is caused by a maternal intrauterine candida infection and manifests with symptoms within the first week. Risk factors for invasive fungal infection include the immature innate and adaptive immune response of preterm infants, disruption of epithelial barriers including the use of central venous catheters, and increased colonization rates due to the use of prolonged broad-spectrum antibiotics, parenteral feeding, and corticosteroids [15]. These infections have a high risk of CNS involvement; in previous studies this was reported in approximately 10–25% of the cases [7]. The symptoms are similar to the ones described for bacterial infections and include apnea, temperature instability, lethargy, hypotension, an elevated white blood cell count, and hyperglycemia (below).

13.2.3 Diagnosis

The diagnosis of newborn CNS infection involves a combination of clinical examination, laboratory tests, and imaging of the brain. However, apart from the cases with late-onset sepsis who may present with clear neurologic symptoms, clinical signs are usually non-specific. Therefore, when sepsis is suspected, the possibility of meningitis should always be considered, and appropriate diagnostic tests need to be performed.

Blood laboratory tests that can support the presence of neonatal CNS infection are similar to those performed in suspected sepsis and include a blood culture, white blood cell and neutrophil count, and other inflammatory markers such as C-reactive protein. However, in the initial phase of an infection, these markers may still be within the normal reference values and cannot be used to rule out an infection. Moreover, some newborns with meningitis may have a negative blood culture [8, 23, 24]. Examination and culture of CSF taken by a lumbar puncture (LP) are therefore the gold standard and crucial to either confirm or rule out meningitis and should also be considered in those with (suspected) early onset sepsis who do not present with neurologic symptoms. In bacterial meningitis CSF analysis will often show an elevated white blood cell and neutrophil count, an elevated protein level, and a low glucose level as compared to plasma glucose level. The interpretation of CSF findings can be challenging, and reference values for CSF parameters in newborns should be used; these are different from those in older children and adults and also vary according to post-menstrual age [25–27].

CSF culture is important to determine the causative microorganism and is especially sensitive in newborns who have not yet received antibiotic treatment. Therefore, a LP should be performed preferably before and otherwise soon after antibiotic therapy is initiated. Results are usually available within 48 hours and can also provide information on the antibiotic susceptibility of a cultured microorganism. Meanwhile, gram-stained smears may also be helpful to identify microorganisms.

When a LP cannot be performed due to clinical instability at presentation and needs to be delayed until after the initiation of antibiotic therapy, the culture will usually be negative, and the diagnosis needs to be made based upon other findings such as abnormal CSF parameters in combination with a positive blood culture and/or abnormal neuroimaging findings (see below) [28, 29].

A repeated LP after 48–72 h of treatment to confirm CSF sterilization is generally not recommended for newborns with good clinical recovery, and there is also no agreement about performing a repeat CSF examination 48 h after discontinuation of antibiotic therapy. However, in complicated cases and in cases with *E. coli* meningitis where relapse has been reported more frequently, repeat CSF examination may be considered to document the effectiveness of antibiotic treatment and guide treatment duration. In one study, in three of four cases with *E. coli* meningitis who relapsed, a repeat LP was performed which showed persistent bacterial growth in the CSF 1–3 days after initiation of antibiotics. In none of these cases was another LP repeated later during their course to ensure sterilization of the CSF [30]. In another study of 111 infants with neonatal meningitis, a repeat LP was performed significantly more often (p = 0.001) in infants with gram-negative organisms, with a median LP on day 5 [31]. In these infants, the white blood cell count on the second but not the first CSF sample was predictive of adverse outcomes at the time of discharge from the hospital.

It is important to be aware that infants with candida meningitis can have a negative blood culture and a normal gram stain and cell count of the CSF and that even CSF cultures may only intermittently be positive [15, 23, 24]. Therefore repeated CSF cultures may be necessary, especially in those infants who show the typical signs of infection on neuroimaging but who have normal CSF findings.

In addition to blood, CSF, and urine cultures, abdominal ultrasound to evaluate renal and hepatic involvement and an eye examination should be done in all infants with invasive candidiasis to search for other sites of invasive infection.

13.2.4 Neuroimaging

Cranial ultrasound (cUS) and MRI are the preferred neuroimaging techniques in the evaluation of a newborn with CNS infection. The different neuropathological changes in meningitis can result in different imaging features (see also Table 13.1 and Fig. 13.1).

Table 13.1 Neuropathological features of neonatal bacterial meningitis and imaging appearance

Choroid plexitis and ventriculitis (a–c)
Ventricular lining, intraventricular adhesions and debris, secondary impaired CSF flow and hydrocephalus
Arachnoiditis and leptomeningitis (d–f)
Exudate and extracerebral effusion, empyema, secondary impaired CSF flow and hydrocephalus
Vasculitis with infarction (g–i) and (j–l)
Perforator stroke in deep gray matter, cortical (pial artery) stroke (g–i)
Hemorrhagic/liquefactive necrosis with or without secondary abscess formation (j–l)
Micro abscess formation (m–o)

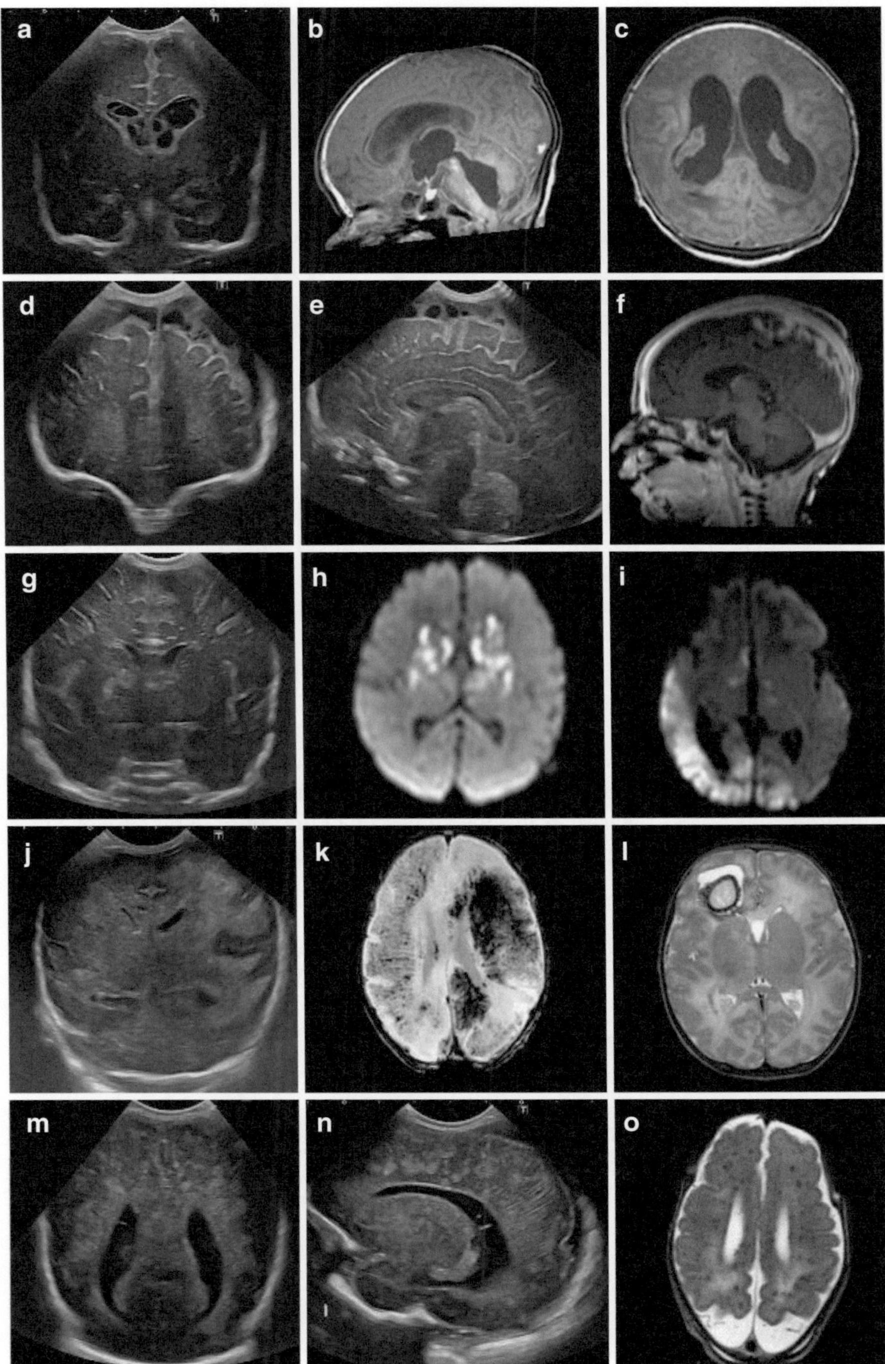

Fig. 13.1 Major neuropathological features in neonatal bacterial meningitis (Table 13.1) and their imaging appearance. (**a–c**) *E. coli* meningitis; (**d–f**) and (**g-i**) group B streptococcal meningitis; (**j, k**) Enterobacteriaceae meningitis; (**l**) *Bacillus cereus*; (**m–o**) *Candida albicans* meningo-encephalitis

As both cUS and MRI have advantages and disadvantages, they are considered complementary.

cUS is the preferred technique for the initial evaluation (see Chap. 14).

The major imaging features of bacterial CNS infection can be depicted by cUS [32, 33]. These include acute findings such as brain swelling and edema with slit-like ventricles and compression of the extracerebral space, ventriculitis, and inflammation of the choroid plexus with echogenic lining of the ventricular ependyma and intraventricular adhesions, stroke-like parenchymal lesions in GBS meningitis, brain abscess and hemorrhagic necrosis in gram-negative meningitis, and micro abscesses in invasive fungal infections. Chronic findings in neonatal meningitis can also be detected by cUS and include tissue loss and atrophy as well as hydrocephalus due to problems with CSF flow.

MRI is more of a burden than cUS for the sick and unstable newborn as it requires transportation to the scanner and it does not allow for frequent and serial imaging. However, it can be difficult to assess the full extent of brain injury by cUS alone. MRI can depict brain lesions in more detail, show their full extent, and also help to visualize areas of the brain that are difficult to assess with cUS such as cortical/subcortical areas at the brain convexity, the extra-cerebral spaces, and the posterior fossa (see Chap. 15) [34–36]. Therefore, every neonate with complicated meningitis (i.e., with neurologic symptoms like seizures and/or with cUS abnormalities) should undergo at least one MRI scan.

Another advantage of early MRI is that it enables the use of diffusion-weighted sequences (DWI). When used within the first week after the onset of illness, DWI is sensitive for the detection of ischemic lesions, for example, stroke-like lesions in GBS, and may also show restricted diffusion in the cortico-spinal tract, although the relation between involvement of the motor pathway and motor outcome in cases with infection is less clear than in other types of brain injury, e.g., stroke. Since newborns and in particular preterm infants have significantly lower glomerular filtration and renal clearance rates than older children and adults, the biologic half-life of MRI contrast agents is prolonged. This may lead to increased exposure of contrast agents like gadolinium in this subgroup, and therefore routine use of contrast enhanced imaging is generally not recommended. As DWI is also helpful in detecting enhancement in cases with brain abscess and/or empyema, it often makes contrast-enhanced imaging redundant [37, 38].

13.2.5 Microorganism

Different microorganisms involved in bacterial CNS infection in the newborn can present with distinctive neuroimaging patterns (Table 13.2). Knowledge of these patterns can support early recognition and treatment. We will therefore discuss the most important patterns below:

Table 13.2 Different microorganisms involved in neonatal bacterial and fungal meningitis and their characteristic brain injury patterns

Microorganism	Neuroimaging pattern
Group B streptococcus	**Stroke-like pattern**, asymmetric distribution – Deep perforator stroke in basal ganglia and/or thalami – Cortical infarctions Can also lead to ventriculitis and hydrocephalus
E. coli	Ventriculitis, adhesions, (late) **hydrocephalus**, isolated segments of the ventricular system, trapped fourth ventricle
Other gram-negative enteric bacteria (including Citrobacter, Serratia, Proteus species)	Severe **hemorrhagic necrosis**, affecting frontal lobes but also often very rapidly spreading to other brain regions, in an asymmetric distribution. Leads to severe destruction of brain tissue Increased risk of **abscess formation**
Listeria monocytogenes	Associated with **green amniotic fluid and preterm birth**. Intraventricular hemorrhage and white matter injury common. Can also lead to small granulomatous lesions in many organs including the brain
Bacillus cereus	**Liquefactive necrosis** in the periventricular and subcortical white matter with an irregular border, usually with an asymmetrical distribution. Followed by cystic degeneration
Candida species	Diffuse **micro abscesses** within the periventricular and subcortical white matter, deep gray matter, cerebellum, and brainstem, sometimes followed by central cystic degeneration and/or glial scarring. May also evolve into macro abscesses and/or cause late hydrocephalus

13.2.5.1 Group B Streptococcus (GBS)

Despite the use of antibiotic prophylaxis, which has led to a decline in incidence of early onset neonatal GBS sepsis and meningitis, GBS is still the most common cause of bacterial CNS infections in newborns [1, 3, 39].

In newborns, GBS meningitis can lead to several neuroimaging abnormalities including edema, ventriculitis, and hydrocephalus. The most distinctive feature is that of arterial involvement and focal ischemic brain infarction. Two patterns of infarction are seen in GBS: (1) perforator strokes in the territories of the lenticulo-striate and thalamostriate arteries affecting the basal ganglia and thalami (see Chap. 9 focal arterial infarction and lobar hemorrhage); (2) patchy focal cortical infarction(s). Abnormalities are often bilateral but can have an asymmetric distribution, and deep gray matter and superficial cortical patterns can also occur together [34, 36] (Fig. 13.2).

Early cUS is less sensitive for the detection of ischemic brain lesions unless there is secondary hemorrhagic transformation, but on follow-up scans beyond 48–72 h, abnormal echogenicity in the deep gray matter and abnormal echogenicity and demarcation of the cortical and subcortical areas can be seen. Smaller cortical infarcts, lesions in the occipital and temporal lobes, and lesions in the cerebellum are often beyond the scope of cUS. MRI with DWI within the first 7–10 days is useful and will show a typical pattern of restricted diffusion with increased signal intensity in affected areas.

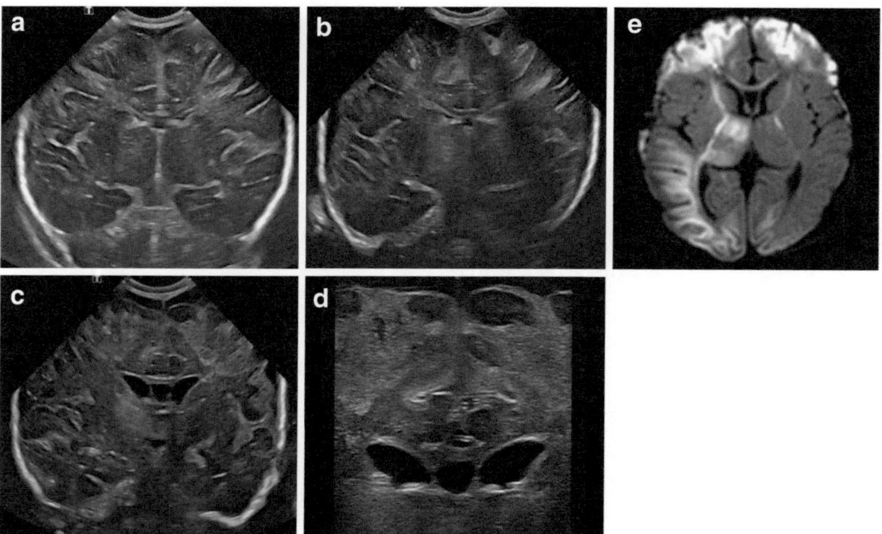

Fig. 13.2 Late-onset group B streptococcal meningitis. Preterm infant, readmitted 4 weeks postnatally. Cranial ultrasound on readmission (**a**) and follow-up scans on day 3 (**b**) and day 10 (**c**) after readmission show the evolution of a stroke-like pattern with asymmetric abnormal echogenicity in multiple cortical areas due to cortical infarctions as well as in the right thalamus due to a perforator stroke. Cranial ultrasound using a high-frequency linear transducer (**d**) on day 10 provides detailed visualization of the cortex and subcortical white matter and now shows cystic evolution in the affected areas emphasizing the importance of dedicated follow-up imaging. Diffusion-weighted MRI on day 6 after readmission (**e**) shows bilateral asymmetric restricted diffusion in cortical areas, the right thalamus, and the posterior limb of the internal capsule on both sides, but more pronounced on the right

13.2.5.2 *Escherichia coli (E. Coli)*

E. coli is the second most common causative microorganism in neonatal meningitis. Infections can be of early or late onset. The most characteristic feature of *E. coli* meningitis is that it carries a high risk of subsequent hydrocephalus [36].

Ventricular dilatation occurs in approximately 20% of cases due to inflammation with an increase in CSF production, obstruction of CSF flow, and reduced CSF resorption secondary to arachnoiditis [28]. Debris and adhesions may develop within the ventricles, and these strands can lead to compartmentalization and entrapment of parts of the ventricular system (Fig. 13.3). It is important to be aware that ventricular dilatation can occur early but can also still develop weeks after the onset of the infection. It is therefore crucial to perform follow-up cUS scans and follow head growth until at least 2 months after the infection. A distinctive type of ventricular dilatation and entrapment in *E. coli* meningitis may be seen at the level of the fourth ventricle and is due to obstruction of both the in- and outflow foramina. This can result in a severe dilatation of an

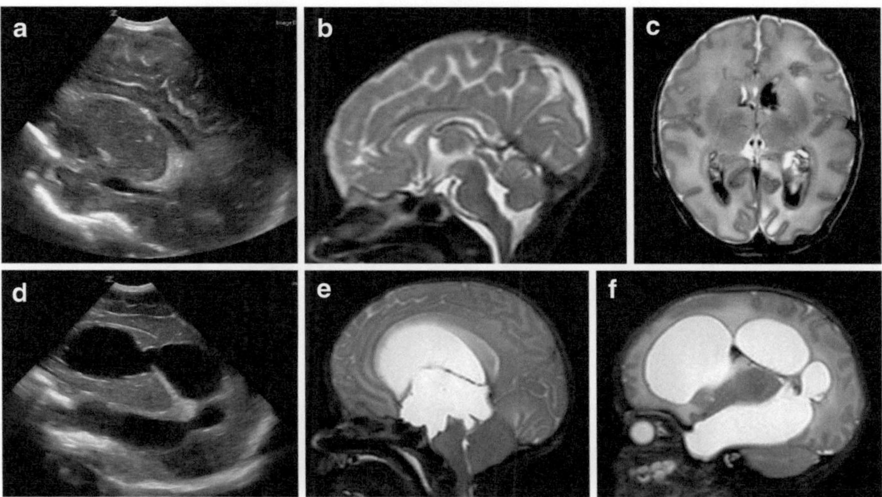

Fig. 13.3 *E. coli* meningitis. Preterm infant, born at 32 weeks gestation with grade 2 intraventricular hemorrhage (IVH) and *E. coli* meningitis. Cranial ultrasound during the first week (**a**) showing normal dimensions of the lateral ventricle with a small echogenicity at the level of the germinal matrix. MRI on day 7, showing normal dimensions of the third and fourth ventricles in the mid-sagittal plane (**b**) and of the lateral ventricles on the transverse plane (**c**) with bilateral IVH and a focal periventricular hemorrhagic infarction adjacent to the left frontal horn. Follow-up cranial ultrasound at 38 weeks gestation (**d**) now showing ventricular dilatation with multiple adhesions leading to isolated dilated segments of the lateral ventricle. Follow-up MRI at 38 weeks gestation, showing a severely dilated third ventricle in the mid-sagittal plane most like due to an obstruction at the level of the aqueduct (**e**) and the multiple adhesions leading to isolated dilated segments of the lateral ventricle in the parasagittal plane (**f**)

"isolated" fourth ventricle, resulting in a high pressure on the adjacent brain stem and cerebellum. Recognition of this severe complication is important for prompt and appropriate treatment; surgical intervention can however be complex [40, 41].

13.2.5.3 Gram-Negative Enterobacteriaceae (Other than *E. coli*)

Other gram-negative microorganisms that may be involved in neonatal meningitis include *Enterobacter* species, *Pseudomonas aeruginosa*, *Klebsiella*, *Proteus*, and *Serratia* species. Infections are usually of late onset, and for some of these microorganisms, outbreaks in neonatal intensive care units have been reported.

Typical for gram-negative enteric bacteria is that they may lead to hemorrhagic and liquefactive necrosis followed by abscess formation and thereby result in rapid and severe cerebral destruction (Fig. 13.4). Brain abscesses usually occur in the frontal lobes, although other brain regions may also be affected [11, 42].

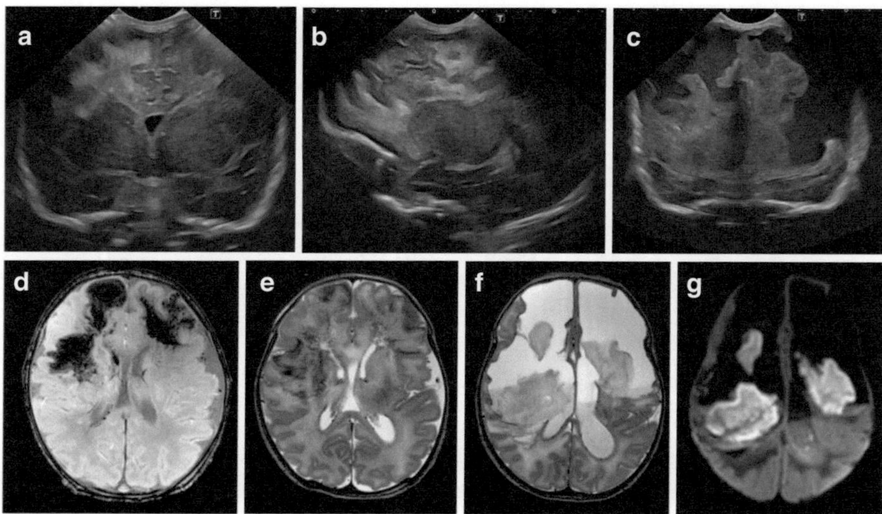

Fig. 13.4 Citrobacter meningitis. Full-term infant, admitted at day 5 with seizures. Cranial ultrasound on admission showing, on a coronal (**a**) and right parasagittal (**b**) view extensive areas of increased echogenicity, most prominent in the frontal lobes, with an asymmetric distribution and irregular demarcation, extending out toward the subcortical white matter. Follow-up cranial ultrasound (**c**) 14 days after admission showing the extensive bilateral tissue destruction due to necrosis and possible abscess formation. MRI on admission showing, on the susceptibility-weighted image (**d**) and T2-weighted image (**e**), hemorrhagic necrosis in the affected areas. An MRI 14 days after admission shows, on a T2-weighted image, (**f**) severe tissue destruction due to liquefactive necrosis and possible infectious debris with restricted diffusion inside the destructed areas (**g**)

In the early stages, cUS can show irregular and asymmetric areas of increased echogenicity within the white matter as well as a mass effect on the surrounding brain tissue. This can evolve into extensive necrosis and destruction of brain tissue. In the case of abscess formation, a focal area of necrosis may subsequently develop in the center of the lesion, and this area becomes echolucent. Diffusion-weighted MR imaging is also very helpful for the detection of abscesses with enhancement in the center of the lesion, reflecting restricted diffusion due to infected brain tissue.

13.2.5.4 *Listeria monocytogenes*

Listeria monocytogenes is a relatively rare cause of meningitis with an incidence of 0.61 per 100,000 live births [43]. Infection with this gram-positive rod may occur in outbreaks and is often related to food contamination. Transplacental infection of the fetus can occur and lead to stillbirth or preterm birth [44]. Characteristic for *Listeria* is a green coloration of the amniotic fluid in the absence of meconium. Intra-uterine, early-onset infection usually presents as a fulminating sepsis and meningitis with small granulomatous lesions in many organs including the brain which can evolve into multiple small brain abscesses. This is associated with high mortality rates. When the neonate is infected during labor or after birth, symptoms may not start till 8–30 days after birth. Late-onset infection usually also results in meningitis [19].

13.2.5.5 *Bacillus cereus*

Bacillus cereus is a gram-positive food bacterium. It is a rare cause of meningitis in neonates but it can have devastating consequences [45]. From the bloodstream, the organism itself invades the brain tissue where its toxins cause a liquefactive necrosis. Extensive brain abnormalities may become visible during the first days after the start of illness although clinical signs may only be subtle. On cUS widespread areas of echogenicity of the periventricular and subcortical white matter with an irregular border can be seen, usually with an asymmetrical distribution. The cortical gray matter is usually spared. Serial scanning can show central necrosis and subsequent cyst formation within hours to days [46] (see also Fig. 13.11).

13.2.5.6 *Candida* Species

The small size of the *Candida* species facilitates its access to the microcirculation and the formation of micro abscesses [47, 48]. In invasive candidiasis cUS is particularly important for recognition and follow-up of these typical lesions [49, 50]. The scattered small round echogenic micro abscesses usually appear within a week after the onset of infection and can be present in the subcortical, periventricular, and deep gray matter and sometimes also in the cerebellum and brainstem [51]. Usually during the course of infection, they start to develop a hypoechoic center and echogenic rim, but they may also become confluent and form macro abscesses. Another important feature of CNS involvement in systemic candidiasis is ventriculitis, seen on cUS as a hyperechoic ventricle wall, presence of intraventricular septae and debris in the ventricles and posterior fossa CSF spaces. Sometimes ventriculitis and meningitis lead to obstructive hydrocephalus. This may occur early but can also still develop weeks after the onset of the infection.

MRI can help to show the full extent of the micro abscesses, also throughout the subcortical areas, cerebellum, and brain stem. During the first weeks, the diffusion-weighted sequences are especially sensitive for the detection of lesions. After 2–4 weeks of successful treatment, the DWI changes may disappear, and cystic evolution of the abscesses and focal signal changes become more prominent on T1- and T2-weighted images (Fig. 13.5).

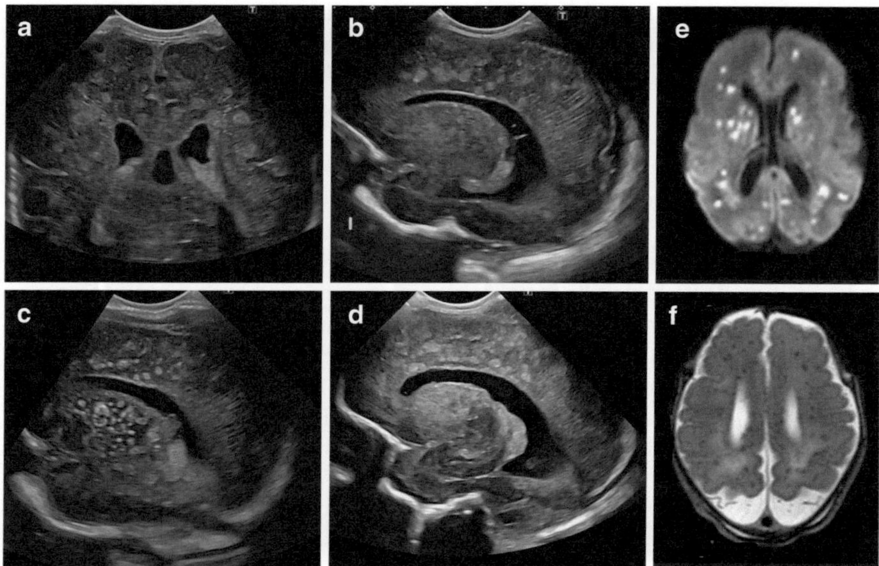

Fig. 13.5 Extremely preterm infant who developed Candida sepsis and meningitis, 14 days after birth. Cranial ultrasound 3 days after onset of illness (**a**, **b**) shows multiple, bilateral round areas of increased echogenicity in the periventricular white and deep gray matter. Follow-up ultrasound 10 days after onset of illness shows a clearer demarcation of microabcesses in the deep gray matter (**c**) together with the formation of a macroabcess on one side (**d**). The MRI within the first week after the onset of illness shows multiple rounded small lesions with restricted diffusion, due to micro abscesses (**e**) and similar lesions on T2 weighted image at two weeks (**f**)

13.2.6 Management

Early recognition and adequate treatment are crucial in newborns with CNS infection as these infections can cause rapid deterioration and lead to irreversible brain damage and even death. This includes supportive treatment, rapid initiation of broad-spectrum antibiotics/antifungal therapy, and treatment of possible neurologic complications (see below).

13.2.6.1 Supportive Treatment

Newborns with meningitis often present with signs of systemic illness and/or septic shock and require additional supportive care. This includes adequate respiratory support, management of circulatory failure and shock, and attention to fluid balance, nutrition, and metabolic state (including glucose homeostasis) and coagulation. Meningitis can lead to cerebral edema and to inappropriate antidiuretic hormone secretion. The latter may result in oliguria, hypo-osmolality, and hyponatremia. Therefore, careful fluid therapy and avoiding both hypo-and hypervolemia and hypo- and hypernatremia are important. Management of shock and systemic hypotension is essential. Impaired cerebrovascular autoregulation and cerebral edema can easily lead to impaired cerebral perfusion and thereby increase the risk of secondary brain injury. Also, the hypercoagulable state of newborns with sepsis and/or meningitis may be a risk factor for the development of cerebral sinovenous thrombosis [52]. In a previous study in preterm infants, cerebral sinovenous thrombosis was related to meningitis in a number of cases [53].

13.2.6.2 Antibiotics

In newborns with suspected sepsis/meningitis, intravenous broad-spectrum antibiotics must be administered as soon as possible. After laboratory tests and blood cultures have been taken and preferably after an LP has been performed, antibiotic treatment should be started immediately without awaiting the results (see also diagnosis). At first, empiric antibiotic therapy should be aimed at the most likely pathogens causing meningitis. The regimen depends on the timing of infection, either early- or late-onset, on whether or not an infection is hospital acquired, and on local resistance patterns within the hospital and the community. Therefore, we strongly recommend following national and local hospital guidelines.

In general, for early-onset sepsis/meningitis in the Western world, the most likely pathogens are GBS and *E. coli*, and when a newborn is admitted with signs of sepsis, the first treatment therefore often consists of ampicillin and an aminoglycoside (typically gentamicin). When meningitis is either suspected (based on CSF analysis) or cannot be excluded, the aminoglycoside needs to be replaced by another agent (such a third-generation cephalosporin) for CSF coverage of possible ampicillin-resistant gram-negative microorganisms. Once the causative microorganism and the antimicrobial susceptibility results are known, empiric antimicrobial therapy can be adjusted and targeted. This usually takes 24–48 h.

The duration of antibiotic treatment depends on the microorganism and on possible complications during illness. In general, a newborn with uncomplicated GBS meningitis is treated for 14 days, and a newborn with *E. coli* or other gram-negative meningitis needs to be treated for a minimum of 21 days. In cases with complicated meningitis, for example, with brain abscess or empyema, the duration of treatment needs to be longer and individualized and can take, for example, up to 6–8 weeks. As mentioned previously, a repeat LP to confirm CSF sterilization is generally not recommended. However, in complicated cases and in cases with *E. coli* meningitis, where relapse has been documented in 2–21% of cases despite antibiotic treatment, a repeat LP may be considered after 48 h to document the effectiveness of antibiotic treatment and guide treatment duration [30].

For invasive fungal infections, the first important step is prevention by limiting the use of broad-spectrum antibiotics and indwelling vascular catheters. In some units with higher rates of infection, it was shown that fluconazole prophylaxis can reduce the incidence of colonization and invasive candida infections without a clear increase in fungal resistance. However, the benefit of this regime for long-term outcome remains a topic of debate [54–57]. Any suspected invasive fungal infection should be treated immediately with empirical antifungal therapy until an invasive fungal infection has been ruled out. The choice of drugs depends on the most common species, their susceptibility, and whether the infant already received fluconazole prophylaxis. Traditionally conventional amphotericin B is the drug of choice for systemic candidiasis; however it can have toxic side effects. Fluconazole has fewer side effects and good CSF penetration; however most *Candida* species, including *Candida glabrata* and *krusei*, are resistant to fluconazole. Lipid formulation amphotericin B was previously recommended as a treatment option but should be used with caution as it has been associated with higher rates of treatment failure, likely due to inadequate concentration in the kidney [16]. Newer drugs like echinocandins should not be used for cases with (possible) meningitis because they do not have good penetration in CSF [16]. Before making a treatment decision, it is important to be aware of the commonly isolated *Candida* species and local susceptibility patterns within the hospital and community and to follow national and local hospital guidelines. Another key component of treatment is the removal of central lines and other foreign material as *Candida* species can form a biofilm on these materials which makes effective clearance of the infection difficult.

13.2.7 Neurologic Complications

Treatment for neurologic complications in newborn meningitis includes the treatment of seizures, hydrocephalus, brain abscess, and inappropriate antidiuretic hormone secretion.

Newborns with a CNS infection are at risk for developing seizures, especially in the acute period of the infection, and these may be difficult to control. Seizures can occur in both early- and late-onset infection but are more common as a neurologic manifestation in late-onset. When seizures are suspected or when the newborn is very ill, (a)EEG monitoring should be used to detect seizures early and provide appropriate treatment (Neurophysiology; see Chap. 16).

Hydrocephalus can be an acute complication in neonatal CNS infection, but more often it develops in the subacute phase, after 2 or 3 weeks, especially in cases with *E. coli* infection. When hydrocephalus is acute and severe, newborns may present with signs of increased intracranial pressure and require prompt treatment. Also in those without clinical signs but with progressive ventriculomegaly seen on cUS scans, treatment is required to prevent secondary injury to the periventricular white matter. The first step includes temporary measures like repeated LPs or taps from a subcutaneous ventricular reservoir. In infants, particularly with *E. coli* meningitis, it is recommended to check with cUS for ventricular compartmentalization and a trapped fourth ventricle as LPs will not be successful in these cases. When hydrocephalus persists weeks to months after the reservoir placement, a ventriculoperitoneal shunt may be required (see also Chap. 3; GMH-IVH).

A brain abscess is a severe complication and occurs especially in newborns with gram-negative infection, in particular in cases with Citrobacter, Serratia, or Proteus infection. There is no consensus on the optimal approach. Apart from antibiotic therapy, neurosurgical drainage and lavage may be warranted and performed by aspiration or open surgical drainage, when the brain abscess becomes larger than 2.5 cm in diameter. It can be considered to perform an ultrasound-guided needle aspiration and lavage [58, 59].

13.2.8 Prognosis

The prognosis of newborn CNS infection depends on several factors including the causative microorganism; the time between onset of infection, diagnosis, and the initiation of appropriate antibiotic therapy; the gestational age of the infant (with a negative effect of preterm birth and/or low birth weight); the timing of infection (early- or late-onset); and the co-occurrence and evolution of brain injury and other complications. In general, newborns who are systemically ill on presentation and need respiratory support, those with a severely abnormal neurologic exam, who develop refractory seizures and/or have a persistently abnormal background pattern on aEEG, are at increased risk for an adverse outcome [60]. Not surprisingly, this risk is greater in those who have abnormal MRI findings or develop complications like hydrocephalus or a brain abscess.

In a study of 113 infants with bacterial meningitis in the first 90 days after birth and with GBS and *E. coli* as the most common pathogens, clinically significant sequelae were seen in 74%, including 8 deaths (7%). Adverse outcome in survivors consisted of hearing loss, visual problems, motor impairments, and/or cognitive delay and was more likely in infants who had seizures during admission, those with a high CSF protein level (>5 g/L), and those with hydrocephalus. Outcomes were similar between early-, late-, and extremely late-onset cases. However, motor deficits (spasticity or paresis) were more common among preterm infants than term infants [3].

In another study describing the outcomes of 50 infants with GBS meningitis, 10 infants died (20%), 39% of survivors had abnormal cognitive outcomes, and 26% had abnormal motor outcomes. In this study, an abnormal cUS scan and extensive white matter lesions on MRI correlated with abnormal motor outcome, while extensive bilateral deep gray matter lesions on MRI correlated with both abnormal cognitive outcome and motor outcome. Of note, only the most severe MRI findings correlated with adverse outcomes [61]. Two other studies investigating smaller groups of infants with GBS meningitis also described a high risk of adverse outcome in those with stroke like lesions on MRI. In the first study, 6/8 (75%) cases with extensive MRI abnormalities had impaired outcomes, including cerebral paresis, visual impairment, global delay, epilepsy, and/or hydrocephalus [34]. In the second study, 4/8 (50%) of cases with ischemic lesions on MRI had adverse outcome [62].

In general, infants with brain abscesses have poor outcomes, with overall mortality rates of approximately 15% and learning disabilities in 75% and epilepsy in 60% of the survivors [3–22].

Invasive candidiasis is associated with significant mortality and a high rate of impaired neurodevelopmental outcomes among extremely preterm infants [15, 63]. With prompt diagnosis and therapy, survival rates have increased over the past years; however approximately half of the survivors will have later neurodevelopmental impairments.

13.3 Conclusion

Bacterial and fungal infections of the CNS in newborns are serious and potentially life-threatening conditions. Early recognition is crucial as these infections can lead to rapid deterioration, followed by irreversible brain damage and even death. Knowledge of the most common microorganisms involved in early- and late-onset infections and their characteristic patterns on neuroimaging is important as this can help the clinician toward a prompt diagnosis followed by adequate treatment which plays an important role in improving outcome.

References

1. Okike IO, Johnson AP, Henderson KL, Blackburn RM, Muller-Pebody B, Ladhani SN, et al. Incidence, etiology, and outcome of bacterial meningitis in infants aged <90 days in the United Kingdom and Republic of Ireland: prospective, enhanced, national population-based surveillance. Clin Infect Dis. 2014;59(10):e150–e7.
2. Stoll BJ, Puopolo KM, Hansen NI, Sanchez PJ, Bell EF, Carlo WA, et al. Early-onset neonatal sepsis 2015 to 2017, the rise of Escherichia coli, and the need for novel prevention strategies. JAMA Pediatr. 2020;174(7):e200593.
3. Ouchenir L, Renaud C, Khan S, Bitnun A, Boisvert AA, McDonald J, et al. The epidemiology, management, and outcomes of bacterial meningitis in infants. Pediatrics. 2017;140:1.
4. Hallmaier-Wacker LK, Andrews A, Hope R, Demirjian A, Lamagni TL, Collin SM. Incidence of infant gram-negative invasive bacterial infections in England, 2011–2019: an observational study using population-wide surveillance data. Arch Dis Child. 2023;108(9):762–7.
5. Giannoni E, Agyeman PKA, Stocker M, Posfay-Barbe KM, Heininger U, Spycher BD, et al. Neonatal sepsis of early onset, and hospital-acquired and community-acquired late onset: a prospective population-based cohort study. J Pediatr. 2018;201:106–14. e4
6. Singh T, Barnes EH, Isaacs D. Australian Study Group for Neonatal I. Early-onset neonatal infections in Australia and New Zealand, 2002–2012. Arch Dis Child Fetal Neonatal Ed. 2019;104(3):F248–F52.
7. Linda S, de Vries Volpe JJ. Bacterial and fungal intracranial infections. In: Volpe JJ, editor. Volpe's neurology of the newborn. 7. Philadelphia: Elsevier; 2024. p. 1209–49.

8. Stoll BJ, Hansen N, Fanaroff AA, Wright LL, Carlo WA, Ehrenkranz RA, et al. To tap or not to tap: high likelihood of meningitis without sepsis among very low birth weight infants. Pediatrics. 2004;113(5):1181–6.

9. Renier D, Flandin C, Hirsch E, Hirsch JF. Brain abscesses in neonates. A study of 30 cases. J Neurosurg. 1988;69(6):877–82.

10. de Oliveira RS, Pinho VF, Madureira JF, Machado HR. Brain abscess in a neonate: an unusual presentation. Childs Nerv Syst. 2007;23(2):139–42.

11. Messerschmidt A, Prayer D, Olischar M, Pollak A, Birnbacher R. Brain abscesses after Serratia marcescens infection on a neonatal intensive care unit: differences on serial imaging. Neuroradiology. 2004;46(2):148–52.

12. Tsutsumi S, Arai H, Hishii M, Suzuki K, Sato K. A case of neonatal cerebellar abscess. Childs Nerv Syst. 2003;19(9):683–5.

13. Howell A, Isaacs D, Halliday R, Australasian Study Group For Neonatal I. Oral nystatin prophylaxis and neonatal fungal infections. Arch Dis Child Fetal Neonatal Ed. 2009;94(6):F429–33.

14. Oeser C, Vergnano S, Naidoo R, Anthony M, Chang J, Chow P, et al. Neonatal invasive fungal infection in England 2004-2010. Clin Microbiol Infect. 2014;20(9):936–41.

15. Weimer KED, Smith PB, Puia-Dumitrescu M, Aleem S. Invasive fungal infections in neonates: a review. Pediatr Res. 2022;91(2):404–12.

16. Kilpatrick R, Scarrow E, Hornik C, Greenberg RG. Neonatal invasive candidiasis: updates on clinical management and prevention. Lancet Child Adolesc Health. 2022;6(1):60–70. https://doi.org/10.1016/s2352-4642(21)00272-8.

17. Edwards JM, Watson N, Focht C, Wynn C, Todd CA, Walter EB, et al. Group B streptococcus (GBS) colonization and disease among pregnant women: a historical cohort study. Infect Dis Obstet Gynecol. 2019;2019:5430493.

18. Charlier C, Disson O, Lecuit M. Maternal-neonatal listeriosis. Virulence. 2020;11(1):391–7.

19. Charlier C, Kermorvant-Duchemin E, Perrodeau E, Moura A, Maury MM, Bracq-Dieye H, et al. Neonatal listeriosis presentation and outcome: a prospective study of 189 cases. Clin Infect Dis. 2022;74(1):8–16.

20. Schwarze R, Bauermeister CD, Ortel S, Wichmann G. Perinatal listeriosis in Dresden 1981-1986: clinical and microbiological findings in 18 cases. Infection. 1989;17(3):131–8.

21. Shane AL, Sanchez PJ, Stoll BJ. Neonatal sepsis. Lancet. 2017;390(10104):1770–80.

22. Dong Y, Glaser K, Speer CP. Late-onset sepsis caused by gram-negative bacteria in very low birth weight infants: a systematic review. Expert Rev Anti-Infect Ther. 2019;17(3):177–88.

23. Cohen-Wolkowiez M, Smith PB, Mangum B, Steinbach WJ, Alexander BD, Cotten CM, et al. Neonatal Candida meningitis: significance of cerebrospinal fluid parameters and blood cultures. J Perinatol. 2007;27(2):97–100.

24. Benjamin DK Jr, Stoll BJ, Fanaroff AA, McDonald SA, Oh W, Higgins RD, et al. Neonatal candidiasis among extremely low birth weight infants: risk factors, mortality rates, and neurodevelopmental outcomes at 18 to 22 months. Pediatrics. 2006;117(1):84–92.

25. Ahmed A, Hickey SM, Ehrett S, Trujillo M, Brito F, Goto C, et al. Cerebrospinal fluid values in the term neonate. Pediatr Infect Dis J. 1996;15(4):298–303.

26. Rodriguez AF, Kaplan SL, Mason EO Jr. Cerebrospinal fluid values in the very low birth weight infant. J Pediatr. 1990;116(6):971–4.

27. Thomson J, Sucharew H, Cruz AT, Nigrovic LE, Freedman SB, Garro AC, et al. Cerebrospinal fluid reference values for young infants undergoing lumbar puncture. Pediatrics. 2018;141:3.

28. Kralik SF, Kukreja MK, Paldino MJ, Desai NK, Vallejo JG. Comparison of CSF and MRI findings among neonates and infants with E coli or group B streptococcal meningitis. AJNR Am J Neuroradiol. 2019;40(8):1413–7.

29. Kralik SF, Vallejo JG, Kukreja MK, Salman R, Orman G, Huisman T, et al. Diagnostic accuracy of MRI for detection of meningitis in infants. AJNR Am J Neuroradiol. 2022;43(9):1350–5.

30. Vissing NH, Monster MB, Nordly S, Dayani GK, Heedegaard SS, Knudsen JD, et al. Relapse of neonatal Escherichia coli meningitis: did we miss something at first? Children (Basel). 2021;8:2.

31. Ting JY, Roberts A, Khan S, Bitnun A, Hawkes M, Barton M, et al. Predictive value of repeated cerebrospinal fluid parameters in the outcomes of bacterial meningitis in infants <90 days of age. PLoS One. 2020;15(8):e0238056.

32. Yikilmaz A, Taylor GA. Sonographic findings in bacterial meningitis in neonates and young infants. Pediatr Radiol. 2008;38(2):129–37.

33. Gupta N, Grover H, Bansal I, Hooda K, Sapire JM, Anand R, et al. Neonatal cranial sonography: ultrasound findings in neonatal meningitis-a pictorial review. Quant Imaging Med Surg. 2017;7(1):123–31.

34. Hernandez MI, Sandoval CC, Tapia JL, Mesa T, Escobar R, Huete I, et al. Stroke patterns in neonatal group B streptococcal meningitis. Pediatr Neurol. 2011;44(4):282–8.

35. Schneider JF, Hanquinet S, Severino M, Rossi A. MR imaging of neonatal brain infections. Magn Reson Imaging Clin N Am. 2011;19(4):761–75. vii-viii

36. Jaremko JL, Moon AS, Kumbla S. Patterns of complications of neonatal and infant meningitis on MRI by organism: a 10 year review. Eur J Radiol. 2011;80(3):821–7.

37. Schneider JF. Neonatal brain infections. Pediatr Radiol. 2011;41(Suppl 1):S143–S8.

38. Mao J, Li J, Chen D, Zhang J, Du YN, Wang YJ, et al. MRI-DWI improves the early diagnosis of brain abscess induced by Candida albicans in preterm infants. Transl Pediatr. 2012;1(2):76–84.

39. Horvath-Puho E, van Kassel MN, Goncalves BP, de Gier B, Procter SR, Paul P, et al. Mortality, neurodevelopmental impairments, and economic outcomes after invasive group B streptococcal disease in early infancy in Denmark and The Netherlands: a national matched cohort study. Lancet Child Adolesc Health. 2021;5(6):398–407.

40. Harter DH. Management strategies for treatment of the trapped fourth ventricle. Childs Nerv Syst. 2004;20(10):710–6.

41. El Damaty A, Eltanahy A, Unterberg A, Baechli H. Trapped fourth ventricle: a rare complication in children after supratentorial CSF shunting. Childs Nerv Syst. 2020;36(12):2961–9.

42. Masand R, Ali A, Purohit A. Neonatal brain abscess: an atypical presentation. J Pediatr Neurosci. 2015;10(3):282–4.

43. Koopmans MM, Bijlsma MW, Brouwer MC, van de Beek D, van der Ende A. Listeria monocytogenes meningitis in The Netherlands, 1985-2014: a nationwide surveillance study. J Infect. 2017;75(1):12–9.

44. Charlier C, Kermorvant-Duchemin E, Perrodeau E, et al. Neonatal Listeriosis Presentation and Outcome: A Prospective Study of 189 Cases. Clin Infect Dis. 2022;74:8–16. https://doi.org/10.1093/cid/ciab337.

45. Tokieda K, Morikawa Y, Maeyama K, Mori K, Ikeda K. Clinical manifestations of Bacillus cereus meningitis in newborn infants. J Paediatr Child Health. 1999;35(6):582–4.

46. Lequin MH, Vermeulen JR, van Elburg RM, Barkhof F, Kornelisse RF, Swarte R, et al. Bacillus cereus meningoencephalitis in preterm infants: neuroimaging characteristics. AJNR Am J Neuroradiol. 2005;26(8):2137–43.

47. Kilpatrick R, Scarrow E, Hornik C, Greenberg RG. Neonatal invasive candidiasis: updates on clinical management and prevention. Lancet Child Adolesc Health. 2022;6:60–70. https://doi.org/10.1016/s2352-4642(21)00272-8.

48. Weimer KED, Smith PB, Puia-Dumitrescu M, Aleem S. Invasive fungal infections in neonates: a review. Pediatric research. 2022;91:404–12. https://doi.org/10.1038/s41390-021-01842-7.

49. Huang CC, Chen CY, Yang HB, Wang SM, et al. Central nervous system candidiasis in very low-birth-weight premature neonates and infants: US characteristics and histopathologic and MR imaging correlates in five patients. Radiology. 1998;209:49–56.

50. Tung KT, MacDonald LM, Smith JC. Neonatal systemic candidiasis diagnosed by ultrasound. Acta Radiol 1990;31(3):293–5.

51. Pahud BA, Greenhow TL, Piecuch B, Weintrub PS. Preterm neonates with candidal brain microabscesses: a case series. Journal of perinatology: official journal of the California Perinatal Association. 2009;29:323–6. https://doi.org/10.1038/jp.2008.201.

52. Steggerda SJ, de Vries LS. Neonatal stroke in premature neonates. Semin Perinatol. 2021;45(7):151471.

53. Kersbergen KJ, Groenendaal F, Benders MJ, de Vries LS. Neonatal cerebral sinovenous thrombosis: neuroimaging and long-term follow-up. J Child Neurol. 2011;26(9):1111–20.
54. Benjamin DK Jr, Hudak ML, Duara S, Randolph DA, Bidegain M, Mundakel GT, et al. Effect of fluconazole prophylaxis on candidiasis and mortality in premature infants: a randomized clinical trial. JAMA. 2014;311(17):1742–9.
55. Manzoni P, Stolfi I, Pugni L, Decembrino L, Magnani C, Vetrano G, et al. A multicenter, randomized trial of prophylactic fluconazole in preterm neonates. N Engl J Med. 2007;356(24):2483–95.
56. Ericson JE, Kaufman DA, Kicklighter SD, Bhatia J, Testoni D, Gao J, et al. Fluconazole prophylaxis for the prevention of candidiasis in premature infants: a meta-analysis using patient-level data. Clin Infect Dis. 2016;63(5):604–10.
57. Healy CM, Campbell JR, Zaccaria E, Baker CJ. Fluconazole prophylaxis in extremely low birth weight neonates reduces invasive candidiasis mortality rates without emergence of fluconazole-resistant Candida species. Pediatrics. 2008;121(4):703–10.
58. Frazier JL, Ahn ES, Jallo GI. Management of brain abscesses in children. Neurosurg Focus. 2008;24(6):E8.
59. Bonfield CM, Sharma J, Dobson S. Pediatric intracranial abscesses. J Infect. 2015;71(Suppl 1):S42–S6.
60. ter Horst HJ, van Olffen M, Remmelts HJ, de Vries H, Bos AF. The prognostic value of amplitude integrated EEG in neonatal sepsis and/or meningitis. Acta Paediatr. 2010;99(2):194–200.
61. Martis JMS, Bok LA, Halbertsma FJJ, van Straaten HLM, de Vries LS, Groenendaal F. Brain imaging can predict neurodevelopmental outcome of Group B streptococcal meningitis in neonates. Acta Paediatr. 2019;108(5):855–64.
62. Choi SY, Kim JW, Ko JW, Lee YS, Chang YP. Patterns of ischemic injury on brain images in neonatal group B Streptococcal meningitis. Korean J Pediatr. 2018;61(8):245–52.
63. Friedman S, Richardson SE, Jacobs SE, O'Brien K. Systemic Candida infection in extremely low birth weight infants: short term morbidity and long term neurodevelopmental outcome. Pediatr Infect Dis J. 2000;19(6):499–504.

## Part V

Neuro-Imaging and Neuro-Monitoring

Cranial Ultrasonography

Gerda Meijler and Sylke J. Steggerda

Abbreviations

AF	Anterior fontanel
cUS	Cranial ultrasound
MF	Mastoid fontanel
PF	Posterior fontanel
RI	Resistance index
TW	Temporal window

G. Meijler (✉)
Department of Neonatology, Isala Women and Children's Hospital, Zwolle, The Netherlands
e-mail: gmeijler@gmail.com

S. J. Steggerda
Department of Pediatrics, Division of Neonatology, Willem-Alexander Children's Hospital, Leiden University Medical Center (LUMC), Leiden, The Netherlands
e-mail: S.J.Steggerda@lumc.nl

© The Author(s) 2024
G. Meijler, K. Mohammad (eds.), *Neonatal Brain Injury*,
https://doi.org/10.1007/978-3-031-55972-3_14

14.1 For Parents

Cranial (or head) ultrasound is a safe and patient-friendly imaging technique. It is portable and can be performed at the bedside, without moving the infant. Most infants are hardly disturbed by a cranial ultrasound examination. Cranial ultrasound is routinely used on the neonatal unit to follow brain growth and brain development in preterm infants, and to look for brain abnormalities in preterm and sick term-born infants. As cranial ultrasound is safe and patient-friendly, it can be repeated when necessary. It is a reliable technique for detecting the most frequent and important forms of brain injury and variants of brain development in both preterm and term-born infants and is the first brain imaging tool used in neonatal intensive care units and other neonatal wards. It helps to detect lesions that may have impact on the infant's outcome in terms of development and to provide the infant with optimal care, also after discharge. With some findings or some clinical situations, it can be helpful to additionally do a brain MRI scan to obtain even more detailed images of the brain.

14.1.1 How Does Ultrasound Work?

Ultrasound uses soundwaves to produce an image. The ultrasound machine sends soundwaves through the transducer (also called probe) to the brain. These waves are reflected by the brain tissue, sent back to the transducer in the form of an echo, and then transformed into signals that become visible on a monitor as an image of the brain. In newborns, cranial ultrasound can be used to make images of the infant's brain. Ultrasound waves travel well through soft tissue but not through the bone. However, the skull of the newborn and young infant has unique properties: the fontanels (soft spots in the middle of the top of the head) and some of the sutures (the connections between the bones of the skull) are still open (Fig. 14.1) and can therefore be used as windows to look into the brain.

Using ultrasound, we can see:

- How the baby's brain is developing—how mature it looks in relation to its age and if it is growing well.
- Whether there is a congenital abnormality—this is a problem in development that has been there from early on in the pregnancy.
- If there are any injuries, like bleedings or effects from infections or lack of oxygen. In most cases problems in the brain are first detected using cranial ultrasound. In the case of abnormalities, the images help us to predict how the baby will progress in the future, particularly in relation to motor skills but also learning, understanding, talking, seeing, and behavior, i.e., what is often called neurodevelopmental progress.

14.1.2 Procedure

The investigator will come to your baby with the scanner. He/she will put some ultrasound gel on the ultrasound transducer and will then place the transducer on the fontanel (see Fig. 14.2).

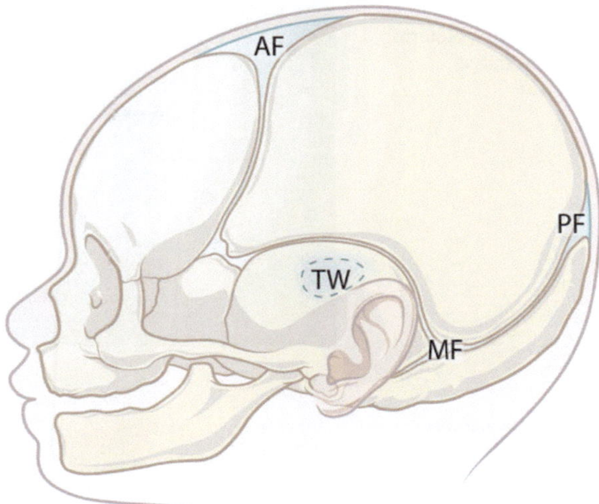

Fig. 14.1 The acoustic windows of the infant's skull, allowing a cranial ultrasound examination. *AF* anterior fontanel (allowing views of the whole brain), *PF* posterior fontanel (allowing more detailed views of the back parts of the brain and of the cerebellum), *TW* temporal window (allowing views of the brainstem and the large vessels around the brainstem), *MF* mastoid fontanel = fontanel behind the ear (allowing detailed views of the cerebellum and the structures around the cerebellum: the "posterior fossa"). From: Meijler G. and Steggerda S.J. Neonatal Cranial Ultrasonography, Springer 2019

Fig. 14.2 Preterm infant, undergoing a cranial ultrasound examination through the anterior fontanel

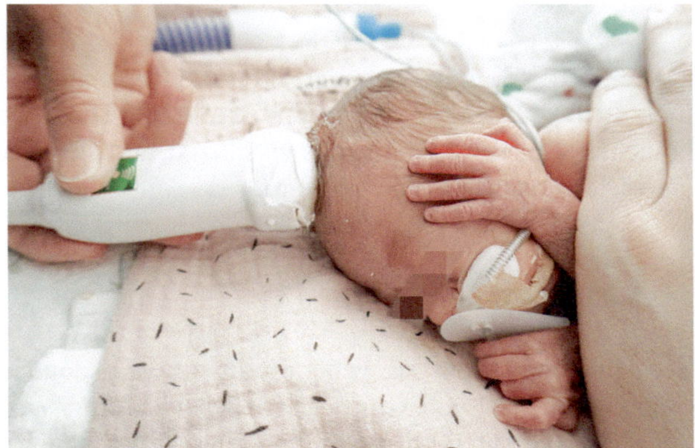

By carefully moving the transducer, almost the whole brain can be visualized in detail. The cerebrum (large brain) is best seen through the anterior and posterior fontanels, while the cerebellum (small brain) is better seen through the fontanels behind the ears (the mastoid fontanels) (Figs. 14.1, 14.2, 14.3, and 14.4).

The investigator will always scan through the anterior fontanel. Depending on whether the lower and back parts of the brain are clearly seen and/or there are specific questions, he/she will use other fontanels as well.

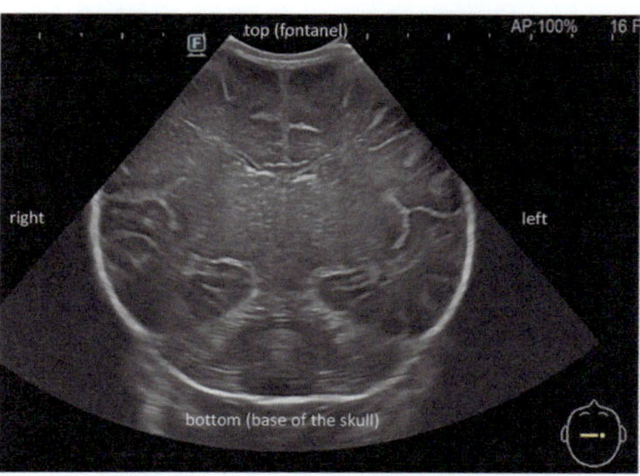

Fig. 14.3 Example of a brain ultrasound scan performed in a preterm infant, scanned before discharge (3 weeks before due date)

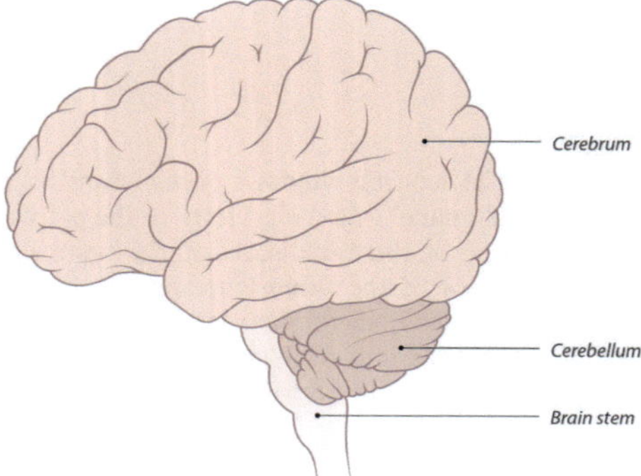

Fig. 14.4 Illustration of the cerebrum, cerebellum, and brain stem. (© Amanda Gautier-Ronopawiro)

While performing a cranial ultrasound examination, the investigator can also look at the vessels in and around the brain. The large vessels and even smaller branches of these vessels can be visualized, and the blood flow velocity within these vessels can be measured and heard.

14.1.3 Results

The ultrasound scans are generally interpreted soon (within 1 or 2 days) after the examination, and you will hear the results from your baby's doctor or physician assistant. As cranial ultrasound is a routine procedure in almost all neonatal units, the results are typically discussed during planned parental meetings with the medical team.

14.2   For Professionals

Cranial ultrasonography (cUS) was introduced into neonatology in the 1970s. Since then, the technique, quality, and analysis of images have improved tremendously. It now enables a detailed view of the neonatal brain, including the cerebellum, brainstem, and the major vessels. As it is safe and can be done at the bedside while hardly disturbing the infant, it is the primary neuro-imaging technique for the neonate and can be used to follow brain growth and maturation and to detect and follow lesions in high-risk neonates.

When the proper system, transducers, and presets are used by a person experienced in neonatal cUS, most forms of preterm brain injury can be reliably detected, especially germinal matrix-intraventricular hemorrhage and its complications, limited and extensive cerebellar hemorrhage, arterial infarction, and cystic white matter injury (see Chaps. 3, 4, 5, and 6 on these topics). cUS may be somewhat less reliable for brain injuries in the full-term infant, especially for the early stages of hypoxic-ischemic injury and arterial infarction (see Chaps. 8 and 9 on Brain Injury in the (Near)Term Neonate). However, again, if performed by an experienced person, using the proper equipment and settings, and if well-timed, it is also extremely useful in the sick full-term infant, as transportation to an MRI unit for early and/or serial imaging is often strenuous and not in the best interest of these vulnerable patients. For optimal timing of cUS examinations and technical details, we refer to our recent book on neonatal cranial ultrasonography [1].

14.2.1 How Ultrasound Works

Ultrasound is a non-invasive diagnostic technique. Ultrasound transducers produce sound waves and operate at high frequencies (in the megahertz (MHz) range), beyond the threshold of human hearing. The sound waves travel through brain tissue and are reflected back to the transducer, in the form of echoes, when they meet boundaries between tissues in the path of the ultrasound beam (e.g., the boundary between fluid and tissue). When these echoes are detected by the transducer, they are converted into electrical signals that are sent to the ultrasound scanner. The scanner calculates the distance from the transducer to the tissue boundary. These distances are then used to generate images of tissue (in case of cranial ultrasonography of the neonatal brain).

14.2.2 The Procedure

Gel is put on the transducer, which is then placed on one of the fontanels. This prevents the forming of air pockets between the transducer and the skin, which can block ultrasound waves from passing into the brain.

For a routine, standard cUS examination the anterior fontanel is used as the acoustic window, allowing a complete overview of the supratentorial brain

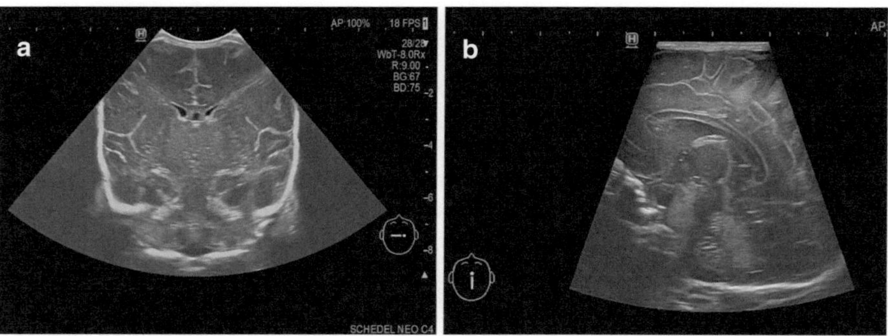

Fig. 14.5 Midcoronal (**a**) and midsagittal (**b**) plane in preterm infant, born at 31 weeks gestation scan performed at postmenstrual age of 35 weeks. Normal findings for this age

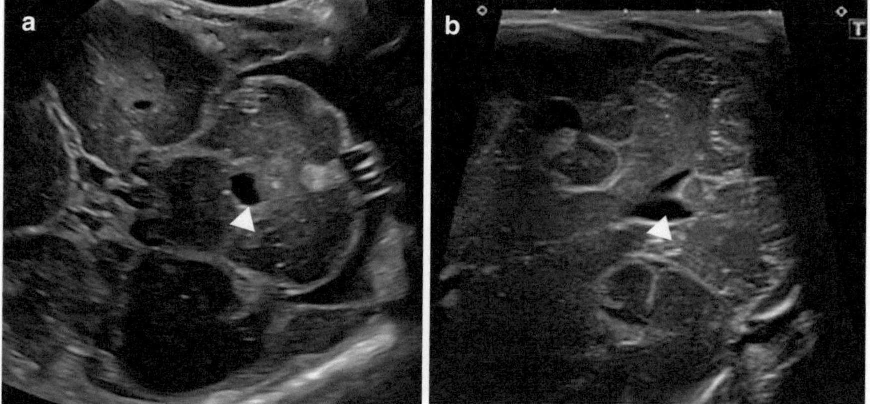

Fig. 14.6 cUS scans using the mastoid fontanel as acoustic window. The cerebellum is shown in more detail. Arrowhead indicates the fourth ventricle. Normal findings. (**a**) Midaxial view and (**b**) midcoronal view in two preterm infants at 25 and 33 weeks' gestation

structures in two directions, scanning the whole brain and saving images in six standard coronal and seven standard sagittal planes [1] (Fig. 14.5).

In smaller infants the anterior fontanel also enables visualization of the infratentorial structures. The infratentorial structures are, however, better visualized through the mastoid fontanel (see Fig. 14.1), which allows a detailed view of the cerebellum, cisterna magna, and the transverse sinuses of the venous dural system, using three standard coronal and three standard axial planes (Fig. 14.6).

The posterior fontanel (see Fig. 14.1) is used to obtain a better view of the occipital horns of the lateral ventricles and the occipital lobes. This view is generally done

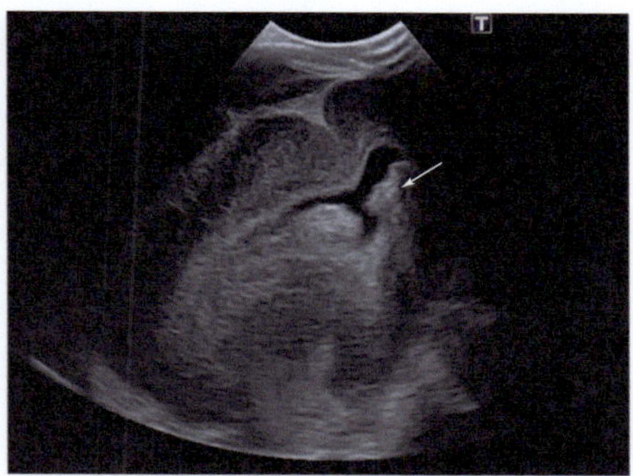

Fig. 14.7 cUS scan using the posterior fontanel window, parasagittal image in preterm infant, showing a hemorrhagic clot in the occipital horn of the lateral ventricle (arrow)

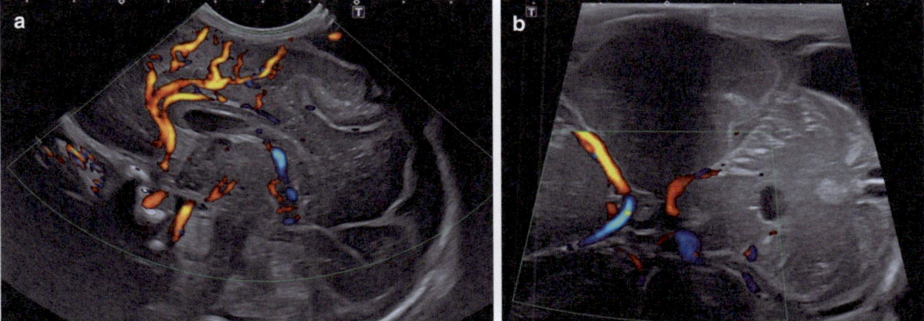

Fig. 14.8 Color Doppler images in a preterm infant. (**a**) In the midsagittal plane through the anterior fontanel, demonstrating flow in the internal carotid artery, basilar artery, anterior cerebral artery, pericallosal artery, and its branches. (**b**) In a transverse plane obtained through the temporal window, showing the circle of Willis

when pathology (e.g., hemorrhagic clot in the occipital horns and/or occipital parenchymal injury) is suspected or present (Fig. 14.7).

The temporal window (see Fig. 14.1) enables visualization of the brainstem and the circle of Willis (Fig. 14.8). In some centers the foramen magnum is additionally used to visualize the cerebellum and the other infratentorial structures.

To obtain proper experience and expertise in performing and interpreting cUS, we recommend reading the several textbooks that are available and to follow (hands-on) courses that are organized on this subject [1, 2].

Timing and frequency of cUS are important for reliable diagnosis and prognosis. Guidelines for timing of cUS examinations vary between centers, with a tendency toward more examinations in European versus North American centers [1, 3, 4]. In general, it is recommended to perform cUS examinations on a regular basis in all very preterm infants until discharge or term-equivalent age and in all other newborn infants at risk for brain abnormalities and/or with neurological symptoms.

When performing cUS, transcranial color Doppler sonography can be performed. With this technique the venous sinuses, main cerebral arteries, and their vascular branches can be depicted, thereby providing useful information about cerebral

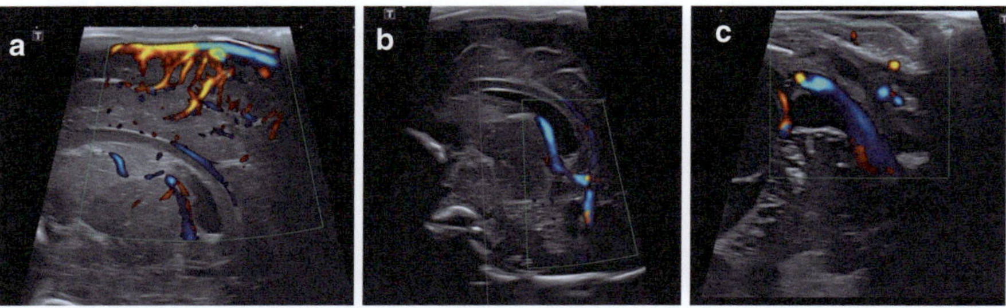

Fig. 14.9 Color Doppler images in a preterm infant (**a**, **b**) in the midsagittal plane through the anterior fontanel, demonstrating flow in the superior sagittal sinus (**a**) and deep venous system (**b**), and (**c**) in a coronal plane obtained through the mastoid fontanel demonstrating flow in the transverse sinus

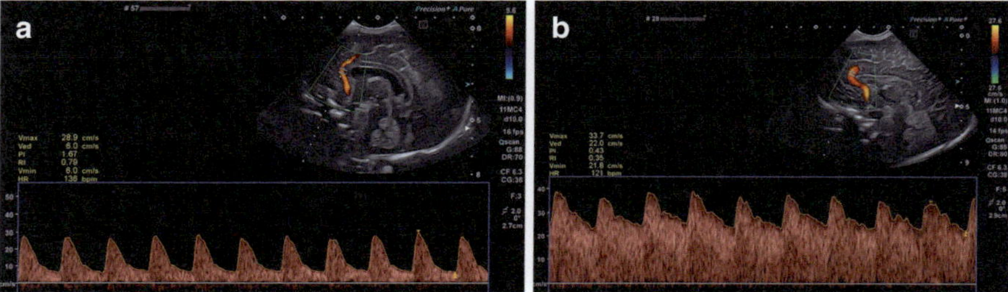

Fig. 14.10 Doppler measurement of resistance index (RI) on the pericallosal artery, in the midsagittal plane through the anterior fontanel. On the left a normal flow pattern and RI in a healthy newborn infant; on the right hyperluxury perfusion and abnormal RI value in an infant with hypoxic-ischemic encephalopathy

vascular anatomy (see Figs. 14.8 and 14.9). This enables the detection of arterial and venous thrombosis, several types of vascular malformations, such as vein of Galen malformation and developmental venous anomalies, and some rare brain tumors [5–7]. In addition, this technique can be used to study alterations in blood flow patterns over time and in various clinical situations, such as increased intracranial pressure, hypo- and hypercarbia, systemic blood pressure fluctuations, hypovolemia, and severe respiratory failure. This is important while many cerebral lesions in the newborn are of circulatory origin. The assessment of cerebral blood flow velocity can thereby provide information about the risk of brain injury, for example, an increased risk of intraventricular hemorrhage or ischemic injury. Doppler sonography also plays a role in determining the severity of brain injury in cases with hypoxic-ischemic encephalopathy, as moderate to severe asphyxia is often followed by a reduction in cerebrovascular resistance and a period of hyperperfusion. This so-called luxury perfusion leads to a rise in diastolic flow velocity and can be measured by the resistance index (RI) (Fig. 14.10). In cases with perinatal asphyxia and hypothermia treatment, a persisting low RI after rewarming is an indicator of poor outcome [8–10].

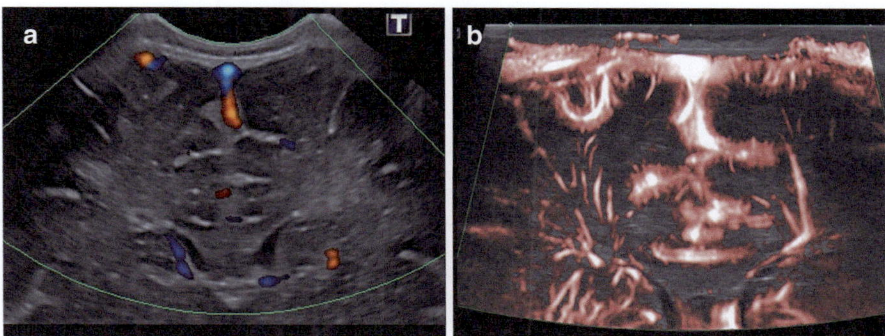

Fig. 14.11 Comparison of power Doppler images obtained with a microconvex transducer (**a**) and microvascular imaging performed with a high-frequency linear transducer (**b**). Same infant and in both examples scanned from the anterior fontanel in the coronal plane. The use of the high-frequency linear ultrasound probe and a more sensitive microvascular imaging technique shows that although directional information is lost, visualization of smaller and superficial vessels can be clearly improved by using this approach

Transcranial Doppler sonography can be performed through different fontanels, depending on the vessels of interest. A routine microconvex ultrasound probe can be used to depict the main cerebral arteries and the venous sinuses. Visualization of smaller and superficial vessels can be improved by using a high-frequency linear ultrasound probe (Fig. 14.11). For more information on the anatomy of the cerebral vasculature and technical aspects of Doppler measurements, we recommend the following papers and textbooks [1, 11–18].

References

1. Meijler G, Steggerda SJ. Neonatal Cranial Ultrasonography. Switzerland: Springer; 2019.
2. Govaert P, Vries LS. An atlas of brain sonography. Cambridge University Press; 2010.
3. Dudink J, Steggerda SJ, Horsch S, Eur. US. brain group. State-of-the-art neonatal cerebral ultrasound: technique and reporting. Pediatr Res. 2020;87(Suppl 1):3–12.
4. Mohammad K, Scott JN, Leijser LM, Zein H, Afifi J, Piedboeuf B, de Vries LS, van Wezel-Meijler G, Lee SK, Shah PS. Consensus approach for standardizing the screening and classification of preterm brain injury diagnosed with cranial ultrasound: a Canadian perspective. Front Pediatr. 2021;9:618236.
5. Horsch S, Govaert P, Cowan FM, Benders MJ, Groenendaal F, Lequin MH, Saliou G, de Vries LS. Developmental venous anomaly in the newborn brain. Neuroradiology. 2014;56(7):579–88.
6. Geraldo AF, Messina SS, Tortora D, Parodi A, Malova M, Morana G, Gandolfo C, D'Amico A, Herkert E, Govaert P, Ramenghi LA, Rossi A, Severino M. Neonatal developmental venous anomalies: clinicoradiologic characterization and follow-up. AJNR Am J Neuroradiol. 2020;41(12):2370–6.
7. Raets M, Dudink J, Raybaud C, Ramenghi L, Lequin M, Govaert P. Brain vein disorders in newborn infants. Dev Med Child Neurol. 2015;57(3):229–40.
8. Elstad M, Whitelaw A, Thoresen M. Cerebral resistance index is less predictive in hypothermic encephalopathic newborns. Acta Paediatr. 2011;100(10):1344–9.

9. Skranes JH, Elstad M, Thoresen M, Cowan FM, Stiris T, Fugelseth D. Hypothermia makes cerebral resistance index a poor prognostic tool in encephalopathic newborns. Neonatology. 2014;106(1):17–23.
10. Gerner GJ, Burton VJ, Poretti A, Bosemani T, Cristofalo E, Tekes A, Seyfert D, Parkinson C, Leppert M, Allen M, Huisman TAGM, Northington FJ, Johnston MV. Transfontanellar duplex brain ultrasonography resistive indices as a prognostic tool in neonatal hypoxic-ischemic encephalopathy before and after treatment with therapeutic hypothermia. J Perinatol. 2016;36(3):202–6.
11. Govaert P. Sonographic stroke templates. Semin Fetal Neonatal Med. 2009;14(5):284–98.
12. Couture A, Veyrac C, Baud C, Saguintaah M, Ferran JL. Advanced cranial ultrasound: transfontanellar Doppler imaging in neonates. Eur Radiol. 2001;11(12):2399–410.
13. Veyrac C, Couture A, Saguintaah M, Baud C. Brain ultrasonography in the premature infant. Pediatr Radiol. 2006;36(7):626–35.
14. Steggerda SJ, de Vries LS. Neonatal stroke in premature neonates. Semin Perinatol. 2021;45(7):151471.
15. Deeg K-H. Sonographic and Doppler sonographic diagnosis of neonatal ischemic stroke. Ultraschall Med. 2017a;38:360–76.
16. Deeg K-H. Duplex sonographic diagnosis of perinatal hemorrhagic stroke. Ultraschall Med. 2017b;38:484–98.
17. Miller E, Daneman A, Doria AS, Blaser S, Traubici J, Jarrin J, Moineddin R, Moore A, Shroff M. Color Doppler US of normal cerebral venous sinuses in neonates: a comparison with MR venography. Pediatr Radiol. 2012;42(9):1070–9.
18. Horsch S, Schwarz S, Arnaez J, Steggerda S, Arena R, Govaert P, EurUS. Brain group. Cerebral Doppler imaging in neonates: A guide for clinical application and diagnosis. Dev Med Child Neurol. 2024;66(12):1570–89.

Magnetic Resonance Imaging (MRI)

15

Miriam Martinez-Biarge and Frances M. Cowan

Abbreviations

ADC	Apparent diffusion coefficient
BGT	Basal ganglia and thalami
CST	Corticospinal tract
CT	Computerized tomography
cUS	Cranial ultrasound
DWI	Diffusion-weighted imaging
FLAIR	Fluid-attenuated inversion recovery
HIE	Hypoxic-ischemic encephalopathy
IVH	Intraventricular hemorrhage
MRA	Magnetic resonance angiography
MRI	Magnetic resonance imaging
MRS	Magnetic resonance spectroscopy
MRV	Magnetic resonance venography
PLIC	Posterior limb of the internal capsule
RF	Radio frequency
SI	Signal intensity
SWI	Susceptibility-weighted imaging
T	Tesla
TCD	Transcerebellar diameter
TE	Times of echo
TR	Times of repetition
W	Weighted
WM	White matter

M. Martinez-Biarge (✉)
Department of Paediatrics, Imperial College Healthcare NHS Trust, London, UK
e-mail: miriam.martinez-biarge@nhs.net

F. M. Cowan
Department of Paediatrics, Imperial College London, London, UK
e-mail: f.cowan@imperial.ac.uk

© The Author(s) 2024
G. Meijler, K. Mohammad (eds.), *Neonatal Brain Injury*,
https://doi.org/10.1007/978-3-031-55972-3_15

15.1 For Parents

Magnetic resonance imaging (MRI) of the brain allows us to see the baby's brain in great detail. Because MRI does not involve radiation (unlike a computerized tomography or CT scan), it is the best method to use in newborn babies and young children. But MRI involves moving the baby to the scanner, and it takes time and cannot be done quickly, so most scanning of the baby's brain is done using ultrasound, a safe method than can be done at the bedside. Often babies will have one or two MRI scans to obtain additional information besides the information that is obtained from the bedside ultrasound scans.

15.1.1 How Does MRI Work?

Water makes up 92–95% of the brain in newborn babies, and this water is free to move to different extents in different tissues within the brain. An MRI scanner is a big magnet that produces a strong magnetic field. Using these magnetic fields, the MR scanner maps the water and its movement in the different regions and tissues and produces an accurate image of different parts of the brain. MRI is also very good at detecting blood in tissues, as blood contains iron and the MR scanner is very sensitive to it.

Using MRI we can see the following:

- How the baby's brain is developing, i.e. how mature it looks in relation to the baby's age and if it is growing in a typical or in an atypical way.
- Whether there is a congenital malformation—this is a problem that has been there from early on in the pregnancy.
- If there are any injuries, bleeding (hemorrhage) or effects from infections or lack of oxygen.

The way the images look helps us to predict how your child will progress, particularly in relation to movements but also learning, understanding, talking, seeing, and behavior, i.e. what is often called neurodevelopmental progress. In many cases problems in the brain are first detected using cranial ultrasound. MRI can be used to confirm these findings and to show regions of the brain or very small abnormalities that are not so easily seen with cranial ultrasound.

Although MRI is a very low-risk procedure, you should understand why your baby's doctor wants to obtain the MRI scan, what information he/she is seeking and how that information will be used to improve the care of your child. In some cases you may prefer that your baby does not have an MRI.

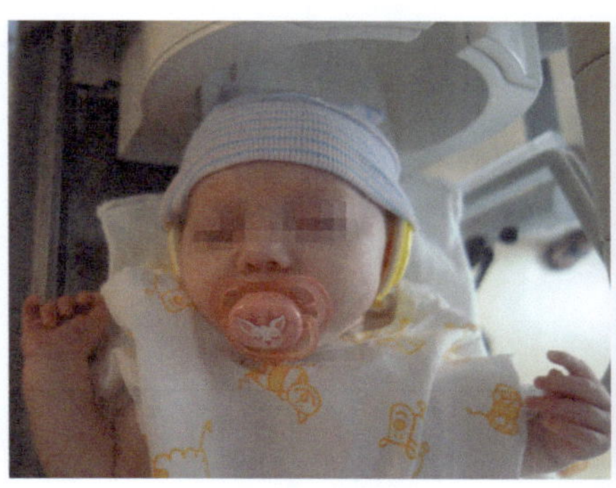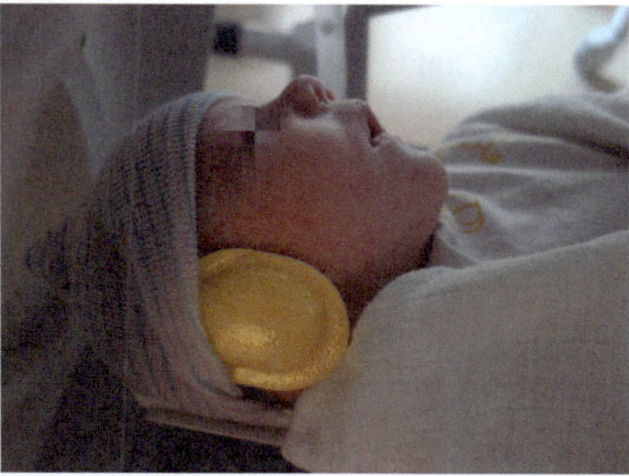

Fig. 15.1 A baby asleep, with ear protection in place, then swaddled and ready to go into the scanner (parental permission given for use)

15.1.2 Procedure

MRI scanners are made so adults can fit in them and thus they are quite large. For babies there are special small mattresses that fit snuggly around them, and your baby will lie on this inside a special tube or coil which fits inside the bigger magnet. Because MRI scanners are noisy, your baby will have protection for their hearing, either headphones or patches over the ears as shown in Fig. 15.1. Babies need to lie fairly still for the 30–60 minutes that the scan takes.

In some centers the "feed and wrap" method is used. This means that the baby is fed (with breast milk or formula) and then swaddled in a blanket. After falling asleep naturally, the baby is placed in the special mattress that fits snuggly to limit too much movement. In some centers babies are scanned in special incubators that can go into the scanner. This has the advantage that the baby can fall asleep in the baby unit and does not need to be moved again when being put into the scanner. Whichever method is used, it is sometimes necessary to use a mild sedative (administered orally or as a suppository into the rectum) particularly if it is vital for diagnosis that very precise images with no sign of movement are obtained.

During a scan, your baby will be continuously monitored to check the heart rate, breathing, and oxygen levels, and someone trained in looking after babies will be there. If your baby wakes and moves, it becomes very difficult to get good images, and your baby will be taken out of the scanner and settled, and they will try to scan again. If this is not effective, then the scan will be done another time.

It is very important that your baby does not have any metal objects attached to them or metal buttons in their clothing, as metal is attracted to the magnet and can cause damage to the magnet or even harm the baby. Therefore, both the nurse and the MR technician will carefully check for any metal objects. Special MRI-compatible monitors, ventilators, and IV pumps are used, in order to be able to continue the monitoring and all the care your baby needs.

15.1.3 Results

Interpreting an MRI scan can require some time, and the technician running the scanner is not the radiologist who does the reporting. In some cases the radiologist may send the images to another specialist for a second opinion before the report is written and then sent to your baby's doctor.

It is important that you have time to discuss the results with your doctor and that you understand everything they say. If you wish to see the images, you can ask your doctor who may be able to arrange this. For some parents this is very helpful, but many parents chose not to do this.

15.2 For Professionals

15.2.1 How MRI Works

MRI uses the electromagnetic properties of the protons contained in the hydrogen nuclei. Hydrogen nuclei can absorb and re-emit radiofrequency (RF) energy when they are inside a magnetic field. As the newborn infant brain contains 92–95% water (by comparison, the adult brain contains 75%), and water contains two hydrogen atoms (and one oxygen atom), hydrogen is by far the most abundant chemical element in the newborn brain (also in the rest of the human body).

Inside the hydrogen nuclei, the proton is comparable to a tiny bar magnet (Fig. 15.2). MR scanners employ powerful magnets which produce a strong magnetic field such that the protons in the body align with that field—this is called longitudinal magnetization. The strength of the magnetic field is measured in tesla (T). Most clinical scanners are 1.5 or 3.0 T. The magnetic field produced by a 1.5 T scanner is 30,000 times stronger than the earth's magnetic field, and that of a 3.0 T scanner is twice as strong again [1]. In order to generate images, a radiofrequency (RF) current is then pulsed across the patient at an angle to the main alignment of the magnetic field, stimulating the protons to spin out of equilibrium, straining against the pull of the main magnetic field, and sending back their own RF energy, which is detected by the receiver—this is called transverse magnetization (see Fig. 15.2). When the RF field is turned off, the protons will realign again with the main magnet field. This process is then repeated many times, and the average time needed for realignment is known as the relaxation time. The relaxation time as well as the amount of energy released is different depending on the molecular structure of each tissue type. MR software uses mathematical formulas to convert this information to images [2].

The two ways of measuring the time it takes for the protons to realign with the magnetic field (relaxation times) are called T1 and T2 relaxation times. The information they provide is reflected in how much brightness or darkness we see in each area of the brain on MRI on T1- and T2-weighted images (Table 15.1).

T1 relaxation time. This depends on the rate at which protons realign with the magnetic field after the RF pulse has been turned off and is the time needed to reach 63% of the maximum longitudinal magnetization. T1 values depend on the strength of the magnetic field (i.e. units of Tesla) and on the type of tissue.

T2 relaxation time. The rate at which the transverse magnetization decreases 63% from its maximum value following the application of an RF pulse. T2 values also depend on the type of tissue, but less on the magnetic field strength.

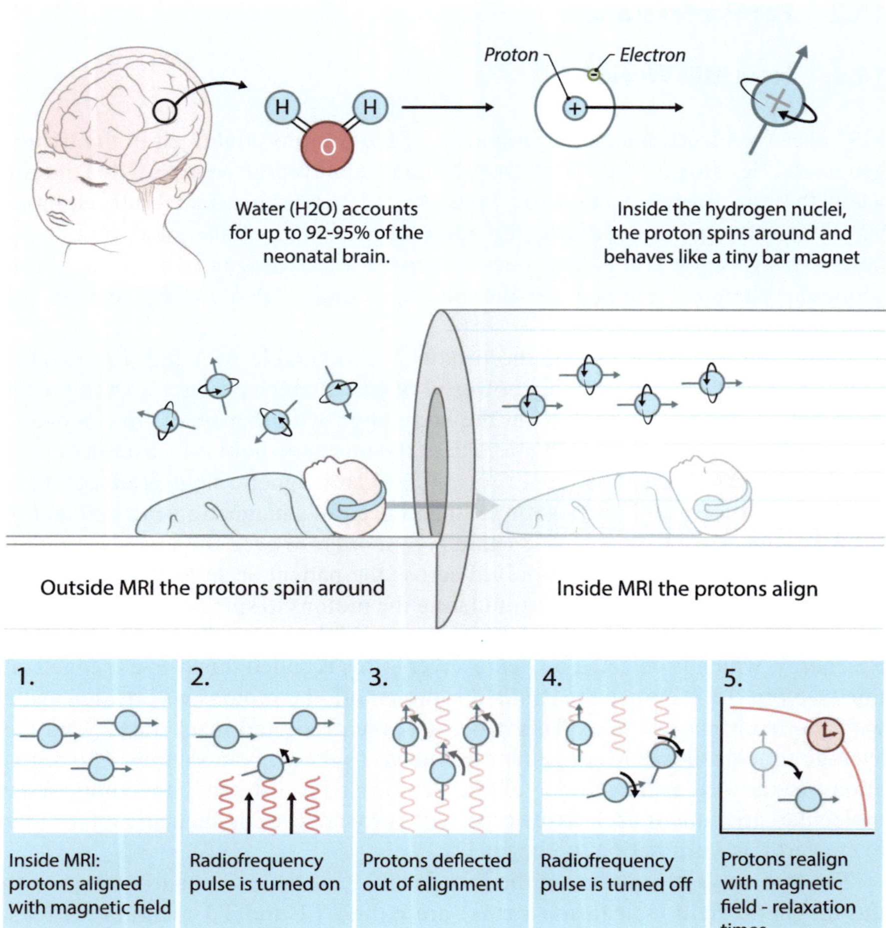

Fig. 15.2 This figure shows how the water molecules in the brain, which are always moving to different extents in different tissues, become aligned in a parallel fashion once the baby lies in the MR scanner. They are deflected from that alignment when the RF pulse is turned on and return to their original position once the RF pulse is turned off. The time it takes for this to happen as well as the amount of energy released is measured and varies depending on the molecular structure of each tissue type. (© Amanda Gautier-Ronopawiro)

15.2.2 MRI Sequences

MR images of the same tissue obtained using different sequences have different appearances giving complementary information. Each sequence has been designed for the optimal visualization of a specific region of the brain or type of lesion. The combination of several sequences optimizes the diagnostic and prognostic capacity of MRI. Almost all MRI examinations include three or more sequences. MRI units

Table 15.1 Appearance (brightness or darkness) of each area of the brain and type of lesion on T1- and T2-weighted images

	White	Gray	Black
T1	Fat Myelinated tissue Sub-acute parenchymal hemorrhage Acute and subacute extra-cerebral hemorrhage, Acute hypoxic-ischemic injury	Gray matter (GM) Unmyelinated white matter (WM) (darker than GM) Pus or debris in cysts or ventricles Germinal matrix	Fluid: CSF and watery fluid-filled cysts Air Bone
T2	Fluid: CSF and fluid-filled cysts Subacute parenchymal hemorrhage (10d–6w)	Fat Gray matter Unmyelinated WM (less dark than GM) Pus in cysts Germinal matrix	Air Myelinated WM (dark gray) Blood vessels Acute hypoxic-ischemic injury Acute and subacute (<10d) parenchymal hemorrhage

usually have pre-defined protocols (combination of sequences), for different ages and suspected conditions, although extra sequences can be added for an individual patient. When requesting an MRI, it is important to give the precise gestational age of the baby even for "term" infants as the brain matures considerably between 37 and 42 weeks and also their corrected age if they were born pre-term and also to mention whether a particular sequence might be helpful in the clinical circumstances. It is also important to provide all relevant clinical and sonographic information when requesting an MRI.

The immature brain has a higher water content and much less myelin than the brain at term age which in turn has much more water and less myelin than in young children of 2 years. A consequence of this is that relaxation times are much longer in newborns than later, and hence the time it takes to acquire images is also longer. It is very important that dedicated neonatal sequences and not standard protocols for adults or older children are used when imaging preterm and term infants; otherwise the image quality will be very poor [3]. It is also important that when calculating an infant's age (so that correct sequences are used), correction is made for prematurity. Another consequence of immaturity is that signal intensities are different in newborns compared to older children, e.g. gray matter on T2 is dark and becomes paler gray with age. Unmyelinated white matter is of high signal, i.e. whiter on T2, but when it myelinates it is dark. Hence neonatal images look very different to those of older children. Around 6 months post-term age as myelination is becoming more widespread, the signals in white and gray matter change, and there is a timepoint where the contrast between the two tissues is less than earlier and later.

The commonest sequences are called conventional MRI sequences: T1- and T2-weighted (W) images. T1-W and T2-W images are obtained using different times of repetition (TR) and times of echo (TE). TR is the time between the application of a RF excitation pulse and the start of the next RF pulse to the same area of tissue. The echo time is the time between the application of the RF pulse and the peak of the echo detected. TE and TR are parameters chosen aiming to maximize contrast between tissues. TR affects contrast on T1-W images; TE affects contrast on T2-W images.

T1-weighted images are obtained using short TR and short TE. On T1-weighted images, tissue containing fat is highlighted and white; clear fluid is dark.

T2-weighted images are obtained using long TR and long TE. On T2-weighted images, clear fluid is highlighted and white (Table 15.1).

Other sequences commonly used in neonatal brain imaging are as follows (see Table 15.2):

15.2.2.1 Diffusion-Weighted Imaging (DWI)

Acute areas of ischemia are seen as bright or high signal reflecting restricted diffusion of water in the tissue.

Normal white matter tracts show greater restricted diffusion in a direction near or at right angles to the tract and then down the length of the tracts where water is freer to move. Hence normal DW images vary depending on whether the direction in which the image is obtained is parallel to or at right angles to the orientation of the tract. This directional information is lost in injured or swollen tissue.

Apparent Diffusion Coefficient (ADC) maps combine the diffusion information obtained in different orientations, and areas of acutely injured or swollen tissue are seen as low signal or dark. From these images an ADC value can be measured; the lower the value, the more injured the tissue. ADC values differ between tissue types, with postmenstrual age and with the age of injury and between scanners (to some extent), so care needs to be taken in their interpretation.

DWI and ADC images are usually evaluated at the same time.

DWI and associated advanced MRI techniques are also used in research to measure the progression of connectivity and maturation in the white matter.

15.2.2.2 Other sequences

Susceptibility-weighted imaging (SWI) quantifies paramagnetic non-heme iron and is now a fairly standard sequence used to detect (small) hemorrhage (this can also be well seen on T2* gradient echo images, but SWI is more sensitive). SWI detects the accumulation of iron in otherwise normal-appearing white matter in infants after IVH and can show even very small punctate white matter lesions and cerebellar hemorrhages [4]. Although SWI images can depict the venous system and also detect calcifications, an MR venogram should also be done to better assess the venous system; and of note cUS is more sensitive for detecting calcifications. When assessing SWI images, the so-called blooming-artifact should be taken into account; this means that the size of a hemorrhage is exaggerated, appearing larger than it really is.

MR Angiography (MRA). These sequences assess blood flow in arteries and are mostly used when an arteriovenous malformation or an arterial obstruction (e.g. in stroke) is suspected. The moving blood in the vessel gives a different signal to the surrounding tissue.

Table 15.2 Summary of the general uses of different imaging sequences

	T1-W	T2-W	DWI and ADC	SWI	MRA/MRV	MRS
Good for	Anatomy, HI lesions, hemorrhage, early myelination	Anatomy, HI lesions, hemorrhage, WM maturity, migration disorders	Recent HI injury (in HIE, stroke, preterm acute WM injury), acute inflammation, assessment of maturation	Identifying hemorrhagic lesions; calcifications, and abnormal vessels	Visualizing arteries/blood flow in veins	HIE Metabolic diseases
How lesions are seen	Acute HI and hemorrhage—both bright (high SI)	Acute HI and acute hemorrhage—both dark (low SI)	Acute HI. Bright/high SI on DWI, low SI on ADC Hemorrhage is generally dark	Blood and vessels are seen as low SI (black)		Abnormal metabolites levels or ratios
When they are used	Used routinely in all conditions	Used routinely in all conditions	Used routinely in all conditions	Used routinely for suspected tissue, ventricular and extracerebral hemorrhage, and calcifications	Arterial hemorrhagic stroke/identifying CSVT Suspected vascular malformation	HIE and suspected metabolic diseases

ADC apparent diffusion coefficient, *CSVT* cerebral sinus venous thrombosis, *DWI* diffusion-weighted imaging, *HI* hypoxia-ischemia, *HIE* hypoxic-ischemic encephalopathy, *IVH* intraventricular hemorrhage, *MRI* magnetic resonance imaging, *MRS* magnetic resonance spectroscopy, *MRA/V* magnetic resonance arteriogram/venogram, *SWI* susceptibility-weighted imaging, *WM* white matter, *WMI* white matter injury

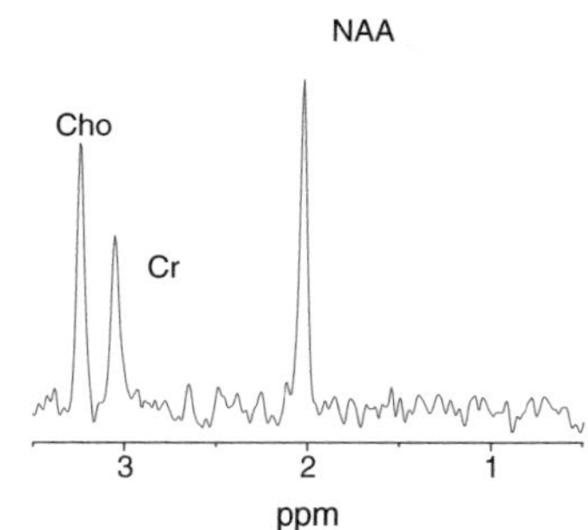

Fig. 15.3 Normal proton spectrum (TE 135) from the central gray matter in a newborn term infant. If lactate were present, it would be seen as a doublet peak at 1.3 ppm. *NAA* N-acetyl aspartate, *Cho* choline, *Cr* creatine, *ppm* parts per million

MR Venography (MRV). These sequences assess blood flow in the veins and are mainly used in neonates to visualize the absence of venous flow suggestive of venous thrombosis.

FLAIR (Fluid Attenuated Inversion Recovery) Images. This sequence is not much used in the neonatal period but can be useful to visualize scar tissue in the white matter a few weeks or months after acute lesions have occurred. It is much more commonly used in older children and adults.

MR Proton Spectroscopy (Fig. 15.3). MR information can also be depicted in a spectral form, giving data on some metabolites in the brain that are present and resonate near to the signal from water, though in much lower quantities. Such metabolites are N-acetyl aspartate (NNA), considered a neuronal marker which is involved in myelination; creatine, which is necessary for the regulation of energy supply and correlates with neuronal cell mass; total choline (marker of membrane turnover); myo-inositol (an osmolyte controlling fluid movement in the cell and hence ionic balance and a glial marker); and glutamate-glutamine (marker of neurogenesis and maturation) [5]. Lactate is a marker of hypoxia or energy failure [4]. MR proton spectroscopy provides useful information in hypoxic, metabolic, and neurodegenerative conditions.

MR phosphorous spectroscopy can also be done, giving more information about energy metabolites, but this is rarely clinically available.

15.2.3 Assessment of Brain Structures on Neonatal MRI

In this section we show illustrated diagrams of the three imaging planes used when presenting MRI brain scans (Fig. 15.4), detail anatomy in a mid-sagittal view (Fig. 15.5), the anatomy of the central gray matter, and corticospinal tracts as seen in different planes (Figs. 15.6, 15.7, and 15.8), the appearance of other brain structures on MRI (Figs. 15.9, 15.10, and 15.11), and differences in MRI signals in relation to infant prematurity (Fig. 15.12).

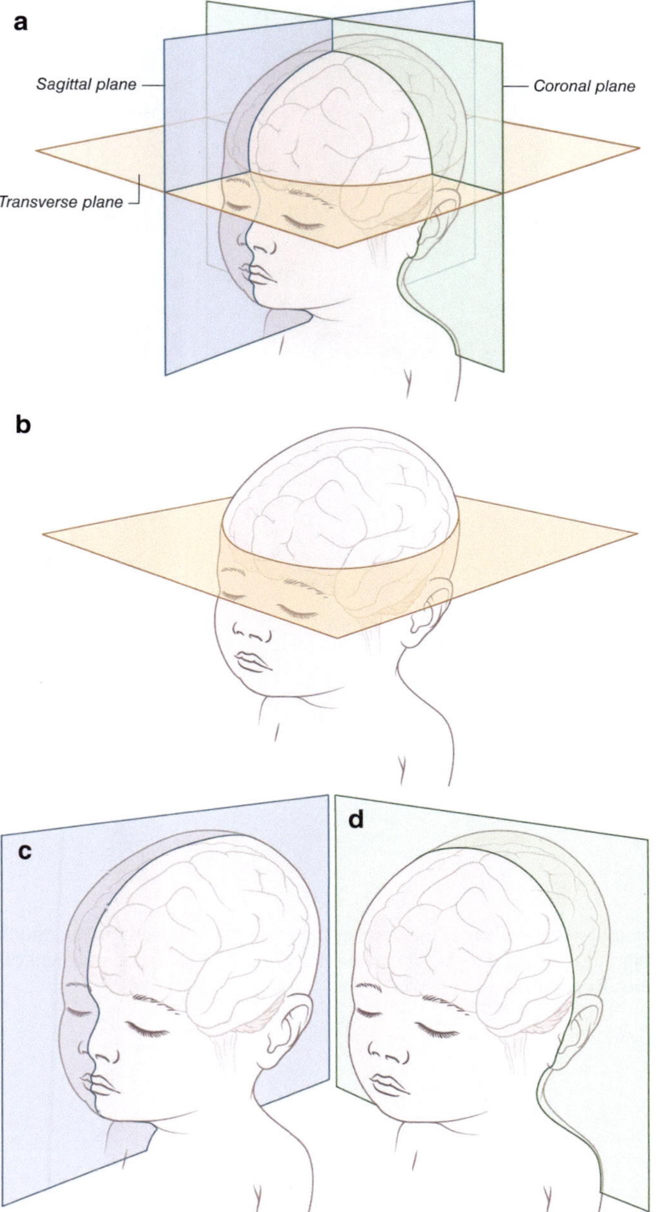

Fig. 15.4 (**a–d**) The MR scanner usually generates three orientations of the human brain
  – Coronal planes are in the direction shown by the green slice. The brain is seen from front to back
  – Transverse (also called axial or horizontal) planes are in the direction shown by the orange slice. The brain is seen from the top down
  – Sagittal and parasagittal planes are in the direction shown by the blue slice. The brain can be viewed in the midline and parallel to this from side to side
MR images in the axial and coronal planes are conventionally orientated with the left side on the right of the image and vice versa. (© Amanda Gautier-Ronopawiro)

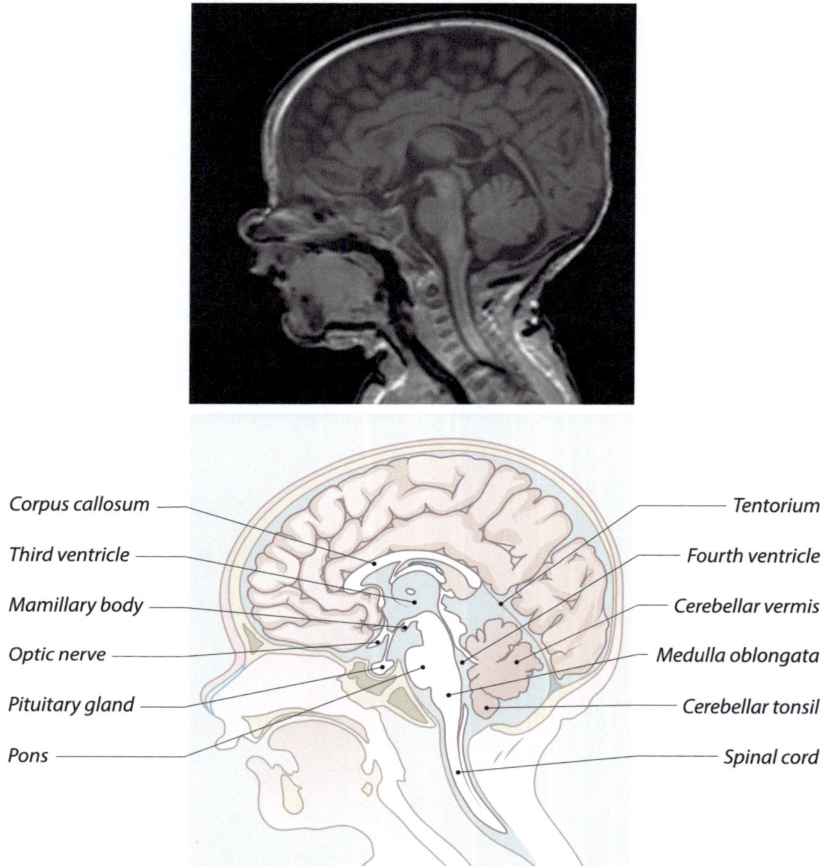

Fig. 15.5 The mid-sagittal plane is the one sagittal plane that is exactly in the middle of the brain dividing the brain into left and right. This plane is very useful for the assessment of anatomy. (© Amanda Gautier-Ronopawiro)

Fig. 15.6 (**a, b**) Basal ganglia and thalami (also called central gray matter): these structures are actively myelinating at term age and have a high-concentration of glutamate receptors and a high metabolic rate; they are therefore very vulnerable to acute hypoxia-ischemia around term age. The basal ganglia (made up of the caudate nucleus, putamen, and globus pallidus) and the thalami play an important role in motor control and coordination, learning, executive function, and behavior. *ALIC* anterior limb of internal capsule, *PLIC* posterior limb of internal capsule. (© Amanda Gautier-Ronopawiro)

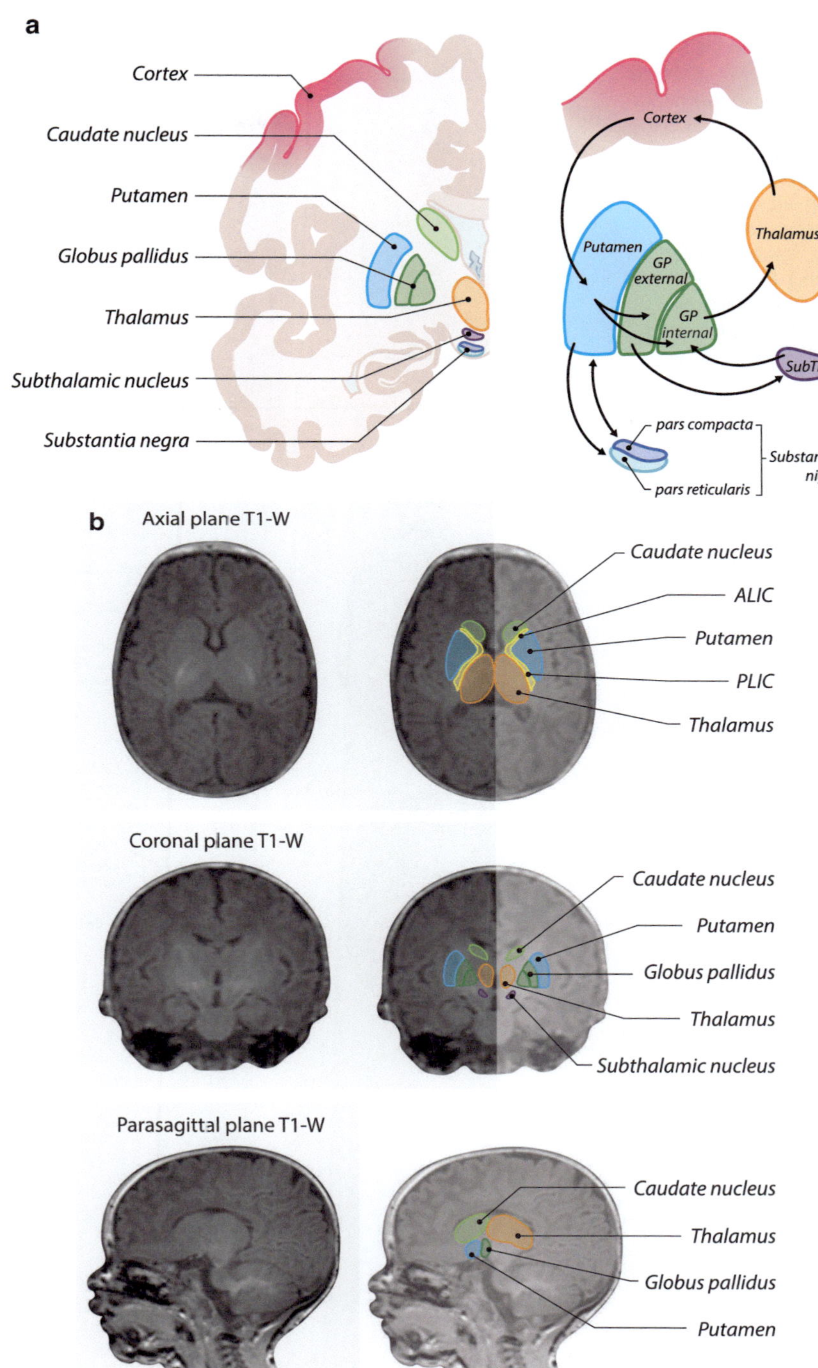
a
Cortex
Caudate nucleus
Putamen
Globus pallidus
Thalamus
Subthalamic nucleus
Substantia negra
Cortex
Thalamus
Putamen
GP external
GP internal
SubTh
pars compacta
pars reticularis
Substantia nigra
b
Axial plane T1-W
Caudate nucleus
ALIC
Putamen
PLIC
Thalamus
Coronal plane T1-W
Caudate nucleus
Putamen
Globus pallidus
Thalamus
Subthalamic nucleus
Parasagittal plane T1-W
Caudate nucleus
Thalamus
Globus pallidus
Putamen

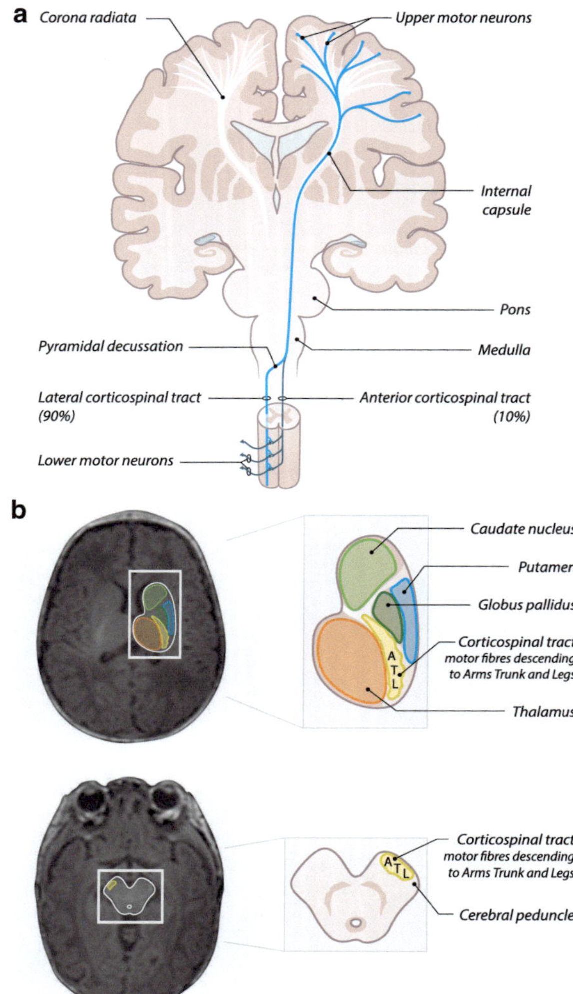

Fig. 15.7 (**a**) The corticospinal tract (CST) is the major pathway involved in voluntary movements: (**a**) gross motor movements (e.g. sitting, walking, running, jumping, riding, swimming) and (**b**) fine motor movements (e.g. writing, typing, drawing, cutting, threading, buttoning). (**b**) All of the corticospinal tract (CST) can be visualized on MRI. Two locations are especially important in neonatal neuroimaging and for prognostication: the posterior limb of the internal capsule (PLIC) at the level of the basal ganglia and the cerebral peduncles at the level of the midbrain. (© Amanda Gautier-Ronopawiro)

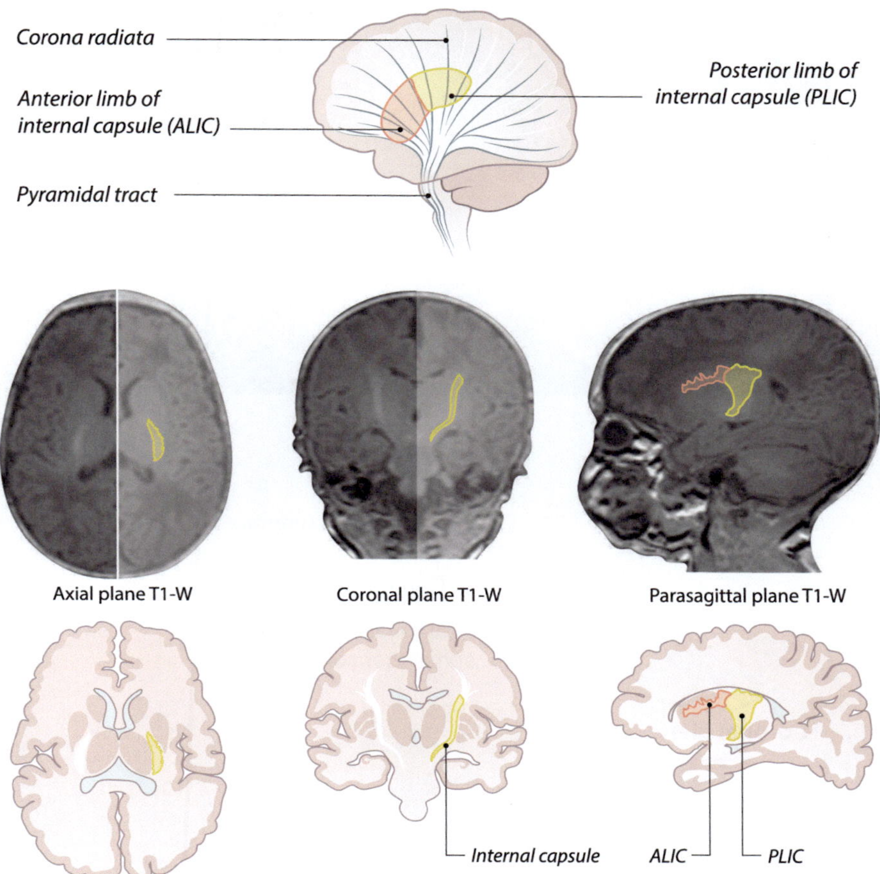

Fig. 15.8 Figure showing all tracts in the white matter converging in the anterior limb (ALIC) and posterior limb (PLIC) of the internal capsule. The PLIC can be seen in different planes, as shown here. Myelination of the PLIC starts around 32–35 weeks gestational age and can be seen on MRI from 36–38 weeks gestational age. Myelination of the ALIC starts later and is only seen from about 6 weeks post term age. (© Amanda Gautier-Ronopawiro)

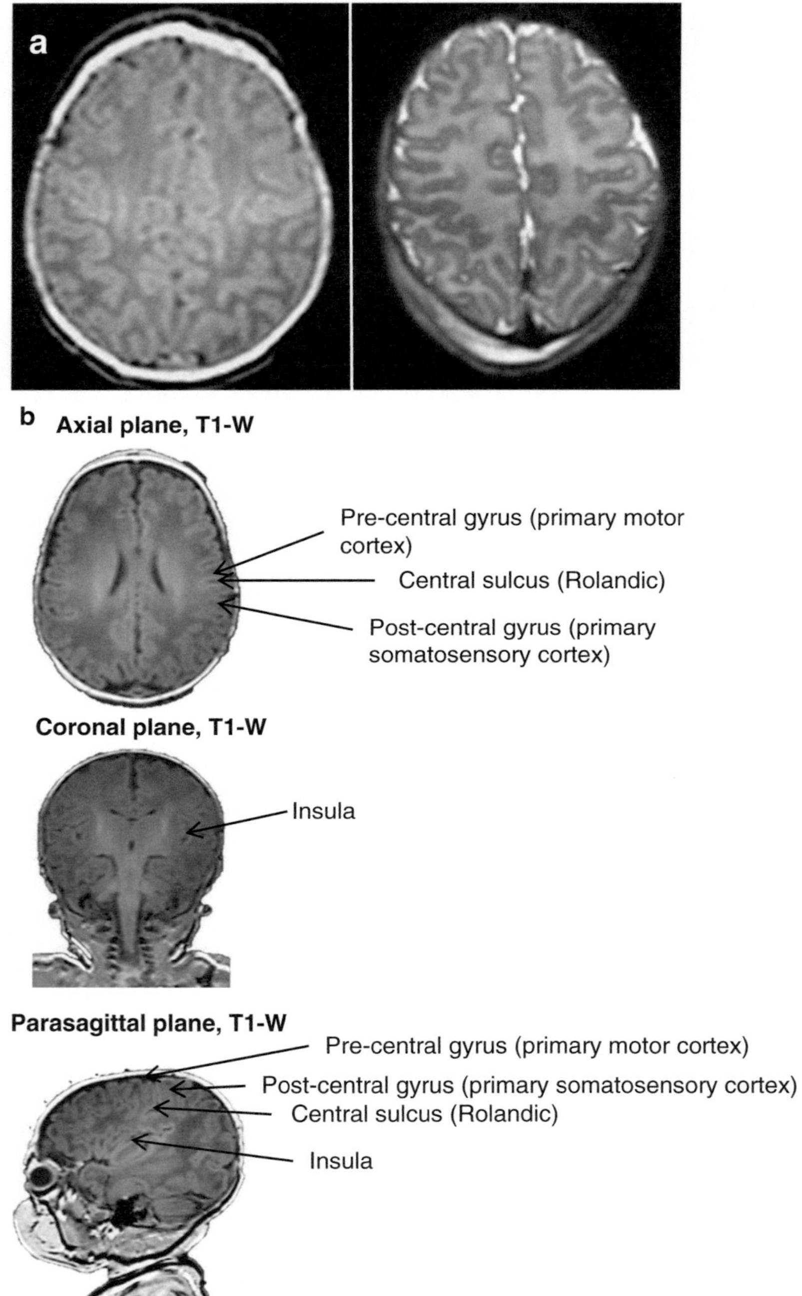

Fig. 15.9 (**a**) The neonatal cortex is of high SI (brighter than the white matter) on T1-W imaging (**a**, left image) and low SI (darker than the white matter) on T2-W imaging (**a**, **right image**). (**b**) Three cortical areas are especially important in the neonatal period, the perirolandic cortex, the insula, and the hippocampus, as all are highly susceptible to perinatal hypoxia-ischemia. The perirolandic cortex is the main origin of the corticospinal tract. Injury to this tract has a significant impact on motor outcomes.

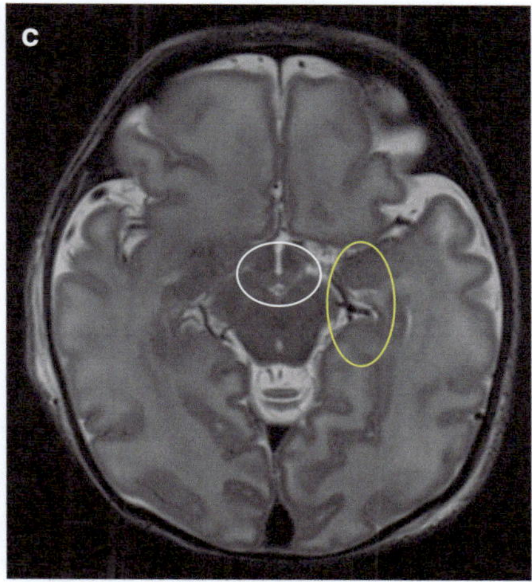

Fig. 15.9 (continued)   (c) Hippocampus and mammillary bodies. The hippocampus, located in the medial temporal lobe (shown in the yellow circle) is very vulnerable to hypoxic-ischemic stress, malnutrition, and steroids. The mammillary bodies, located centrally (in the red circle), at a similar level, are very vulnerable to hypoxia-ischemia. They both play a major role in learning and memory. To image the small mammillary bodies, thin 2mm T2-W axial slices are required and these should be added to the routine protocol for imaging an infant with HIE [6]

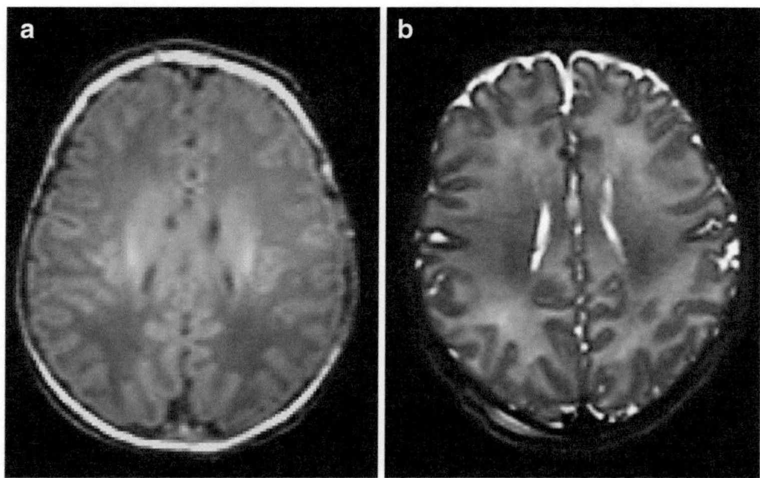

Fig. 15.10 In the neonatal period and until 6 months, unmyelinated white matter (WM) is seen as low SI (darker than cortex and the basal ganglia and thalami (BGT)) on T1-W (**a**) and high SI (brighter than cortex and the BGT) on T2-W (**b**). T1-W imaging is better for identification of myelinated tracts in WM, whereas T2-W imaging allows for better delineation between WM and gray matter and for the assessment of WM maturity. Advanced MRI techniques (volumetric MRI, diffusion-weighted imaging, diffusion tensor imaging, functional MRI) are being used in research studies to examine WM microstructure, maturation, and connectivity in preterm infants and infants with perinatal brain injury. These studies have shown a good correlation between these imaging markers and later cognitive and behavioral outcomes at a population level. However these population level values are not used at present to predict cognitive outcomes in individual patients in a clinical setting

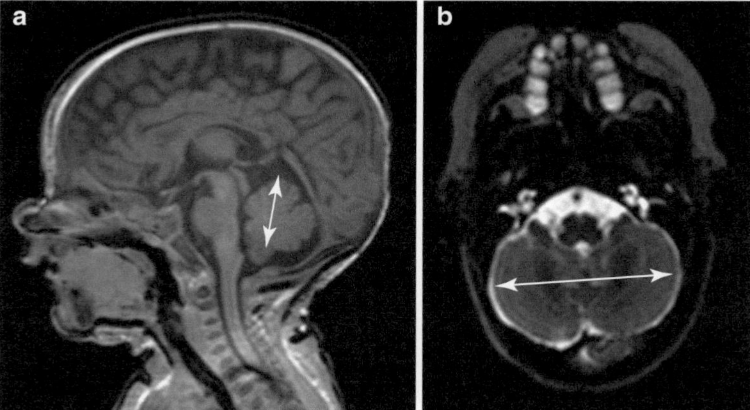

Fig. 15.11 Cerebellar hemorrhage and impaired cerebellar growth are not uncommon in preterm infants, and both conditions can be detected easily using MRI. Linear measures of the cerebellar vermis height (**a**) and the transverse cerebellar diameter (TCD, **b**) can be used to assess overall size and growth of the cerebellum. Mean vermis height at 40 weeks gestation is 23 mm; mean width (TCD) at 40 weeks gestation is 53 mm in term born infants

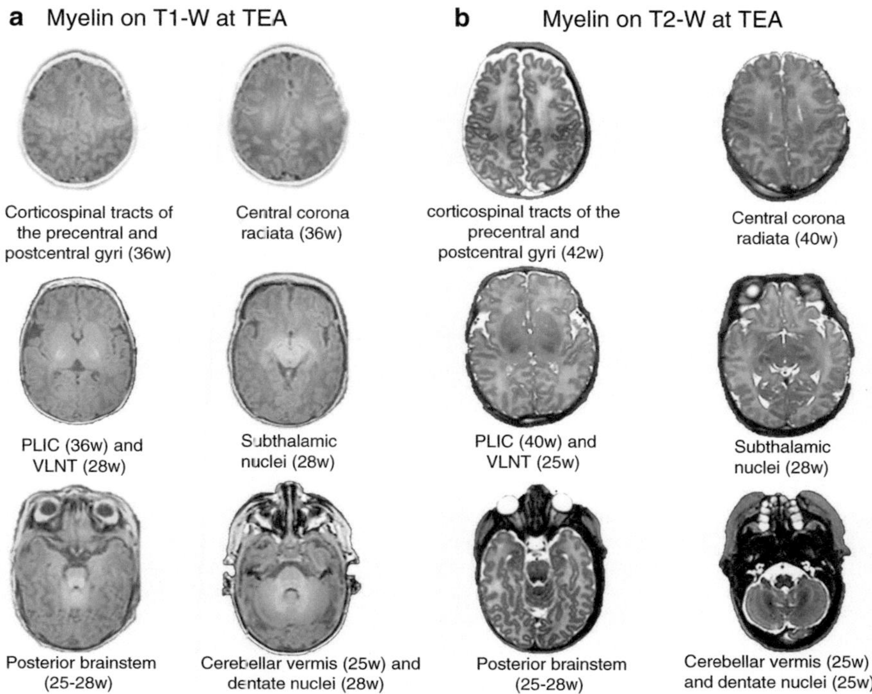

Fig. 15.12 Myelination at term age: myelin is seen as high SI (white or brighter than cortex) on T1-W images mainly because of accumulation of fat and as low SI (black or darker than cortex) on T2-W images mainly because of loss of water. Myelin in white matter (WM) tracts is better visualized on T1-W imaging, whereas myelin in gray matter is better visualized on T2-W imaging. Myelination progresses from bottom to top, from posterior to anterior, and from deep structures to superficial ones. Myelination is seen histologically before being seen on MRI. Myelin can be seen on MRI from the 20th postmenstrual week in the posterior brainstem (lower) tracts

15.2.4 Clinical Indications of MRI (Table 15.3)

Table 15.3 Clinical Indications of Neonatal MRI

	Role in diagnosis	Role in prognosis	Optimal timing
Neonatal HIE	Identify patterns of injury consistent with acute HI and support clinical diagnosis Identify conditions additional to HIE Identify metabolic conditions that may masquerade as or co-exist with HIE Identify prenatal or established injury and aid timing of acute injury	Excellent in prediction of motor impairment and its severity Rather good for predicting visual and cognitive impairment	DWI-ADC: 1–6 days from acute injury T1 and T2 from day 2 but injury not fully seen still later in 1–2 weeks Best to perform soon after re-warming when DW changes should still be well seen.
Neonatal arterial ischemic infarction	Confirms diagnosis Defines infarcted area Aids timing the onset of stroke MRA can show arterial changes (occlusion, stenosis, absent branches, focal flow defect, increased distal flow)	Excellent in the prediction of hemiplegia Good for predicting minor motor dysfunction, visual, cognitive, and language impairment, and later epilepsy	DWI-ADC: 1 (from birth or onset of symptoms)–6 days T1 and T2 from days 1–2 Best to perform 1–6 days after the event
Cerebral sinus venous thrombosis (CSVT)	MRV can show decreased venous flow, sometimes intraluminal clots (confirm absent flow with Doppler ultrasound) MRI identifies associated parenchymal abnormalities	Depends on the associated parenchymal lesions	Early (first week) to decide if anticoagulant treatment (LMWH) is needed After first week to delineate parenchymal lesions
Premature infants	Confirms or excludes lesions seen on cUS Shows punctate lesions in white matter and/or cerebellum Shows maturation and myelination of the white matter Shows sequelae of preterm birth on brain development in infants with and without major lesions	Excellent for prediction of motor, cognitive, and visual outcomes in infants with major WM lesions Not yet for individual cognitive prognosis in the absence of major WM lesions Assessment of BGT lesions in HIE and stroke has similar predictive value to that in term infants	Any time in the neonatal period when: – Suspicion that WM injury cannot be fully delineated by cUS alone – Suspected underlying or concomitant condition – Redirection of care considered At term-equivalent age (TEA) to assess growth and myelination and evolution of previous lesions If 1 MRI is done, TEA is the preferred moment

(continued)

Table 15.3 (continued)

	Role in diagnosis	Role in prognosis	Optimal timing
Neonatal seizures of unknown origin (excluding HIE and stroke)	Along with cUS, can help to identify underlying cause	Depends on the underlying cause	As soon as possible, to identify potential treatable conditions Include MRA and MRV to rule out AV malformations and CSVT
Meningitis	Identifies pattern and severity of injury—Can suggest likely pathogen Identifies associated complications	Useful for predicting outcomes depending on the site of lesions but not as definitive and with less available data than for HIE and stroke	Early: To decide if surgery for hydrocephalus or cyst drainage is required; to help to decide duration of antibiotic therapy After the acute phase: To help to predict motor and cognitive outcomes
Congenital infections	Identifies pattern and severity of injury and associated developmental abnormality typical of specific pathogens	Good in the prediction of outcomes after congenital CMV Not so well described in other congenital infections	At any moment in the neonatal period Fetal MRI if prenatal diagnosis
Congenital malformations	Identifies type and severity of malformation	Depends on the specific malformation	At any moment in the neonatal period Fetal MRI if prenatal US suggestive
Metabolic disorders	Can show abnormalities suggestive or pathognomonic of some specific inborn errors of metabolism (note calcium and small cysts not as well seen on MRI as on cUS)	Depends on the specific disorder	As soon as the condition is suspected, to identify potentially treatable disorders
Congenital heart disease (CHD)	Can identify associated abnormal brain development and fetal and postnatally acquired brain injury, especially if performed pre- and post-surgery	Prognosis depends on the combination of brain development + type and extent of brain lesion + systemic factors associated with heart disease	Whenever there are abnormal neurological signs, dysmorphic features, known genetic anomalies associated with brain abnormalities, or signs of parenchymal injury on cUS Pre- and post-operative MRI should be considered in infants with critical CHD[a]

ADC apparent diffusion coefficient, *AV* arterio-venous, *CHD* congenital heart disease, *CMV* cytomegalovirus, *CSVT* cerebral sinus venous thrombosis, *cUS* cranial ultrasound, *DWI* diffusion-weighted imaging, *HI* hypoxia-ischemia, *HIE* hypoxic-ischemic encephalopathy, *LMWH* low-molecular-weight heparin, *IVH* intraventricular hemorrhage, *MRA/V* magnetic resonance arteriogram/venogram, *MRI* magnetic resonance imaging, *MRS* magnetic resonance spectroscopy, *SWI* susceptibility-weighted imaging, *TEA* term-equivalent age, *WM* white matter, *WMI* white matter injury

[a]British Association of Perinatal Medicine. Fetal and Neonatal Brain Magnetic Resonance Imaging: Clinical Indications, Acquisitions and Reporting—A Framework for Practice, 2023. Available at: https://hubble-live-assets.s3.amazonaws.com/bapm/file_asset/file/53/BAPM_MRI_standards_for_fetal_neonatal_brain_imaging_FINAL_SUBMISSION_080216.pdf

References

1. Currie S, Hoggard N, Craven IJ, Hadjivassiliou M, Wilkinson ID. Understanding MRI: basic MR physics for physicians. Postgrad Med J. 2013;89(1050):209–23. https://doi.org/10.1136/postgradmedj-2012-131342. Epub 2012 Dec 7
2. Bitar R, Leung G, Perng R, Tadros S, Moody AR, Sarrazin J, McGregor C, Christakis M, Symons S, Nelson A, Roberts TP. MR pulse sequences: what every radiologist wants to know but is afraid to ask. Radiographics. 2006;26(2):513–37. https://doi.org/10.1148/rg.262055063.
3. Rutherford M, Malamateniou C, Zeka J, Counsell S. MR imaging of the neonatal brain at 3 Tesla. Eur J Paediatr Neurol. 2004;8(6):281–9. https://doi.org/10.1016/j.ejpn.2004.08.003.
4. Dubois J, Alison M, Counsell SJ, Hertz-Pannier L, Hüppi PS, Benders MJNL. MRI of the neonatal brain: a review of methodological challenges and neuroscientific advances. J Magn Reson Imaging. 2021;53(5):1318–43. https://doi.org/10.1002/jmri.27192. Epub 2020 May 18. PMID: 32420684; PMCID: PMC8247362
5. Robertson NJ, Cox IJ. Magnetic resonance spectroscopy of the neonatal brain. In: Rutherford MA, editor. On MRI of the neonatal brain. W.B. Saunders; 2002. Available at: https://www.mrineonatalbrain.com/ch04-16.php.
6. Lequin MH, Steggerda SJ, Severino M, Tortora D, Parodi A, Ramenghi LA, Groenendaal F, Meys KME, Benders MJNL, de Vries LS, Vann SD. Mammillary body injury in neonatal encephalopathy: a multicentre, retrospective study. Pediatr Res 2022;92(1):174–9.

Neurophysiological Monitoring

16

Mohamed El-Dib and Linda S. de Vries

Abbreviations

aEEG	Amplitude-integrated EEG
ASM	Anti-seizure medications
BS	Burst suppression
C	Continuous
cEEG	Conventional EEG
CHD	Congenital heart disease
CNS	Central nervous system
DC	Discontinuous
ECMO	Extracorporeal membrane oxygenation
FT	Flat trace
IVH	Intraventricular hemorrhage
LV	Low voltage
NICU	Neonatal intensive care unit
PPHN	Persistent pulmonary hypertension of the neonate
SWC	Sleep wake cycling

M. El-Dib (✉)
Neonatal Neurocritical Care, Department of Pediatrics, Division of Newborn Medicine, Brigham and Women's Hospital, Boston, MA, USA

Department of Pediatrics, Harvard Medical School, Boston, MA, USA
e-mail: mel-dib@bwh.harvard.edu

L. S. de Vries
Department of Neonatology, University Medical Center Utrecht (UMCU), Utrecht, The Netherlands

Department Pediatrics, Division Neonatology, Willem Alexander's Children Hospital, Leiden University Medical Center (LUMC), Leiden, The Netherlands
e-mail: l.s.de_vries@lumc.nl

© The Author(s) 2024
G. Meijler, K. Mohammad (eds.), *Neonatal Brain Injury*,
https://doi.org/10.1007/978-3-031-55972-3_16

16.1 For Parents

16.1.1 What Is EEG

An EEG is a test that measures the brain electric activity. It monitors the brain's electrical waves similar to how an EKG monitors the heart's electrical rhythm.

16.1.2 What Are the Types of EEG Devices?

aEEG (amplitude integrated EEG) or the brain monitor is a bedside tool that is usually applied by NICU nurses and physicians to give an overview of brain electric activity over time. It needs a limited number of electrodes (2–4).

cEEG (conventional EEG) needs more training to place many electrodes on your baby's head using a special glue. The cEEG machine usually also has a video camera, so your baby's brain waves and movements can be recorded simultaneously. If there are abnormal brain waves, the doctors can see whether, if any, abnormal movements happened at the same time.

16.1.3 Why Is My Baby on the EEG Device?

The main reasons why an infant needs an EEG monitor are as follows:

1. To check the presence of neonatal seizures. Seizures are abnormal brain activities that are sometimes associated with shaking or stiffening of limbs, staring, and unresponsiveness. But most neonatal seizures are silent, which means that they don't cause symptoms or only cause very subtle symptoms that can also be ascribed to other problems. Therefore, most seizures can only be detected by EEG. In addition, since babies do a lot of shaking movements that are not seizures, having an EEG to confirm if these movements are seizures is very important.
2. To look at the general activity of the brain and to assess the presence of encephalopathy: a general term for abnormal brain function. Such assessment can help decide which baby needs therapy, e.g., body cooling, and if treated, EEG can help monitor the recovery of brain activity.
3. To evaluate the overall health of the brain, especially in high-risk conditions, e.g., complicated birth, infection of the central nervous system, intracranial bleeding, or other serious conditions.

16.1.4 How Is it Applied?

This is done by attaching small electrodes to the baby's scalp. The electrodes can take different forms, which include disks attached by paste or glue, hydrogel stickers, or thin needles which are inserted into the skin. These electrodes are connected to a box that can record the baby's brain activity. Sometimes a cap is used, with the electrodes built into it. This is especially helpful when using many electrodes (Fig. 16.1).

Fig. 16.1 Demonstration of EEG application: (**a**) aEEG 5 hydrogel electrodes and (**b**) cEEG cap. (© Amanda Gautier-Ronopawiro)

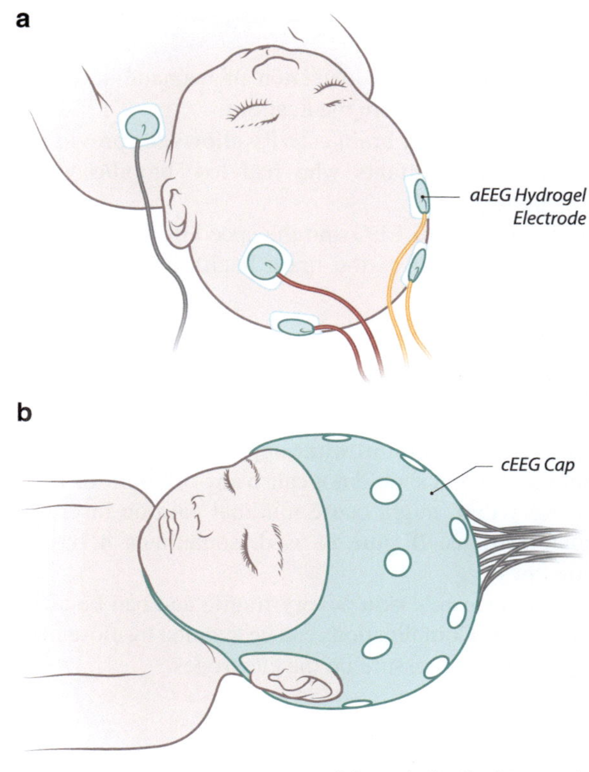

16.1.5 What Is Normal

The expectation of EEG in term infants is to be "continuous" which means there are no pauses in electric activity. In addition, the EEG should be of good voltage and symmetric on both brain halves. Also, EEG should be able to detect changes during sleep. A normal sleep-wake cycle on the EEG suggests a healthy brain.

When EEG is done in preterm babies, it should be compared to EEG of infants born at the same gestational age. It is normal for EEG of preterm babies to be "discontinuous," which means there are short periods of low voltage. These periods become shorter as infants advance in gestational age.

16.1.6 How Will the Reading Affect Management?

1. Accurate and fast detection of neonatal seizures allows for the early start of proper anti-seizure medications.
2. Assessment of brain activity allows for providing proper treatment, e.g., body cooling in infants who had low blood/oxygen reaching the brain around delivery.
3. Evaluation of EEG and the speed of recovery allow the doctors to understand the condition of the brain health and to be able to predict the outcome of the baby.

16.1.7 Does EEG Cause Complications?

Apart from discomfort while applying the EEG electrodes, EEG monitoring itself is not painful and should not cause any discomfort. If needles are used, these needles are very thin, might cause minimal pain on insertion only, and typically have no complications. If glue is used, sometimes it has an intense smell that rapidly goes away.

The neonate's skin is very fragile and can be affected by the attachment of the electrodes. Complications can be avoided by close monitoring of the skin and avoiding excessive pressure on the electrodes.

16.2   For Professionals

16.2.1   General EEG Principles

EEG allows for detecting cortical cerebral electric activity using electrodes applied to the scalp. Although the conventional EEG (cEEG) implies applying 21 electrodes according to the International 10–20 System, in neonates 9 electrodes can be used, and this is sufficient to characterize the neonatal EEG [1]. In the NICU, EEG is often displayed at the bedside as a simplified, time-compressed trend called amplitude-integrated EEG (aEEG). Stand-alone aEEG systems use fewer electrodes (typically three to five) to facilitate easy application and use. With aEEG, visual inspection of the raw or source EEG recording is essential for confirming aEEG findings. For clarity in this paper, we will use "aEEG" when referring to aEEG trends and their source EEG signals and "cEEG" when referring to multichannel conventional EEG recordings.

cEEG tracings show different morphologies in waveform, amplitude (μV), and frequency (Hz). EEG waveforms are classified by frequency into four types: delta (<4 Hz), theta (4–7 Hz), alpha (8–13 Hz), and Beta (>13 Hz).

Analysis of cEEG tracings includes evaluation of three main components: the background, sleep-wake cycling, and the presence of specific patterns. The cEEG background is distinguished based on the continuity of electrical activity into continuous or discontinuous patterns. Cycling between sleep and wakefulness and differentiation between the two sleep states (quiet sleep and active sleep) are maturational characteristics that can be evaluated in the neonatal cEEG. Finally, specific patterns and characteristics have been shown to play a role in detecting brain functional and metabolic state, degree of maturation, response to ischemia, seizures, and neurologic outcome in neonates [2–4].

Abnormal cEEG features can present either in the form of electrical excitability as seen in seizures or in the form of electrical depression and flat tracings. Thus, the cEEG tracing provides a wide range of information about the neurological integrity of the brain. The American Clinical Neurophysiology Society (ACNS) has published guidelines for the use and standardization of terminology of neonatal cEEG [5, 6].

aEEG is complimentary to cEEG and has the advantage of being easier to apply and to interpret by non-neurophysiologists. aEEG gives an overview of trends in cerebral activity (including recovery from injury) and easy identification of sleep-wake cycling and can screen for seizures [7–10]. aEEG emphasizes the amplitude of the EEG signal as its central feature. In this technique, the "raw" EEG signal is significantly processed and filtered and then presented in a highly compressed time scale, typically at a rate of 6 cm/h. Thus, a full minute of EEG is represented by only a single millimeter of aEEG display. It allows for longer trend recording as fewer electrodes are more easily maintained, and the compressed time scale enables ease of interpretation. However, aEEG has limitations, including lower sensitivity for detecting seizures and increased susceptibility to artifacts as compared to cEEG.

Fig. 16.2 Common classification used to describe aEEG tracing, especially in term infants: continuous (C) with SWC, discontinuous (DC), burst suppression (BS), low voltage (LV), and inactive, flat trace (FT)

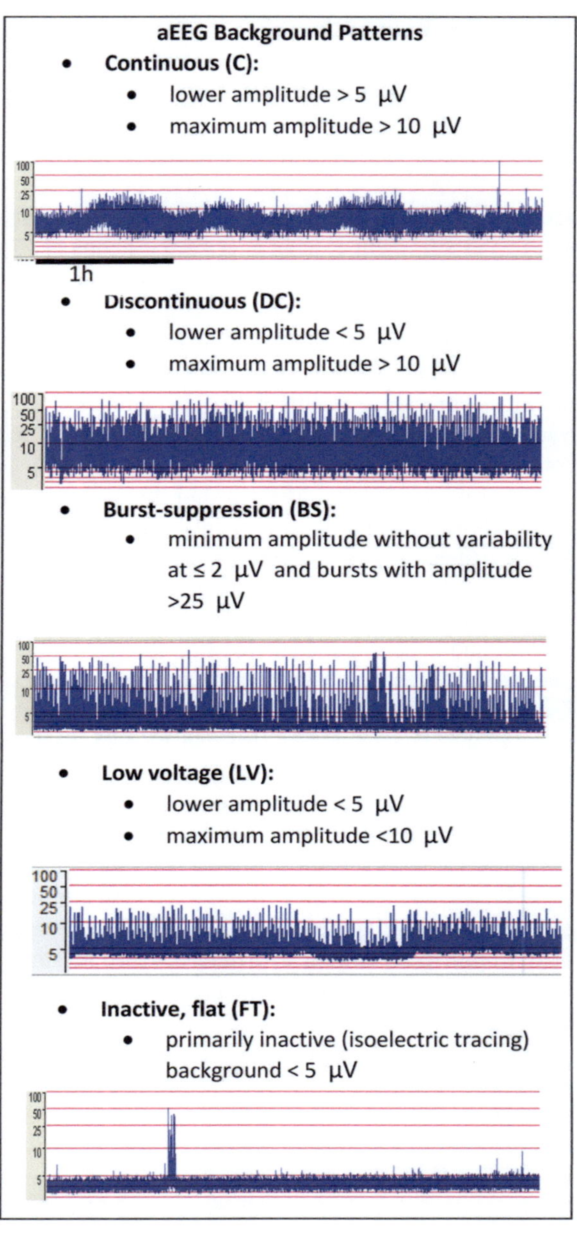

The most commonly used system for aEEG interpretation and classification uses visual pattern recognition to classify aEEG into five distinct patterns. These patterns are continuous (C), discontinuous (DC), burst suppression (BS), low voltage (LV), and inactive or flat (FT) [11] (Fig. 16.2).

Table 16.1 Examples of high-risk clinical scenarios eligible for cEEG monitoring

- Clinical syndrome of acute neonatal encephalopathy
- Cardiac or pulmonary risks for acute brain injury and clinical encephalopathy
- Congenital heart defects requiring early surgery using cardiopulmonary bypass
- CNS infection
- CNS trauma
- Inborn errors of metabolism (suspected or confirmed)
- Perinatal stroke (suspected or confirmed)
- Sinovenous thrombosis (suspected or confirmed)
- Premature infants with additional risk factors
- Genetic/syndromic disease involving CNS

Adopted from [5]

16.2.2 Indications of Use of Continuous EEG in the NICU

The American Clinical Neurophysiology Society has published guidelines for the use of continuous EEG in infants [5] (Table 16.1).

16.2.3 Value of Continuous EEG in the NICU

While initial EEG work relied on brief (30–60 min) EEG recordings, longer recording (hours to days) is essential for more accurate identification of seizures and can provide real-time information regarding changes in brain function [12, 13]. The use of continuous EEG monitoring in the NICU has been associated with better identification of seizures, timely initiation of anti-seizure medications (ASM), reduction in progression to status epilepticus, decrease of seizure burden, reduction in use of ASM, shortening of length of NICU stay, and reduction of discharge on ASM [14–18].

16.2.4 EEG in Neonatal Seizures

Basic science data show that electrographic-only seizures contribute to neonatal brain injury [19, 20]. Early recognition of electroclinical phenotypes, such as the channelopathies, allows for targeted treatment and guides diagnostic approaches [21, 22]. Optimal seizure detection may increase ASM efficacy, since seizures stop more easily when treated earlier [23, 24]. Moreover, studies suggest that seizure burden is independently associated with worse neurodevelopmental outcomes and that minimizing seizure burden may improve these outcomes [18, 25–27].

16.2.4.1 cEEG Is the Gold Standard for Diagnosing Seizures in Neonates

Clinical diagnosis of seizures in critically ill infants is insufficient because the majority of seizures are electrographic only [28–32]. In addition, ASM can cause electroclinical uncoupling, in which clinical signs of seizures are suppressed even as electrographic seizures continue [33, 34].

Prolonged cEEG monitoring, rather than a brief 60-min recording, is needed to capture seizures because an abnormal or normal background or interictal activity cannot confirm or exclude a diagnosis of seizures. Once seizures are detected, cEEG monitoring should be continued for at least 24 h after the last seizure [5].

16.2.4.2 aEEG for the Detection of Neonatal Seizures

While aEEG can detect seizures, it is less sensitive and specific than cEEG. Fewer than half of all seizures are detected when only the aEEG trend is inspected [35–37]. However, when the accompanying limited channel source EEG is inspected along with the aEEG trend by highly experienced users, 76% of seizures [38] and up to 80–90% of patients with seizures [35, 37] may be identified. Having access to a seizure detection algorithm further improves the ability to detect neonatal seizures [38].

aEEG has limited ability to adequately characterize neonatal seizures due to numerous factors. First, aEEG is a very compressed trend: in standard displays, each millimeter of aEEG represents up to a minute of recording. Very brief seizures are thus not easily seen. In addition, by definition aEEG is dependent on changes in amplitude, so it is more likely to miss low-voltage seizures. In contrast to aEEG, cEEG is capable of detecting brief (<30 s) and low-amplitude seizures [36, 38–40]. Also, aEEG typically has very few EEG electrodes, which may limit ability to record focal seizures in all brain regions [41]. Sensitivity is also impacted by placement of the aEEG electrode. Since the majority of neonatal seizures originate from central and temporal regions, they might not be detected by frontally placed leads [35, 37]. The generally recommended aEEG leads placement should be biparietal (P3-P4) if one channel is used and preferably parieto-central if two channels are used (C3-P3 and C4-P4). An alternative for the two channels is to use fronto-parietal channels (F3-P3 and F4-P4). Finally, it's worth noting that the accuracy of interpreting aEEG readings relies heavily on the clinician's level of experience. Using statistical modeling, improved utility of aEEG for neonatal seizure screening was demonstrated when used in highest risk population and interpreted by an expert [42]. aEEG is a better alternative to relying solely on clinical assessment when cEEG is unavailable for diagnosing neonatal seizures [27]. It can also serve as a screening tool while waiting for cEEG to become available. Moreover, displaying the aEEG trend alongside cEEG recording at the bedside can aid NICU care providers in promptly detecting seizures.

16.2.5 EEG in Neonatal Encephalopathy

16.2.5.1 aEEG in Neonatal Encephalopathy

aEEG is used as a bedside tool in infants with neonatal encephalopathy (NE) to identify and classify the severity of encephalopathy and to inform prognostication. In infants with encephalopathy not undergoing hypothermia treatment, an abnormal aEEG pattern predicts adverse neurodevelopmental outcome within 3–12 h of birth [43–47]. The predictive value of aEEG improves when combined with clinical examination [45]. While aEEG has been included in the criteria for some hypothermia trials as evidence of encephalopathy [48, 49], its use as an entry criterion has been challenged [50]. The predictive values of aEEG patterns differ based on whether an infant received hypothermia. At 6 h after birth, an abnormal aEEG pattern has a sensitivity of 95–96% and specificity of 39–61% for predicting death and moderate/severe disability in the setting of hypothermia, compared to sensitivity of 84% and a specificity of 79% in normothermia [51, 52]. The altered predictive value of an early abnormal aEEG trace is expected since hypothermia modifies/improves the outcome. This high sensitivity supports the use of aEEG as a screening tool to identify those at risk for poor outcomes who warrant hypothermia treatment. However, an early normal aEEG should still be used cautiously since 20% of infants may experience worsening of the aEEG between 3 and 6 h [47] and the negative predictive value of a normal aEEG at 6 h is only 77% [51]. Therefore, proper aEEG monitoring for at least 6 h of life, or even further, is crucial for screening for encephalopathy.

In the pre-hypothermia era, aEEG background recovery within 24 h was associated with a favorable outcome [53], and the onset of sleep-wake cycling (SWC) before 36 h correlated with good neurological outcomes [54]. The positive predictive value of aEEG background changes over the course of hypothermia; aEEG background may gradually improve over the first 48–72 h of cooling [55–57]. The predictive value of an abnormal aEEG is highest at 72 h of life in cooled infants, compared to 36 h, in non-cooled infants [52]. In cooled infants, PPV increases from 66% at 24 h to 85% at 48 h and 89% at 72 h [51]. These findings underscore the importance of monitoring infants throughout the duration of cooling and rewarming to understand the trajectory of recovery or absence of recovery of background over time. Moreover, aEEG can continue to monitor for potential seizures through rewarming especially when cEEG is discontinued after 24 h (see below).

16.2.5.2 cEEG in Neonatal Encephalopathy

Visual review of the cEEG signal is important for neuromonitoring in neonatal encephalopathy. Analyzing the full cEEG offers a more thorough assessment of grading, prognosis, and regional findings like seizures or focal injuries, compared to just observing the aEEG trend. Perinatal brain injury is associated with initial suppression, followed by seizures at around 6–15 h, and finally gradual improvement of background activity after 3 days [58]. These EEG features can help determining the timing and severity of brain injury [59, 60].

Early EEG is a reliable predictor of outcome in neonatal encephalopathy [61]. Without hypothermia, an abnormal cEEG at around 9 h of life can identify infants with abnormal outcomes [62], but the best predictive ability is around 24 h of life [63]. In those who receive therapeutic hypothermia, the greatest prognostic value of cEEG background is even later (48 h after birth) [32]. Similar to aEEG, the trajectory or evolution of the EEG background needs to be followed over time.

There is notable variability in the visual interpretation of cEEG background [64]. This points to the need for consensus training, improved classification systems, and development of clinically applicable automated analysis algorithms. cEEG backgrounds of highest predictive value include burst suppression, low voltage, and inactive trace [65]. Similar to aEEG, sleep-wake cycling on cEEG is a valuable

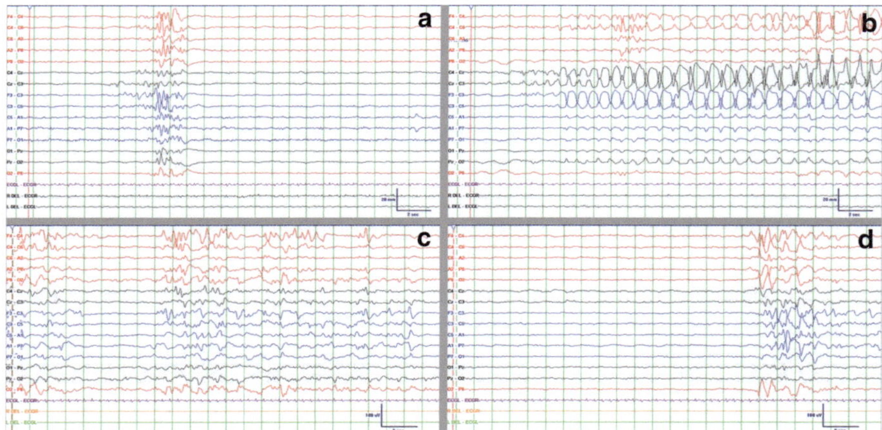

Fig. 16.3 cEEG at age 2 days with (**a**) markedly discontinuous background activity (interburst intervals up to 40 s) and absent sleep-wake cycling, consistent with severe NE. In addition, frequent seizures occurred; here (**b**) starting from the mid to left central region. (**c**) EEG at age 10 days has improved with nearly continuous background activity in wakefulness (interburst intervals up to 5 s), but in sleep (**d**) interburst intervals are still very long (up to 20 s). At day 10, there are still no normal graphoelements seen, and there remains abnormal sleep-wake cycling, which indicates poor neurodevelopmental prognosis. (From: El-Dib et al. [13] with permission)

marker for prognosis: a well-developed sleep-wake cycle at 6–12 h of age predicts a normal outcome, while its absence at 48 h is a poor prognostic sign [63, 66]. Finally, a high seizure burden, and not necessarily presence of seizures, is associated with adverse outcome [26, 67, 68]. A comprehensive assessment that includes all cEEG features could be the most valuable [69].

An example of cEEG over time for a neonate with NE is demonstrated in Fig. 16.3.

For infants who are at a high risk of seizures, including those with neonatal encephalopathy, it is recommended to conduct cEEG monitoring for at least 24 h. This enables the detection of seizures and helps in determining the prognosis [5]. Additionally, infants undergoing therapeutic hypothermia should be monitored during both therapeutic hypothermia and rewarming, as there is a potential risk of seizures in the rewarming phase [70–73]. However, it has been suggested that normal/mildly abnormal cEEG during the first 24 h of therapeutic hypothermia indicates a very low risk of subsequent seizures [71, 74].

16.2.6 EEG in Preterm Infants

Nowadays, the focus in caring for extremely premature babies is on optimizing their long-term neurodevelopment. Although not primary neurologic disorders, complications like respiratory distress syndrome, sepsis, and necrotizing enterocolitis are associated with negative long-term neurodevelopmental outcomes. Proper use of neuromonitoring in extremely premature infants has the potential for neuroprotection and improved outcomes.

16.2.6.1 aEEG in Extremely Preterm Infants in First Days of Life

aEEG can be used easily and safely in extremely preterm infants [75]. With increasing postmenstrual age, aEEG shows predictive maturational changes (Fig. 16.4).

Early aEEG background is predictive of long-term outcomes, and normal features, such as cyclicity indicating emerging SWC, are associated with good prognosis [76–81]. Abnormal aEEG could be associated with IVH as well as later adverse outcomes [77, 78, 82]. Care should be taken in interpreting aEEG in extremely preterm infants, since it can be impacted by sedative and analgesic medications, hemodynamic changes, plasma glucose, and carbon dioxide levels [83–89]. Given the changing background with postmenstrual age and the need to consider multiple factors, additional training may be needed to gain expertise in aEEG for this group. Several studies have shown that early aEEG patterns in extremely preterm infants may indicate unfavorable outcomes. However, there is no evidence to suggest that utilizing aEEG routinely can lead to better outcomes. Experienced users can utilize aEEG to evaluate brain health in extremely preterm infants and make predictions about their prognosis. Further studies are necessary to determine how aEEG can be utilized to guide interventions at the bedside.

16.2.6.2 cEEG in Extremely Preterm Infants

For extremely premature infants, cEEG monitoring is a valuable tool for assessing detailed cortical function. Nevertheless, multichannel recordings can pose difficulties for the youngest preterm infants, necessitating special attention to ensure safety

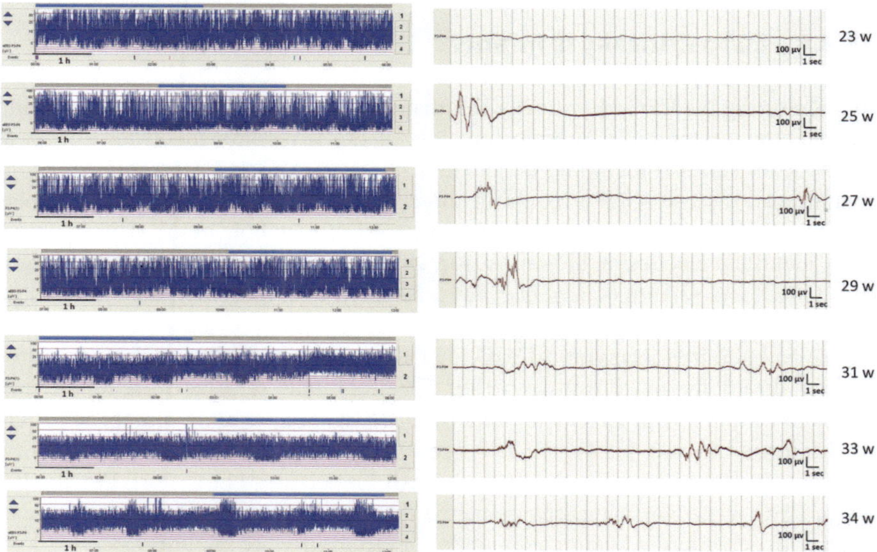

Fig. 16.4 On the right side are single-channel conventional EEGs (about 36 s of recording) plotted with a speed 10 mm/s and voltage of 100 μV/cm, demonstrating a progressive decrease in interburst interval (IBI) with age (represents the most discontinuous part of the aEEG recording). On the left side are corresponding aEEG (about 6 h) from the same recordings in a speed of 6 cm/h. With maturation, the aEEG shows higher amplitude, narrower bandwidth, increased continuity, and evolving sleep-wake cyclicity. (From El-Dib et al. [12] with permission)

and signal quality optimization [83, 90]. Encouragingly, one study of cEEG in 70 neonates <32 weeks gestational age (GA) and another of 50 neonates <30 weeks GA reported no instances of skin injury [91, 92]. In the future, an EEG cap designed for preterm infants can have a significant advantage.

Limited data suggest that cEEG changes may provide early indicators of intraventricular hemorrhage (IVH) in extremely preterm infants, even prior to ultrasound diagnosis [77, 78]. In addition, cEEG has the potential to predict neurodevelopmental outcome starting from the first few days of life, with the highest predictive value being closer to term-equivalent age [93, 94]. Finally, cEEG continues to be the gold standard for detection of seizures in preterm infants. Common causes of acute seizures in preterm infants include high-grade IVH, hypoxia-ischemia, transient metabolic disturbance, or infection [95]. There is great variability in reported incidence of seizures in extremely preterm infants, depending on the method of assessment, ranging from 0.34–5% in studies based on clinical signs alone [96–98] and 0.9–8.7% in studies using cEEG [99–103]. Studies using aEEG have reported higher rates, which may be overestimated due to other rhythmic activities [81, 104, 105]. Rhythmic EEG findings mistaken as seizures may commonly arise from artifacts [87, 88, 100, 106–108]. However, to differentiate these from seizures, these rhythmic activities do not show evolution in amplitude, frequency, or morphology [87, 88]. It is important to be cautious when diagnosing seizures in extremely preterm infants and possibly use cEEG to avoid unnecessary use of ASM, especially when optimal seizure management in extremely preterm infants is not known [109].

16.2.7 EEG in Critically Ill Infants

By monitoring the EEG of critically ill infants, we can detect neonatal seizures and identify any compromise of brain function. cEEG is recommended for infants at high risk for seizures including infants in need for ECMO and newborns with congenital heart disease (CHD) requiring surgery, severe persistent pulmonary hypertension (PPHN), CNS infection, and inborn error of metabolism [5]. A prospective study identified electrographic seizures in 18% of 99 infants and children undergoing ECMO, and seizure occurrence was associated with mortality and unfavorable outcome [110]. Another study identified electrographic seizures in 23% of 70 infants and children receiving ECMO [111]. Infants with CHD are also at risk for seizures during the postoperative period. Electrographic seizures were reported in 8% of 161 infants with CHD who underwent cEEG after cardiac surgery with cardiopulmonary bypass [112]. Other causes of neonatal hemodynamic instability, including PPHN and meningitis, increase risk for seizures [113, 114]. Finally, the use of EEG in neonatal hyperammonemia due to inborn error of metabolism can assist with detection of significant number of electrographic seizures [115, 116].

Apart from detecting seizures, cEEG and aEEG monitoring can also aid in predicting outcomes. A study conducted on 150 infants with CHD who underwent aEEG monitoring after cardiac surgery demonstrated that a prolonged recovery time to a continuous background was linked with higher mortality risk and poorer neurodevelopmental outcomes [117]. Moreover, a retrospective study of 76 neonates with critical CHD demonstrated that postoperative abnormal background pattern and ictal activity on aEEG were associated with new postoperative brain injury on MRI [118]. Similarly, in a study of 30 infants with PPHN and CHD, abnormal aEEG background was associated with adverse neurologic outcome [119]. In a prospective study which included 60 infants undergoing cardiac surgery with cardiopulmonary bypass, after controlling for other risk factors, abnormal postoperative aEEG background pattern and lack of return of sleep-wake cycling independently predicted poorer intelligence quotient at 4 years [120]. In a cohort of 29 infants with bacterial meningitis, those infants with markedly abnormal EEGs died or had severe neurologic impairment [121].

cEEG/aEEG monitoring should be considered in critically ill infants who are at risk for seizures or when additional information on neurologic function is required. Whether such monitoring will lead to interventions capable of improving outcome is yet to be demonstrated.

16.3 Conclusion

In conclusion, EEG, whether in the form of cEEG or aEEG, is a valuable tool for monitoring neonatal brain activity, detecting seizures, and assessing neurological integrity. It aids in timely intervention, reduces seizure burden, and provides important prognostic information in neonatal encephalopathy, extremely preterm, and critically ill infants (Table 16.2).

Table 16.2 Prognostic value of aEEG and cEEG in full-term infants with NE and preterm Infants

aEEG in term NE and HT	Prognosis	
<6 h after birth	Abnormal background predictive of poor outcome	Sensitivity>90% [51, 52]
	Normal background predictive of a normal outcome	NPV 77% [51]
48–72 h after birth	Abnormal background predictive of poor outcome	PPV >85% [51]
72 h after birth	Absence of SWC predictive of a poor outcome	PPV 88% [57]
cEEG in term NE and HT	**Prognosis**	
48–72 h after birth	Abnormal background predictive of poor outcome	Sensitivity 93% [32]
aEEG in preterm infants		
24–72 h after birth	Presence of cyclicity predictive of a normal outcome	NPV 74% [81]
	Abnormal background with long IBI predictive of a poor outcome	Pooled sensitivity 0.83 and pooled specificity 0.83 [122] PPV 76% [81]
Second week after birth	Abnormal background with long IBI predictive of a poor outcome	PPV 95% [82]
	Absence of cyclicity	PPV 96% [82]

aEEG amplitude integrated EEG, *cEEG* continuous EEG, *NPV* negative predictive value, *PPV* positive predictive value, *IBI* interburst interval, *SWC* sleep-wake cycling

References

1. Tekgul H, Bourgeois BFD, Gauvreau K, Bergin AM. Electroencephalography in neonatal seizures: comparison of a reduced and a full 10/20 montage. Pediatr Neurol. 2005;32(3):155–61.
2. Clancy RR, Bergqvist AGC, Dlugos DJ. Neonatal electroencephalography. In: Ebersole J, Pedley T, editors. Current practice of clinical electroencephalography. Philadelphia, PA: Lippincott Williams & Wilkins; 2003. p. 160–234.
3. Holmes GL, Lombroso CT. Prognostic value of background patterns in the neonatal EEG. J Clin Neurophysiol. 1993;10(3):323–52.
4. Hrachovy RA, Mizrahi EM. Atlas of neonatal electroencephalography. Springer Publishing Company; 2015.
5. Shellhaas RA, Chang T, Tsuchida T, Scher MS, Riviello JJ, Abend NS, Nguyen S, Wusthoff CJ, Clancy RR. The American Clinical Neurophysiology Society's guideline on continuous electroencephalography monitoring in neonates. J Clin Neurophysiol. 2011;28(6):611–7.
6. Tsuchida TN, Wusthoff CJ, Shellhaas RA, Abend NS, Hahn CD, Sullivan JE, Nguyen S, Weinstein S, Scher MS, Riviello JJ, Clancy RR. American clinical neurophysiology society standardized EEG terminology and categorization for the description of continuous EEG monitoring in neonates: report of the American Clinical Neurophysiology Society critical care monitoring committee. J Clin Neurophysiol. 2013;30(2):161–73.
7. Durrani NUR, Dinan MH. Amplitude-integrated electroencephalography: a primer for neonatologists and practitioners in the NICU. NeoReviews. 2022;23(2):e96–e107.
8. El-Dib M, Chang T, Tsuchida TN, Clancy RR. Amplitude-integrated electroencephalography in neonates. Pediatr Neurol. 2009;41(5):315–26.
9. Hellstrom-Westas L, de Vries L, Rosen I. Atlas of AMPLITUDE-INTEGRATED EEGs in the NEWBORN. London: CRC Press; 2008.
10. Shah NA, Wusthoff CJ. How to use: amplitude-integrated EEG (aEEG). Arch Dis Child Educ Pract Ed. 2015;100(2):75–81.
11. Hellstrom-Westas L, Rosen I, de Vries LS, Greisen G. Amplitude-integrated EEG classification and interpretation in preterm and term infants. NeoReviews. 2006;7(2):e76–87.
12. El-Dib M, Abend NS, Austin T, Boylan G, Chock V, Cilio MR, Greisen G, Hellström-Westas L, Lemmers P, Pellicer A, Pressler RM, Sansevere A, Szakmar E, Tsuchida T, Vanhatalo S, Wusthoff CJ. Neuromonitoring in neonatal critical care part II: extremely premature infants and critically ill neonates. Pediatr Res. 2023; 94(1):55–63.
13. El-Dib M, Abend NS, Austin T, Boylan G, Chock V, Cilio MR, Greisen G, Hellström-Westas L, Lemmers P, Pellicer A, Pressler RM, Sansevere A, Tsuchida T, Vanhatalo S, Wusthoff CJ. Neuromonitoring in neonatal critical care part I: neonatal encephalopathy and neonates with possible seizures. Pediatr Res. 2023; 94(1):64–73.
14. Bashir RA, Espinoza L, Vayalthrikkovil S, Buchhalter J, Irvine L, Bello-Espinosa L, Mohammad K. Implementation of a neurocritical care program: improved seizure detection and decreased antiseizure medication at discharge in neonates with hypoxic-ischemic encephalopathy. Pediatr Neurol. 2016;64:38–43.
15. Glass HC, Soul JS, Chang T, Wusthoff CJ, Chu CJ, Massey SL, Abend NS, Lemmon M, Thomas C, Numis AL, Guillet R, Sturza J, McNamara NA, Rogers EE, Franck LS, McCulloch CE, Shellhaas RA. Safety of early discontinuation of antiseizure medication after acute symptomatic neonatal seizures. JAMA Neurol. 2021;78(7):817–25.
16. Harris ML, Malloy KM, Lawson SN, Rose RS, Buss WF, Mietzsch U. Standardized treatment of neonatal status epilepticus improves outcome. J Child Neurol. 2016;31(14):1546–54.
17. Jan S, Northington FJ, Parkinson CM, Stafstrom CE. EEG monitoring technique influences the management of hypoxic-ischemic seizures in neonates undergoing therapeutic hypothermia. Dev Neurosci. 2017;39(1–4):82–8.
18. Srinivasakumar P, Zempel J, Trivedi S, Wallendorf M, Rao R, Smith B, Inder T, Mathur AM. Treating EEG seizures in hypoxic ischemic encephalopathy: a randomized controlled trial. Pediatrics. 2015;136(5):e1302–9.

19. Stafstrom CE, Chronopoulos A, Thurber S, Thompson JL, Holmes GL. Age-dependent cognitive and behavioral deficits after kainic acid seizures. Epilepsia. 1993;34(3):420–32.
20. Wasterlain CG. Recurrent seizures in the developing brain are harmful. Epilepsia. 1997;38(6):728–34.
21. Sands TT, Balestri M, Bellini G, Mulkey SB, Danhaive O, Bakken EH, Taglialatela M, Oldham MS, Vigevano F, Holmes GL, Cilio MR. Rapid and safe response to low-dose carbamazepine in neonatal epilepsy. Epilepsia. 2016;57(12):2019–30.
22. Vilan A, Mendes Ribeiro J, Striano P, Weckhuysen S, Weeke LC, Brilstra E, de Vries LS, Cilio MR. A distinctive ictal amplitude-integrated electroencephalography pattern in newborns with neonatal epilepsy associated with KCNQ2 mutations. Neonatology. 2017;112(4):387–93.
23. Painter MJ, Scher MS, Stein AD, Armatti S, Wang Z, Gardiner JC, Paneth N, Minnigh B, Alvin J. Phenobarbital compared with phenytoin for the treatment of neonatal seizures. N Engl J Med. 1999;341(7):485–9.
24. Sharpe C, Reiner GE, Davis SL, Nespeca M, Gold JJ, Rasmussen M, Kuperman R, Harbert MJ, Michelson D, Joe P, Wang S, Rismanchi N, Le NM, Mower A, Kim J, Battin MR, Lane B, Honold J, Knodel E, Arnell K, Bridge R, Lee L, Ernstrom K, Raman R, Haas RH. Levetiracetam versus phenobarbital for neonatal seizures: a randomized controlled trial. Pediatrics. 2020;145:6.
25. Alharbi HM, Pinchefsky EF, Tran MA, Salazar Cerda CI, Parokaran Varghese J, Kamino D, Widjaja E, Mamak E, Ly L, Nevalainen P, Hahn CD, Tam EWY. Seizure burden and neurologic outcomes after neonatal encephalopathy. Neurology. 2023;100(19):e1976–84.
26. Kharoshankaya L, Stevenson NJ, Livingstone V, Murray DM, Murphy BP, Ahearne CE, Boylan GB. Seizure burden and neurodevelopmental outcome in neonates with hypoxic-ischemic encephalopathy. Dev Med Child Neurol. 2016;58(12):1242–8.
27. Van Rooij LGM, Toet MC, Van Huffelen AC, Groenendaal F, Laan W, Zecic A, De Haan T, Van Straaten ILM, Vrancken S, Van Wezel G, Van Der Sluijs J, Ter Horst H, Gavilanes D, Laroche S, Naulaers G, De Vries LS. Effect of treatment of subclinical neonatal seizures detected with aEEG: randomized, controlled trial. Pediatrics. 2010;125(2):e358–66.
28. Bye AME, Flanagan D. Spatial and temporal characteristics of neonatal seizures. Epilepsia. 1995;36(10):1009–16.
29. Helmers SL, Wypij D, Constantinou JE, Newburger JW, Hickey PR, Carrazana EJ, Barlow JK, Kuban KC, Holmes GL. Perioperative electroencephalographic seizures in infants undergoing repair of complex congenital cardiac defects. Electroencephalogr Clin Neurophysiol. 1997;102(1):27–36.
30. Laroia N, Guillet R, Burchfiel J, McBride MC. EEG background as predictor of electrographic seizures in high-risk neonates. Epilepsia. 1998;39(5):545–51.
31. Murray DM, Boylan GB, Ali I, Ryan CA, Murphy BP, Connolly S. Defining the gap between electrographic seizure burden, clinical expression and staff recognition of neonatal seizures. Arch Dis Child Fetal Neonatal Ed. 2008;93(3):F187–91.
32. Nash KB, Bonifacio SL, Glass HC, Sullivan JE, Barkovich AJ, Ferriero DM, Cilio MR. Video-EEG monitoring in newborns with hypoxic-ischemic encephalopathy treated with hypothermia. Neurology. 2011;76(6):556–62.
33. Boylan GB, Rennie JM, Pressler RM, Wilson G, Morton M, Binnie CD. Phenobarbitone, neonatal seizures, and video-EEG. Arch Dis Child Fetal Neonatal Ed. 2002;86(3):F165–70.
34. Scher MS, Alvin J, Gaus L, Minnigh B, Painter MJ. Uncoupling of EEG-clinical neonatal seizures after antiepileptic drug use. Pediatr Neurol. 2003;28(4):277–80.
35. Shellhaas RA, Clancy RR. Characterization of neonatal seizures by conventional EEG and single-channel EEG. Clin Neurophysiol. 2007;118(10):2156–61.
36. Shellhaas RA, Soaita AI, Clancy RR. Sensitivity of amplitude-integrated electroencephalography for neonatal seizure detection. Pediatrics. 2007;120(4):770–7.
37. Zhang L, Zhou YX, Chang LW, Luo XP. Diagnostic value of amplitude-integrated electroencephalogram in neonatal seizures. Neurosci Bull. 2011;27(4):251–7.
38. Shah DK, Mackay MT, Lavery S, Watson S, Harvey AS, Zempel J, Mathur A, Inder TE. Accuracy of bedside electroencephalographic monitoring in comparison with

simultaneous continuous conventional electroencephalography for seizure detection in term infants. Pediatrics. 2008;121(6):1146–54.

39. Rennie JM, Chorley G, Boylan GB, Pressler R, Nguyen Y, Hooper R. Non-expert use of the cerebral function monitor for neonatal seizure detection. Arch Dis Child Fetal Neonatal Ed. 2004;89(1):F37–40.

40. Toet MC, van der Meij W, de Vries LS, Uiterwaal CS, van Huffelen KC. Comparison between simultaneously recorded amplitude integrated electroencephalogram (cerebral function monitor) and standard electroencephalogram in neonates. Pediatrics. 2002;109(5):772–9.

41. Stevenson NJ, Lauronen L, Vanhatalo S. The effect of reducing EEG electrode number on the visual interpretation of the human expert for neonatal seizure detection. Clin Neurophysiol. 2018;129(1):265–70.

42. Sandoval Karamian AG, Wusthoff CJ. How helpful is aEEG? Context and user experience matter. Am J Perinatol. 2022;39(10):1132–7.

43. al Naqeeb N, Edwards AD, Cowan FM, Azzopardi D. Assessment of neonatal encephalopathy by amplitude-integrated electroencephalography. Pediatrics. 1999;103(6 Pt 1):1263–71.

44. Hellstrom-Westas L, Rosen I, Svenningsen NW. Predictive value of early continuous amplitude integrated EEG recordings on outcome after severe birth asphyxia in full term infants. Arch Dis Child Fetal Neonatal Ed. 1995;72(1):F34–8.

45. Shalak LF, Laptook AR, Velaphi SC, Perlman JM. Amplitude-integrated electroencephalography coupled with an early neurologic examination enhances prediction of term infants at risk for persistent encephalopathy. Pediatrics. 2003;111(2):351–7.

46. ter Horst HJ, Sommer C, Bergman KA, Fock JM, van Weerden TW, Bos AF. Prognostic significance of amplitude-integrated EEG during the first 72 hours after birth in severely asphyxiated neonates. Pediatr Res. 2004;55(6):1026–33.

47. Toet MC, Hellstrom-Westas L, Groenendaal F, Eken P, de Vries LS. Amplitude integrated EEG 3 and 6 hours after birth in full term neonates with hypoxic-ischaemic encephalopathy. Arch Dis Child Fetal Neonatal Ed. 1999;81(1):F19–23.

48. Azzopardi DV, Strohm B, Edwards AD, Dyet L, Halliday HL, Juszczak E, Kapellou O, Levene M, Marlow N, Porter E, Thoresen M, Whitelaw A, Brocklehurst P. Moderate hypothermia to treat perinatal asphyxial encephalopathy. N Engl J Med. 2009;361(14):1349–58.

49. Gluckman PD, Wyatt JS, Azzopardi D, Ballard R, Edwards AD, Ferriero DM, Polin RA, Robertson CM, Thoresen M, Whitelaw A, Gunn AJ. Selective head cooling with mild systemic hypothermia after neonatal encephalopathy: multicentre randomised trial. Lancet. 2005;365(9460):663–70.

50. Sarkar S, Barks JD, Donn SM. Should amplitude-integrated electroencephalography be used to identify infants suitable for hypothermic neuroprotection? J Perinatol. 2008;28(2):117–22.

51. Chandrasekaran M, Chaban B, Montaldo P, Thayyil S. Predictive value of amplitude-integrated EEG (aEEG) after rescue hypothermic neuroprotection for hypoxic ischemic encephalopathy: a meta-analysis. J Perinatol. 2017;37(6):684–9.

52. Del Río R, Ochoa C, Alarcon A, Arnáez J, Blanco D, García-Alix A. Amplitude integrated electroencephalogram as a prognostic tool in neonates with hypoxic-ischemic encephalopathy: a systematic review. PLoS One. 2016;11(11):e0165744.

53. van Rooij LG, Toet MC, Osredkar D, van Huffelen AC, Groenendaal F, de Vries LS. Recovery of amplitude integrated electroencephalographic background patterns within 24 hours of perinatal asphyxia. Arch Dis Child Fetal Neonatal Ed. 2005;90(3):F245–51.

54. Osredkar D, Toet MC, van Rooij LG, van Huffelen AC, Groenendaal F, de Vries LS. Sleep-wake cycling on amplitude-integrated electroencephalography in term newborns with hypoxic-ischemic encephalopathy. Pediatrics. 2005;115(2):327–32.

55. Hallberg B, Grossmann K, Bartocci M, Blennow M. The prognostic value of early aEEG in asphyxiated infants undergoing systemic hypothermia treatment. Acta Paediatr. 2010;99(4):531–6.

56. Massaro AN, Tsuchida T, Kadom N, El-Dib M, Glass P, Baumgart S, Chang T. aEEG evolution during therapeutic hypothermia and prediction of NICU outcome in encephalopathic neonates. Neonatology. 2012;102(3):197–202.

57. Thoresen M, Hellström-Westas L, Liu X, De Vries LS. Effect of hypothermia on amplitude-integrated electroencephalogram in infants with asphyxia. Pediatrics. 2010;126(1):e131–9.
58. Gunn AJ, Thoresen M. Neonatal encephalopathy and hypoxic-ischemic encephalopathy. Handb Clin Neurol. 2019;162:217–37.
59. Filan P, Boylan GB, Chorley G, Davies A, Fox GF, Pressler R, Rennie JM. The relationship between the onset of electrographic seizure activity after birth and the time of cerebral injury in utero. BJOG. 2005;112(4):504–7.
60. Obeid R, Sogawa Y, Gedela S, Naik M, Lee V, Telesco R, Wisnowski J, Magill C, Painter MJ, Panigrahy A. The correlation between a short-term conventional electroencephalography in the first day of life and brain magnetic resonance imaging in newborns undergoing hypothermia for hypoxic-ischemic encephalopathy. Pediatr Neurol. 2017;67:91–7.
61. Liu W, Yang Q, Wei H, Dong W, Fan Y, Hua Z. Prognostic value of clinical tests in neonates with hypoxic-ischemic encephalopathy treated with therapeutic hypothermia: a systematic review and meta-analysis. Front Neurol. 2020;11:133.
62. Murray DM, O'Connor CM, Ryan CA, Korotchikova I, Boylan GB. Early EEG grade and outcome at 5 years after mild neonatal hypoxic ischemic encephalopathy. Pediatrics. 2016;138:e20160659.
63. Murray DM, Boylan GB, Ryan CA, Connolly S. Early EEG findings in hypoxic-ischemic encephalopathy predict outcomes at 2 years. Pediatrics. 2009;124(3):e459–67.
64. Massey SL, Shou H, Clancy R, DiGiovine M, Fitzgerald MP, Fung FW, Farrar J, Abend NS. Interrater and intrarater agreement in neonatal electroencephalogram background scoring. J Clin Neurophysiol. 2019;36(1):1–8.
65. Awal MA, Lai MM, Azemi G, Boashash B, Colditz PB. EEG background features that predict outcome in term neonates with hypoxic ischaemic encephalopathy: a structured review. Clin Neurophysiol. 2016;127(1):285–96.
66. Korotchikova I, Connolly S, Ryan CA, Murray DM, Temko A, Greene BR, Boylan GB. EEG in the healthy term newborn within 12 hours of birth. Clin Neurophysiol. 2009;120(6):1046–53.
67. Fitzgerald MP, Massey SL, Fung FW, Kessler SK, Abend NS. High electroencephalographic seizure exposure is associated with unfavorable outcomes in neonates with hypoxic-ischemic encephalopathy. Seizure. 2018;61:221–6.
68. Weeke LC, Boylan GB, Pressler RM, Hallberg B, Blennow M, Toet MC, Groenendaal F, de Vries LS. Role of EEG background activity, seizure burden and MRI in predicting neurodevelopmental outcome in full-term infants with hypoxic-ischaemic encephalopathy in the era of therapeutic hypothermia. Eur J Paediatr Neurol. 2016;20(6):855–64.
69. Bourel-Ponchel E, Querne L, Flamein F, Ghostine-Ramadan G, Wallois F, Lamblin MD. The prognostic value of neonatal conventional-EEG monitoring in hypoxic-ischemic encephalopathy during therapeutic hypothermia. Dev Med Child Neurol. 2023;65(1):58–66.
70. Chalak LF, Pappas A, Tan S, Das A, Sánchez PJ, Laptook AR, Van Meurs KP, Shankaran S, Bell EF, Davis AS, Heyne RJ, Pedroza C, Poindexter BB, Schibler K, Tyson JE, Ball MB, Bara R, Grisby C, Sokol GM, D'Angio CT, Hamrick SEG, Dysart KC, Cotten CM, Truog WE, Watterberg KL, Timan CJ, Garg M, Carlo WA, Higgins RD. Association between increased seizures during rewarming after hypothermia for neonatal hypoxic ischemic encephalopathy and abnormal neurodevelopmental outcomes at 2-year follow-up: a nested multisite cohort study. JAMA Neurol. 2021;78(12):1484–93.
71. Glass HC, Wusthoff CJ, Shellhaas RA, Tsuchida TN, Bonifacio SL, Cordeiro M, Sullivan J, Abend NS, Chang T. Risk factors for EEG seizures in neonates treated with hypothermia: a multicenter cohort study. Neurology. 2014;82(14):1239–44.
72. Lynch NE, Stevenson NJ, Livingstone V, Mathieson S, Murphy BP, Rennie JM, Boylan GB. The temporal characteristics of seizures in neonatal hypoxic ischemic encephalopathy treated with hypothermia. Seizure. 2015;33:60–5.
73. Worden LT, Chinappen DM, Stoyell SM, Gold J, Paixao L, Krishnamoorthy K, Kramer MA, Westover MB, Chu CJ. The probability of seizures during continuous EEG monitoring in high-risk neonates. Epilepsia. 2019;60(12):2508–18.

74. Cornet MC, Pasupuleti A, Fang A, Gonzalez F, Shimotake T, Ferriero DM, Glass HC, Cilio MR. Predictive value of early EEG for seizures in neonates with hypoxic-ischemic encephalopathy undergoing therapeutic hypothermia. Pediatr Res. 2018;84(3):399–402.

75. Davis AS, Gantz MG, Do B, Shankaran S, Hamrick SE, Kennedy KA, Tyson JE, Chalak LF, Laptook AR, Goldstein RF, Hintz SR, Das A, Higgins RD, Ball MB, Hale EC, Van Meurs KP. Serial aEEG recordings in a cohort of extremely preterm infants: feasibility and safety. J Perinatol. 2015;35(5):373–8.

76. Bowen JR, Paradisis M, Shah D. Decreased aEEG continuity and baseline variability in the first 48 hours of life associated with poor short-term outcome in neonates born before 29 weeks gestation. Pediatr Res. 2010;67(5):538–44.

77. Iyer KK, Roberts JA, Hellström-Westas L, Wikström S, Hansen Pupp I, Ley D, Breakspear M, Vanhatalo S. Early detection of preterm intraventricular hemorrhage from clinical electroencephalography. Crit Care Med. 2015a;43(10):2219–27.

78. Iyer KK, Roberts JA, Hellström-Westas L, Wikström S, Hansen Pupp I, Ley D, Vanhatalo S, Breakspear M. Cortical burst dynamics predict clinical outcome early in extremely preterm infants. Brain. 2015b;138(Pt 8):2206–18.

79. Middel RG, Brandenbarg N, Van Braeckel K, Bos AF, Ter Horst HJ. The predictive value of amplitude-integrated electroencephalography in preterm infants for IQ and other neuropsychological outcomes at early school age. Neonatology. 2018;113(4):287–95.

80. Song J, Xu F, Wang L, Gao L, Guo J, Xia L, Zhang Y, Zhou W, Wang X, Zhu C. Early amplitude-integrated electroencephalography predicts brain injury and neurological outcome in very preterm infants. Sci Rep. 2015;5

81. Wikström S, Pupp IH, Rosén I, Norman E, Fellman V, Ley D, Hellström-Westas L. Early single-channel aEEG/EEG predicts outcome in very preterm infants. Acta Paediatr. 2012;101(7):719–26.

82. Klebermass K, Olischar M, Waldhoer T, Fuiko R, Pollak A, Weninger M. Amplitude-integrated EEG pattern predicts further outcome in preterm infants. Pediatr Res. 2011;70(1):102–8.

83. Griesmaier E, Enot DP, Bachmann M, Neubauer V, Hellström-Westas L, Kiechl-Kohlendorfer U, Keller M. Systematic characterization of amplitude-integrated EEG signals for monitoring the preterm brain. Pediatr Res. 2013;73(2):226–35.

84. Helderman JB, Welch CD, Leng X, O'Shea TM. Sepsis-associated electroencephalographic changes in extremely low gestational age neonates. Early Hum Dev. 2010;86(8):509–13.

85. Norman E, Wikström S, Rosén I, Fellman V, Hellström-Westas L. Premedication for intubation with morphine causes prolonged depression of electrocortical background activity in preterm infants. Pediatr Res. 2013;73(1):87–94.

86. ter Horst HJ, Jongbloed-Pereboom M, van Eykern LA, Bos AF. Amplitude-integrated electroencephalographic activity is suppressed in preterm infants with high scores on illness severity. Early Hum Dev. 2011;87(5):385–90.

87. Weeke LC, Dix LML, Groenendaal F, Lemmers PMA, Dijkman KP, Andriessen P, de Vries LS, Toet MC. Severe hypercapnia causes reversible depression of aEEG background activity in neonates: an observational study. Arch Dis Child Fetal Neonatal Ed. 2017a;102(5):F383–8.

88. Weeke LC, van Ooijen IM, Groenendaal F, van Huffelen AC, van Haastert IC, van Stam C, Benders MJ, Toet MC, Hellström-Westas L, de Vries LS. Rhythmic EEG patterns in extremely preterm infants: classification and association with brain injury and outcome. Clin Neurophysiol. 2017b;128(12):2428–35.

89. West CR, Groves AM, Williams CE, Harding JE, Skinner JR, Kuschel CA, Battin MR. Early low cardiac output is associated with compromised electroencephalographic activity in very preterm infants. Pediatr Res. 2006;59(4 Pt 1):610–5.

90. Vanhatalo S, Metsäranta M, Andersson S. High-fidelity recording of brain activity in the extremely preterm babies: feasibility study in the incubator. Clin Neurophysiol. 2008;119(2):439–45.

91. El Ters NM, Mathur AM, Jain S, Vesoulis ZA, Zempel JM. Long term electroencephalography in preterm neonates: safety and quality of electrode types. Clin Neurophysiol. 2018;129(7):1366–71.

92. Lloyd R, Goulding R. Filan P, Boylan G. Overcoming the practical challenges of electroencephalography for very preterm infants in the neonatal intensive care unit. Acta Paediatr. 2015;104(2):152–7.

93. Lloyd RO, O'Toole JM, Livingstone V, Filan PM, Boylan GB. Can EEG accurately predict 2-year neurodevelopmental outcome for preterm infants? Arch Dis Child Fetal Neonatal Ed. 2021;106(5):535–41.

94. Lloyd RO, O'Toole JM, Livingstone V, Hutch WD, Pavlidis E, Cronin AM, Dempsey EM, Filan PM, Boylan GB. Predicting 2-y outcome in preterm infants using early multimodal physiological monitoring. Pediatr Res. 2016;80(3):382–8.

95. Pisani F, Spagnoli C. Outcome in preterm infants with seizures. Handb Clin Neurol. 2019;162:401–14.

96. Lanska MJ, Lanska DJ. Neonatal seizures in the United States: results of the National Hospital Discharge Survey, 1980-1991. Neuroepidemiology. 1996;15(3):117–25.

97. Lanska MJ, Lanska DJ, Baumann RJ, Kryscio RJ. A population-based study of neonatal seizures in Fayette County, Kentucky. Neurology. 1995;45(4):724–32.

98. Ronen GM, Penney S, Andrews W. The epidemiology of clinical neonatal seizures in Newfoundland: a population-based study. J Pediatr. 1999;134(1):71–5.

99. Le Bihannic A, Beauvais K, Busnel A, de Barace C, Furby A. Prognostic value of EEG in very premature newborns. Arch Dis Child Fetal Neonatal Ed. 2012;97(2):F106–9.

100. Lloyd RO, O'Toole JM, Pavlidis E, Filan PM, Boylan GB. Electrographic seizures during the early postnatal period in preterm infants. J Pediatr. 2017;187:18–25.e12

101. Okumura A, Hayakawa F, Kato T, Itomi K, Maruyama K, Kubota T, Suzuki M, Kidokoro H, Watanabe K. Ictal electroencephalographic findings of neonatal seizures in preterm infants. Brain and Development. 2008;30(4):261–8.

102. Pisani F, Copioli C, Turco EC, Sisti L, Cossu G, Seri S. Mortality risk after neonatal seizures in very preterm newborns. J Child Neurol. 2012;27(10):1264–9.

103. Scher MS, Aso K, Beggarly ME, Hamid MY, Steppe DA, Painter MJ. Electrographic seizures in preterm and full-term neonates: clinical correlates, associated brain lesions, and risk for neurologic sequelae. Pediatrics. 1993;91(1):128–34.

104. Shah DK, Zempel J, Barton T, Lukas K, Inder TE. Electrographic seizures in preterm infants during the first week of life are associated with cerebral injury. Pediatr Res. 2010;67(1):102–6.

105. Vesoulis ZA, Inder TE, Woodward LJ, Buse B, Vavasseur C, Mathur AM. Early electrographic seizures, brain injury, and neurodevelopmental risk in the very preterm infant. Pediatr Res. 2013;75(4):564–9.

106. Janáčková S, Boyd S, Yozawitz E, Tsuchida T, Lamblin MD, Gueden S, Pressler R. Electroencephalographic characteristics of epileptic seizures in preterm neonates. Clin Neurophysiol. 2016;127(8):2721–7.

107. Lee SS, El Ters N, Vesoulis ZA, Zempel JM, Mathur AM. Variable association of physiologic changes with electrographic seizure-like events in infants born preterm. J Pediatr. 2023;257:113348.

108. Pisani F, Barilli AL, Sisti L, Bevilacqua G, Seri S. Preterm infants with video-EEG confirmed seizures: outcome at 30 months of age. Brain and Development. 2008;30(1):20–30.

109. Pavlidis E, Lloyd RO, Boylan GB. EEG—a valuable biomarker of brain injury in preterm infants. Dev Neurosci. 2017;39(1–4):23–35.

110. Lin JJ, Banwell BL, Berg RA, Dlugos DJ, Ichord RN, Kilbaugh TJ, Kirsch RE, Kirschen MP, Licht DJ, Massey SL, Naim MY, Rintoul NE, Topjian AA, Abend NS. Electrographic seizures in children and neonates undergoing extracorporeal membrane oxygenation. Pediatr Crit Care Med. 2017;18(3):249–57.

111. Okochi S, Shakoor A, Barton S, Zenilman AR, Street C, Streltsova S, Cheung EW, Middlesworth W, Bain JM. Prevalence of seizures in pediatric extracorporeal membrane oxygenation patients as measured by continuous electroencephalography. Pediatr Crit Care Med. 2018;19:1162.

112. Naim MY, Gaynor JW, Chen J, Nicolson SC, Fuller S, Spray TL, Dlugos DJ, Clancy RR, Costa LV, Licht DJ, Xiao R, Meldrum H, Abend NS. Subclinical seizures identified by postoperative electroencephalographic monitoring are common after neonatal cardiac surgery. J Thorac Cardiovasc Surg. 2015;150(1):169–78. discussion 178-180
113. Klinger G, Chin CN, Otsubo H, Beyene J, Perlman M. Prognostic value of EEG in neonatal bacterial meningitis. Pediatr Neurol. 2001;24(1):28–31.
114. Scher MS, Klesh KW, Murphy TF, Guthrie RD. Seizures and infarction in neonates with persistent pulmonary hypertension. Pediatr Neurol. 1986;2(6):332–9.
115. Olischar M, Shany E, Aygün C, Azzopardi D, Hunt RW, Toet MC, Hamosh A, de Vries LS, Hellström-Westas L, Theda C. Amplitude-integrated electroencephalography in newborns with inborn errors of metabolism. Neonatology. 2012;102(3):203–11.
116. Wiwattanadittakul N, Prust M, Gaillard WD, Massaro A, Vezina G, Tsuchida TN, Gropman AL. The utility of EEG monitoring in neonates with hyperammonemia due to inborn errors of metabolism. Mol Genet Metab. 2018;125(3):235–40.
117. Gunn JK, Beca J, Hunt RW, Olischar M, Shekerdemian LS. Perioperative amplitude-integrated EEG and neurodevelopment in infants with congenital heart disease. Intensive Care Med. 2012;38(9):1539–47.
118. Claessens NHP, Noorlag L, Weeke LC, Toet MC, Breur J, Algra SO, Schouten ANJ, Haas F, Groenendaal F, Benders M, Jansen NJG, de Vries LS. Amplitude-integrated electroencephalography for early recognition of brain injury in neonates with critical congenital heart disease. J Pediatr. 2018;202:199–205.e191
119. El-Naggar WI, Keyzers M, McNamara PJ. Role of amplitude-integrated electroencephalography in neonates with cardiovascular compromise. J Crit Care. 2010;25(2):317–21.
120. Latal B, Wohlrab G, Brotschi B, Beck I, Knirsch W, Bernet V. Postoperative amplitude-integrated electroencephalography predicts four-year neurodevelopmental outcome in children with complex congenital heart disease. J Pediatr. 2016;178:55–60.e51
121. Chequer RS, Tharp BR, Dreimane D, Hahn JS, Clancy RR, Coen RW. Prognostic value of EEG in neonatal meningitis: retrospective study of 29 infants. Pediatr Neurol. 1992;8(6):417–22.
122. Fogtmann EP, Plomgaard AM, Greisen G, Gluud C. Prognostic accuracy of electroencephalograms in preterm infants: a systematic review. Pediatrics. 2017;139:2.

Mohamed El-Dib

Abbreviations

aEEg	Amplitude-integrated EEG
CHD	Congenital heart disease
CNS	Central nervous system
$CrSO_2$	Cerebral regional oxygenation saturation
DWI	Diffusion-weighted imaging
GA	Gestational age
Hb	Hemoglobin
HbO_2	Oxyhemoglobin
MRI	Magnetic resonance imaging
NE	Neonatal encephalopathy
NIRS	Near-infrared spectroscopy

M. El-Dib (✉)
Neonatal Neurocritical Care, Department of Pediatrics, Division of Newborn Medicine,
Brigham and Women's Hospital, Boston, MA, USA

Department of Pediatrics, Harvard Medical School, Boston, MA, USA
e-mail: mel-dib@bwh.harvard.edu

© The Author(s) 2024
G. Meijler, K. Mohammad (eds.), *Neonatal Brain Injury*,
https://doi.org/10.1007/978-3-031-55972-3_17

17.1 For Parents

17.1.1 What Is NIRS

Near-infrared spectroscopy (NIRS) is a technique that measures the amount of oxygen inside the brain tissues. The device has a thin cable attached to a sensor/probe—a small, soft patch on the baby's side of the forehead. The probe uses near-infrared light, which is very safe. The light goes a few centimeters into the brain and measures the color of the red blood cells (the cells that carry oxygen around the body) as it changes according to the amount of oxygen they carry (Fig. 17.1).

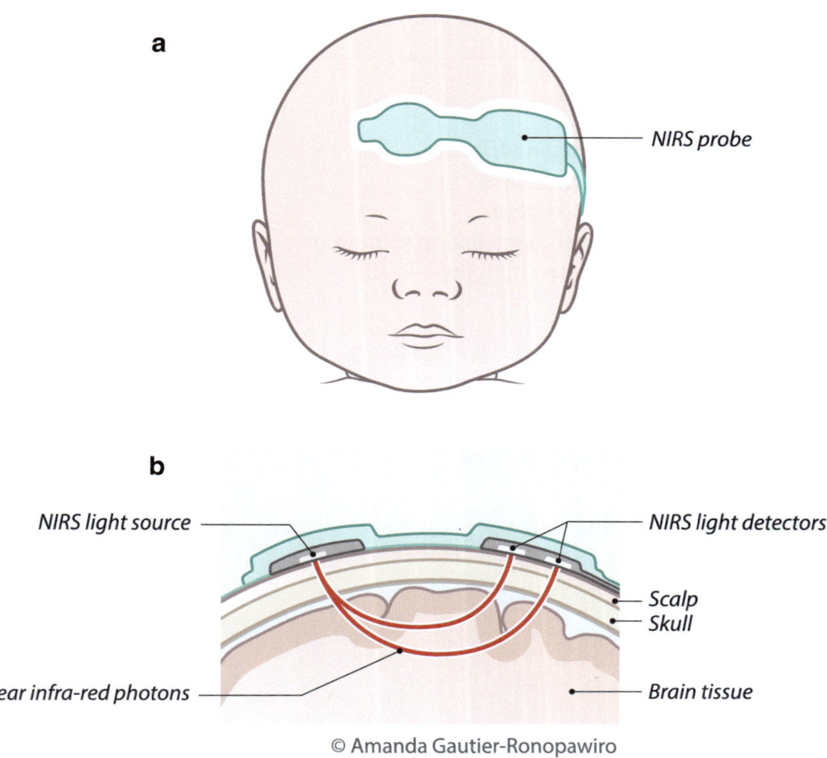

Fig. 17.1 An illustration of a cerebral NIRS probe attached to the forehead of an infant and an illustration of the basic technology used in NIRS. (© Amanda Gautier-Ronopawiro)

17.1.2 Why Is My Baby on the NIRS Device?

The most common reason for using NIRS in babies is the risk of brain injury. This includes preterm infants at risk of developing intraventricular hemorrhage as well as risk of decreased brain perfusion, which means not enough blood and oxygen flowing through the brain. Also, it has an important value when used in term-born infants who suffered decreased oxygen and/or blood to their brain around the time of birth. Aside from these two groups, NIRS has many applications in critically ill infants and infants undergoing surgery where measuring the oxygen in the brain could be beneficial.

17.1.3 How Is it Applied

The probe is put on the sides of the forehead of the infant and held in place by a bandage or sticky hydrogel. One probe is often used, but sometimes two probes are used to measure the amount of oxygen (oxygen saturation) on both sides of the brain. In addition, NIRS is sometimes used on the abdomen to measure oxygen saturation of the kidneys and bowel.

17.1.4 What Is its Value

The oxygen saturation in the brain is affected by many factors. Your baby's doctor will use the NIRS value to assess the following:

1. How much blood goes to the brain: The amount of blood going to the brain could be affected by factors like blood pressure, the flow of blood to other organs, and how much the brain blood vessels are constricted or dilated. Factors that could affect these vessels include how much carbon dioxide or glucose (sugar) is in the blood.
2. How much oxygen is delivered to the brain: This could be affected by the availability of red blood cells carrying this oxygen. Situations with decreased number of red cells (anemia) could be associated with decreased brain oxygenation. In addition, any cause of decreased oxygen going to the body (e.g., lung problems) could affect oxygen going to the brain.
3. How much oxygen is used by the brain: The brain uses oxygen from blood proportionate to its activity. Changes in brain activities could be reflected in the amount of oxygen used.

17.1.5 What Is Normal

The range of normal oxygen saturation of the brain is very wide. Although ranges between 55 and 85 are considered "normal," it is better to use NIRS to monitor trends or changes in oxygen saturation over time. Any acute or prolonged changes in oxygen level need attention.

17.1.6 How Will the Reading Affect the Way My Baby Is Treated?

If the NIRS shows a low value (e.g., oxygen saturation < 50–60% or a decrease from baseline by 20%), the doctor will consider adjusting your baby's treatment and support. The adjustments usually follow a guideline that lists how treatment may respond to low oxygen saturation in the brain. These treatments are all used in routine clinical practice to support respiration, blood circulation, and blood transport of gases (oxygen, carbon dioxide).

17.1.7 Does NIRS Cause Any Complications?

The newborn skin is very fragile and can be affected by the probe attachment. Skin complications are avoided by closely monitoring the skin, avoiding excessive pressure on the probe, and changing the probe's location regularly.

17.2 For Professionals

17.2.1 NIRS Background

Near-infrared spectroscopy (NIRS) measures tissue oxygen saturation in organs 2–3 cm below its sensors, e.g., in the brain, kidney, or intestine. Similar to a peripheral oxygen saturation monitor, NIRS uses the relative transparency of biological tissue to near-infrared light at a wavelength dependent on the absorption characteristics of hemoglobin, which varies with oxygenation. By monitoring the intensity of light passing through the brain at two wavelengths, changes in attenuation can be converted into changes in the cerebral concentrations of oxyhemoglobin (HbO_2) and deoxyhemoglobin (Hb). These two measures provide a regional oxygen saturation measurement (rSO_2) [rSO2% = HbO_2/(HbO_2 + Hb) * 100], essentially a mixed tissue saturation, representing more venous than arterial saturation, with a ratio of approximately 70% venous and 30% arterial blood. When NIRS is used on the scalp, cerebral regional oxygen saturation ($CrSO_2$) can be measured.

Continuous NIRS monitoring has been used in neonates with congenital heart disease (CHD), term infants with neonatal encephalopathy, as well as premature infants and has assisted in the determination of cerebral oxygenation and cerebral autoregulation in the context of systemic hypotension, a hemodynamically significant patent ductus arteriosus (PDA) and the need for blood transfusion [1–4].

17.2.2 Possible Indications for the Use of NIRS in the Neonatal Intensive Care Unit (NICU) [4]

1. Monitoring of extremely premature infants <28 weeks gestational age (GA) for the first 72 h after birth.
2. Infants with neonatal encephalopathy receiving therapeutic hypothermia (throughout cooling and re-warming).
3. Neonates with significant anemia requiring transfusion (before, during, and after).
4. Infants receiving inotropes and/or hydrocortisone for blood pressure support (before, during, and after inotropes).
5. Infants on significant respiratory support (e.g., high airway pressures, high-frequency ventilation, or inhaled nitric oxide).
6. Preterm infants with PDA to evaluate its hemodynamic significance.
7. Infants with hydrocephalus (especially before, during, and after therapeutic lumbar puncture or surgical intervention).
8. Neonates with CNS injury/abnormality, e.g., seizures, infarct/stroke, vascular malformations such as vein of Galen, or other AV malformation.

17.2.3 Normative Value

Normal $CrSO_2$ ranges from 55% to 85% when adult sensors are used (most available clinical studies), while the neonatal sensor measures 10% higher [5].

17.2.4 Factors that Affect NIRS Measurement

Many factors can affect cerebral oxygen saturation, limiting the ability to use the absolute measure of cerebral saturations. These factors include device type, sensor type, sensor position, head position, GA, time after birth, and day-to-day interventions such as endotracheal tube suctioning, handling, and diaper changes [5–11]. There are different types of NIRS devices and probes with significant variability of readings between them. While all devices have similar principles, they differ in their sensors, interface, display, and algorithms [12, 13]. Although the variations in $CrSO_2$ measurements between the left and right cerebral hemispheres are usually insignificant, studies have shown that differences of up to ±18% may be observed when comparing four different sites in the same newborn [11]. Also, while studies have indicated that minor changes in head position do not produce significant changes in $CrSO_2$ [6], it is worth noting that changes in head position can cause movement artifacts in NIRS signals. Furthermore, everyday care procedures like endotracheal tube suctioning, surfactant administration, handling, and diaper changing can result in substantial fluctuations in $CrSO_2$ [7, 14]. Although these fluctuations may indicate real changes in cerebral perfusion and oxygenation, they are often accompanied by significant head and/or body movements in the newborn, introducing movement artifacts that should be taken into consideration when interpreting NIRS changes in this context. This underscores the importance of utilizing $CrSO_2$ as a trend monitor instead of an absolute measure of cerebral oxygenation, especially since sensors will need to be repositioned during NIRS monitoring to accommodate changes in the baby's position and avoid scalp irritation.

17.2.5 Complications of NIRS Monitoring

NIRS monitoring, though non-invasive, requires yet another sensor on the fragile skin and may disturb very preterm infants. Proper training is needed regarding placement of probes and skin protection, as well as appropriate training of providers with the use of a standardized approach to interpretation and subsequent intervention.

Potential complications like skin irritation, skin bruising, or burns are avoided by close skin monitoring, avoiding excessive pressure on the probe, and changing probe position regularly.

17.2.6 Evidence of Use of NIRS in Clinical Practice

While NIRS has been used in many centers for decades as a research tool, it has been adopted and used clinically in specialized centers due to its potential value and low risk. It has been established in extremely preterm infants that the systematic use of NIRS in the first 3 days after birth reduces the burden of cerebral hypoxia [15] and that cerebral hypoxia, regardless of NIRS use, is associated with low brain electric activity and severe intracranial hemorrhage [16]. While the systematic use of

NIRS did not significantly alter early brain imaging findings [17, 18], early EEG or molecular biomarkers of cerebral injury [17, 18], or eventually combined death or severe brain injury at 36 weeks postmenstrual age [19], the use of NIRS in specialized centers could potentially improve personalized brain care and might have an effect on long-term outcome.

17.2.7 Pathological Conditions Affecting CrSO$_2$

17.2.7.1 Factors Associated with Decreased CrSO$_2$

Hypocarbia

Hypocarbia is associated with cerebral vasoconstriction, which can lead to cerebral ischemia and white matter injury [20–23]. An acute decrease in end-tidal CO_2 was associated with decreased CrSO$_2$ [24].

Anemia

The hemoglobin concentration correlates with CrSO$_2$ [25, 26]. Red blood cell transfusion is associated with increased CrSO$_2$ in anemic premature neonates [26, 27] (Fig. 17.2). Improvement in CrSO$_2$ and a reduction in desaturation spells were more significant in those with a pre-transfusion CrSO$_2$ < 55% [27].

Hypotension with Lack of Autoregulation

The positive correlation between cerebral oxygenation and arterial blood pressure has been used as a marker of cerebrovascular pressure passivity which is common in sick premature infants and is associated with intraventricular hemorrhage [28–32]. A decrease of absolute mean blood pressure is not always associated with a decrease in CrSO$_2$ and is not necessarily associated with worse

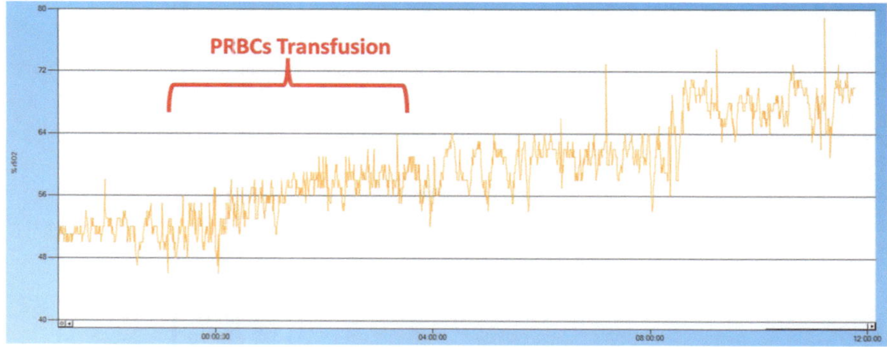

Fig. 17.2 Effect of anemia and transfusion on cerebral saturation. This tracing represents 12 hours of NIRS recording in a 5-day-old neonate, 25 weeks GA and 700 grams. Hematocrit concentration was noted to be 25%. Transfusion of packed red cells was associated with increased cerebral saturation from about 50% to about 70%

neurodevelopmental outcome. Nevertheless, $CrSO_2 < 50\%$ is associated with worse neurodevelopmental outcome [33]. More studies are needed to confirm if $CrSO_2$ can be used as a marker to treat low blood pressure. However, when used, it must be combined with other parameters to fully evaluate the significance of the low blood pressure, e.g., blood lactate, capillary refill, urine output, and cardiac output [34]. Nonetheless, rapid correction of blood pressure and significant fluctuations in blood pressure should be avoided.

Thoracic Hyperinflation

Mechanical ventilation can alter intrathoracic pressure leading to changes in venous return and thereby cardiac output, which can affect cerebral circulation [35, 36]. NIRS has a potential to detect the effects of mechanical respiratory support on the cerebral perfusion [37–39].

Patent Ductus Arteriosus (PDA)

Studies have shown that hemodynamically significant PDA is associated with decreased $CrSO_2$ [40, 41]. However, reports regarding the effect of either medical or surgical treatments of PDA on $CrSO_2$ have been inconsistent [42–44]. Whether NIRS can be used to assess the hemodynamic significance of PDA needs more studies.

Apnea

$CrSO_2$ decreased significantly during apneic spells associated with bradycardia compared to spells with no bradycardia [45]. An example is shown in Fig. 17.3.

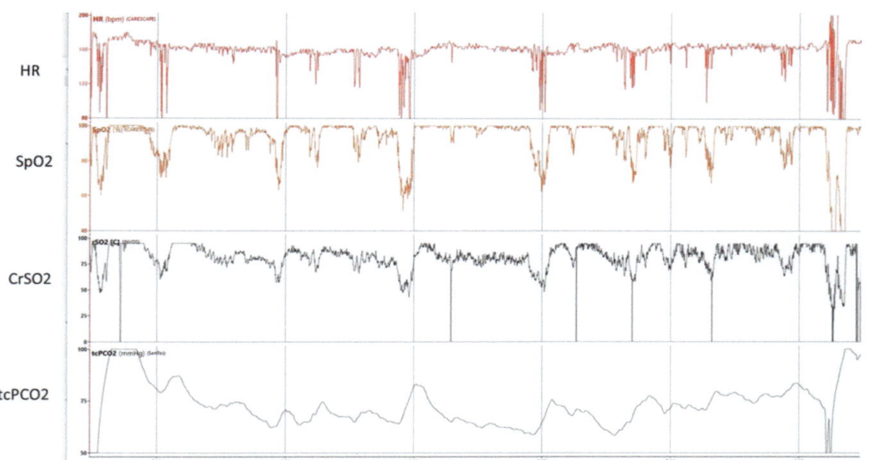

Fig. 17.3 Changes of NIRS during hypoxic events. This multimodal recording demonstrates repeated hypoxic events in a preterm infant 25 5/7 weeks GA, 880 grams, 3 days old, on high-frequency jet ventilation. Repeated hypoxic events (drops SpO_2) are associated with drops in heart rate (HR) and cerebral saturation ($CrSO_2$) and followed by increase in transcutaneous CO_2 ($tcPCO_2$)

Germinal Matrix-Intraventricular Hemorrhage (GM-IVH)

Multiple studies have reported increased $CrSO_2$ in the first hours after birth in premature infants who later developed GM-IVH [46–48]. However, infants already identified with IVH are noted to have lower $CrSO_2$ [3, 49–51].

Post-Hemorrhagic Ventricular Dilatation (PHVD)

In preterm infants with PHVD, ventricular decompression was associated with an increase in $CrSO_2$ [52–54].

A decrease in $CrSO_2$ could be associated with decreased cerebral O2 delivery/perfusion or increased O2 consumption. A patient with significantly decreased $CrSO_2$ relative to baseline or absolute $CrSO_2 < 60\%$ needs to be evaluated for anemia, hypoxia, hypotension, chest hyperinflation, and hypocarbia and treated accordingly (Fig. 17.4).

17.2.7.2 Factors Associated with Increased $CrSO_2$

Hypercarbia

Hypercarbia is associated with cerebral vasodilatation and with the development of GMH-IVH [55, 56]. An acute increase in end-tidal CO_2 was associated with increased $CrSO_2$ [24].

Hyperoxia

$CrSO_2$ correlates with systemic O_2 saturation (SaO_2). Because of the concern for oxygen toxicity, the FiO2 should only be changed to maintain systemic SaO_2 within recommended target ranges [34].

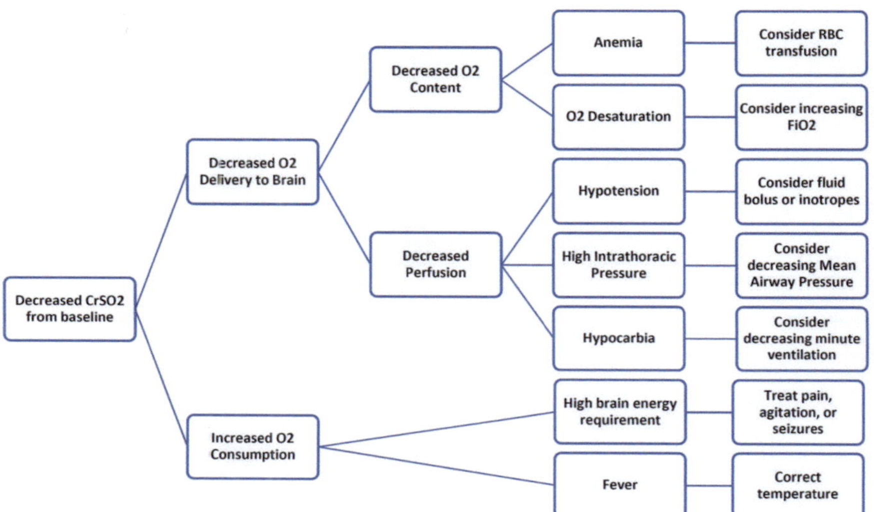

Fig. 17.4 Possible etiologies of decreased cerebral saturation and possible suggested interventions (with permission from El-Dib and Soul [4])

Hypoglycemia

Hypoglycemia can be associated with increased cerebral blood flow [57]. Although studies have demonstrated negative correlation between blood glucose and $CrSO_2$ [58], whether NIRS can be used as a marker of significant hypoglycemia is yet to be determined [59].

Inotropes with Lack of Autoregulation

While of potential benefit, the use of inotropes in premature infants may be associated with increased mortality and morbidity [60]. NIRS was used to monitor increasing cerebral blood flow with the use of inotropes [61]. It can help to monitor the effect of these medications on cerebral perfusion and oxygenation and potentially could lead to interventions to limit their adverse effects.

An increase in $CrSO_2$ could be associated with increased cerebral O_2 delivery/ perfusion or decreased O2 consumption. A patient with significantly increased $CrSO_2$ relative to baseline or absolute $CrSO_2 > 90\%$ needs to be evaluated for hyperoxia, hypercarbia, hypoglycemia, over-sedation, or severe brain injury (Fig. 17.5).

17.2.7.3 Full-Term Neonates with Neonatal Encephalopathy

Among infants with neonatal encephalopathy (NE) undergoing therapeutic hypothermia, NIRS demonstrates patterns of brain oxygenation that are predictive of either favorable or adverse outcomes [62, 63]. The early hours of therapeutic hypothermia, from 1 to 4 h, are characterized by decreased $CrSO_2$ [63], which is hypothesized to reflect decreased oxygen delivery coinciding with the abrupt decrease in body temperature [64]. From 12 h onward, there is an increase in $CrSO_2$. One study found that the increase in $CrSO_2$ from day 1 to day 2 was only significant among those with an abnormal post-rewarming MRI [65]. Similarly, $CrSO_2$ was

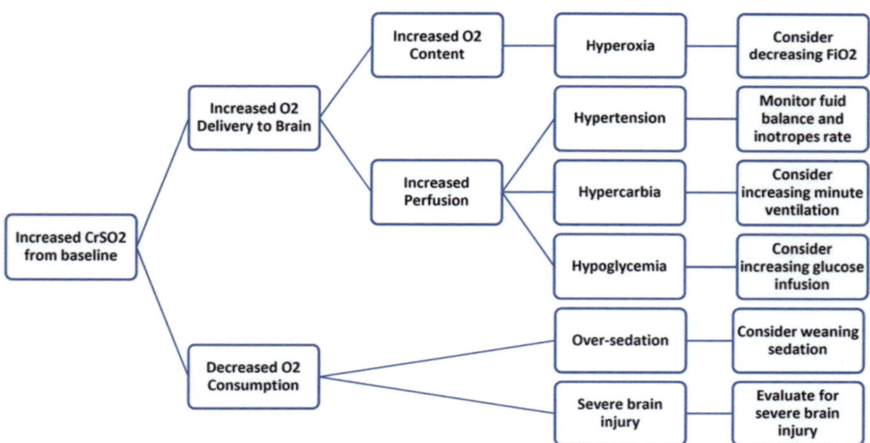

Fig. 17.5 Possible etiologies of increased cerebral saturation and possible suggested interventions (with permission from El-Dib and Soul [4])

significantly higher in infants who had brain injury demonstrated on post-rewarming MRI [65], day 10 MRI, or autopsy [63] or had adverse outcome defined as death or neurodevelopmental impairment at 18 months [62] (Fig. 17.6). Combining $CrSO_2$ and aEEG had the highest predictive value for MRI-detected brain injury and for adverse outcome [62, 66, 67].

17.2.7.4 Congenital Heart Disease

CHD remains a significant risk factor for neurodevelopmental disability and impairment, despite remarkable advances in surgical repair in the last decades [68]. NIRS monitoring has been incorporated for research and also clinical use in many pediatric cardiac ICUs [69, 70]. Newborns with non-cyanotic CHD have an average $CrSO_2$ of

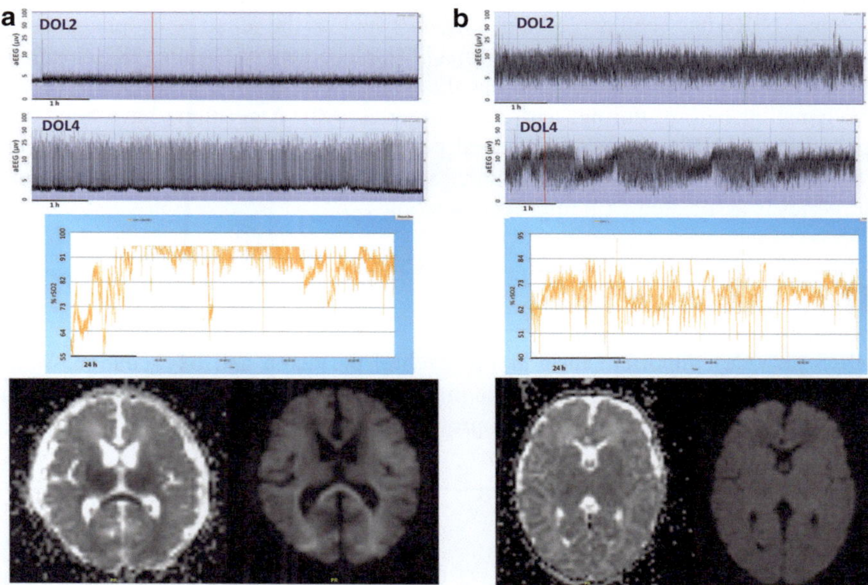

Fig. 17.6 Illustration of the value of NIRS in monitoring neonates receiving therapeutic hypothermia for neonatal encephalopathy. (**a**) aEEG and $CrSO_2$ progression and brain MRI in a term baby with severe encephalopathy (GA 40 1/7 weeks, maternal chorioamnionitis, fetal heart rate decelerations, Apgar scores 2, 2, and cardiopulmonary resuscitation for 20 min, umbilical vein pH = 6.94). aEEG evolved from flat (FT) (upper panel) to burst suppression (BS) background (lower panel) (see Chap. 16 "Neurophysiology"). $CrSO_2$ progressed to maximum measurable level of 95%. Post-rewarming MRI showed extensive brain injury (demonstrated on apparent diffusion coefficient (ADC) map sequence to the left and diffusion-weighted imaging (DWI) sequence to the right) (see Chap. 8 "Hypoxic-Ischemic Encephalopathy"). (**b**) aEEG and $CrSO_2$ progression and brain MRI in a term baby with moderate encephalopathy (GA 39 5/7 weeks, floppy at birth, Apgar score 0, 3 and 3, needed PPV for 10 min before intubation, umbilical artery pH = 6.87). aEEG evolved from discontinuous (DC) (upper panel) to continuous (C) with cycling (lower panel). $CrSO_2$ was stable in the mid 70s during hypothermia and rewarming. Post-rewarming MRI was normal (demonstrated on ADC map sequence to the left and DWI sequence to the right). Adopted from El-Dib et al. [1] with permission

~70%, while those with cyanotic CHD have $CrSO_2$ ranging from 40% to 70% [71]. Monitoring $CrSO_2$ during cardiac surgery and in the peri-operative period may help identify newborns at risk of brain injury and/or adverse neurologic outcome, which could help clinicians use strategies to optimize cerebral oxygenation and perfusion and improve outcome [72]. Several studies have identified that lower $CrSO_2$ is associated with neuronal dysfunction and adverse neurologic outcome [72, 73]. One study showed that a post-operative combination of low $CrSO_2$ and high lactate level was most predictive of death or poor neurodevelopmental outcome up to 21 months [74], with optimal cutoff values <58% and >7.4 mmol/L, respectively (sensitivity 95%).

17.2.7.5 NIRS in Anesthesia and Surgery

Non-cardiac surgeries, especially those conducted under general anesthesia, have also been associated with worse neurodevelopmental outcomes [75]. The use of cerebral NIRS has been explored in surgeries such as the repair of esophageal atresia [76], congenital diaphragmatic hernia [77], placement of G-tube [78], closure of gastroschisis [79], and more, as it has the potential to monitor brain perfusion and oxygenation before, during, and after surgeries [80]. Algorithms have been suggested to use NIRS to correct cerebral perfusion and oxygenation during surgery [81, 82]. However, it is yet to be studied whether the universal use of NIRS during surgeries is associated with improved outcomes.

17.3 Conclusion

NIRS provides important insights on cerebral perfusion and oxygenation. When used, especially as part of multimodal monitoring, it can assist in providing personalized care aiming for cerebral neuroprotection and improved newborn brain care.

References

1. El-Dib M, Abend NS, Austin T, Boylan G, Chock V, Cilio MR, Greisen G, Hellström-Westas L, Lemmers P, Pellicer A, Pressler RM, Sansevere A, Tsuchida T, Vanhatalo S, Wusthoff CJ. Neuromonitoring in neonatal critical care part I: neonatal encephalopathy and neonates with possible seizures. Pediatr Res. 2023;94(1):64–73.
2. El-Dib M, Abend NS, Austin T, Boylan G, Chock V, Cilio MR, Greisen G, Hellström-Westas L, Lemmers P, Pellicer A, Pressler RM, Sansevere A, Szakmar E, Tsuchida T, Vanhatalo S, Wusthoff CJ. Neuromonitoring in neonatal critical care part II: extremely premature infants and critically ill neonates. Pediatr Res. 2023;94(1):55–63.
3. El-Dib M, Munster C, Sunwoo J, Cherkerzian S, Lee S, Hildrey E, Steele T, Bell K, Franceschini MA, Volpe JJ, Inder T. Association of early cerebral oxygen saturation and brain injury in extremely preterm infants. J Perinatol. 2022;42(10):1385–91.
4. El-Dib M, Soul JS. Monitoring and management of brain hemodynamics and oxygenation. Handb Clin Neurol. 2019;162:295–314.
5. Alderliesten T, Dix L, Baerts W, Caicedo A, van Huffel S, Naulaers G, Groenendaal F, van Bel F, Lemmers P. Reference values of regional cerebral oxygen saturation during the first 3 days of life in preterm neonates. Pediatr Res. 2016;79(1):55–64.

6. Ancora G, Maranella E, Aceti A, Pierantoni L, Grandi S, Corvaglia L, Faldella G. Effect of posture on brain hemodynamics in preterm newborns not mechanically ventilated. Neonatology. 2010;97(3):212–7.

7. Limperopoulos C, Gauvreau KK, O'Leary H, Moore M, Bassan H, Eichenwald EC, Soul JS, Ringer SA, Di Salvo DN, Du Plessis AJ. Cerebral hemodynamic changes during intensive care of preterm infants. Pediatrics. 2008;122(5):e1006–13.

8. Roche-Labarbe N, Fenoglio A, Aggarwal A, Dehaes M, Carp SA, Franceschini MA, Grant PE. Near-infrared spectroscopy assessment of cerebral oxygen metabolism in the developing premature brain. J Cereb Blood Flow Metab. 2012;32(3):481–8.

9. Sorensen LC, Greisen G. The brains of very preterm newborns in clinically stable condition may be hyperoxygenated. Pediatrics. 2009;124(5):e958-959e963.

10. Tina LG, Frigiola A, Abella R, Artale B, Puleo G, D'Angelo S, Musmarra C, Tagliabue P, Li Volti G, Florio P, Gazzolo D. Near infrared spectroscopy in healthy preterm and term newborns: correlation with gestational age and standard monitoring parameters. Curr Neurovasc Res. 2009;6(3):148–54.

11. Wijbenga RG, Lemmers PMA, Van Bel F. Cerebral oxygenation during the first days of life in preterm and term neonates: differences between different brain regions. Pediatr Res. 2011;70(4):389–94.

12. Dix LML, Van Bel F, Baerts W, Lemmers PMA. Comparing near-infrared spectroscopy devices and their sensors for monitoring regional cerebral oxygen saturation in the neonate. Pediatr Res. 2013;74(5):557–63.

13. Schneider A, Minnich B, Hofstätter E, Weisser C, Hattinger-Jürgenssen E, Wald M. Comparison of four near-infrared spectroscopy devices shows that they are only suitable for monitoring cerebral oxygenation trends in preterm infants. Acta Paediatr. 2014;103(9):934–8.

14. Kaiser JR, Gauss CH, Williams DK. Surfactant administration acutely affects cerebral and systemic hemodynamics and gas exchange in very-low-birth-weight infants. J Pediatr. 2004;144(6):809–14.

15. Hyttel-Sorensen S, Pellicer A, Alderliesten T, Austin T, Van Bel F, Benders M, Claris O, Dempsey E, Franz AR, Fumagalli M, Gluud C, Grevstad B, Hagmann C, Lemmers P, Van Oeveren W, Pichler G, Plomgaard AM, Riera J, Sanchez L, Winkel P, Wolf M, Greisen G. Cerebral near infrared spectroscopy oximetry in extremely preterm infants: phase II randomised clinical trial. BMJ (Online). 2015;350

16. Plomgaard AM, Alderliesten T, Austin T, van Bel F, Benders M, Claris O, Dempsey E, Fumagalli M, Gluud C, Hagmann C, Hyttel-Sorensen S, Lemmers P, van Oeveren W, Pellicer A, Petersen TH, Pichler G, Winkel P, Greisen G. Early biomarkers of brain injury and cerebral hypo- and hyperoxia in the SafeBoosC II trial. PLoS One. 2017;12(3):e0173440.

17. Plomgaard AM, Hagmann C, Alderliesten T, Austin T, van Bel F, Claris O, Dempsey E, Franz A, Fumagalli M, Gluud C, Greisen G, Hyttel-Sorensen S, Lemmers P, Pellicer A, Pichler G, Benders M. Brain injury in the international multicenter randomized SafeBoosC phase II feasibility trial: cranial ultrasound and magnetic resonance imaging assessments. Pediatr Res. 2016a;79(3):466–72.

18. Plomgaard AM, van Oeveren W, Petersen TH, Alderliesten T, Austin T, van Bel F, Benders M, Claris O, Dempsey E, Franz A, Fumagalli M, Gluud C, Hagmann C, Hyttel-Sorensen S, Lemmers P, Pellicer A, Pichler G, Winkel P, Greisen G. The SafeBoosC II randomized trial: treatment guided by near-infrared spectroscopy reduces cerebral hypoxia without changing early biomarkers of brain injury. Pediatr Res. 2016b;79(4):528–35.

19. Hansen ML, Pellicer A, Hyttel-Sørensen S, Ergenekon E, Szczapa T, Hagmann C, Naulaers G, Mintzer J, Fumagalli M, Dimitriou G, Dempsey E, Tkaczyk J, Cheng G, Fredly S, Heuchan AM, Pichler G, Fuchs H, Nesargi S, Hahn GH, Piris-Borregas S, Širc J, Alsina-Casanova M, Stocker M, Ozkan H, Sarafidis K, Hopper AO, Karen T, Rzepecka-Weglarz B, Oguz SS, Arruza L, Memisoglu AC, Del Rio Florentino R, Baserga M, Maton P, Truttmann AC, de Las Cuevas I, Agergaard P, Zafra P, Bender L, Lauterbach R, Lecart C, de Buyst J, El-Khuffash A, Curley A, Vaccarello OO, Miletin J, Papathoma E, Vesoulis Z, Vento G, Cornette L, Lopez LS, Yasa B, Klamer A, Agosti M, Baud O, Mastretta E, Cetinkaya M,

McCall K, Zeng S, Hatzidaki E, Bargiel A, Marciniak S, Gao X, Huijia L, Chalak L, Yang L, Rao SA, Xu X, Gonzalez BL, Wilinska M, Yin Z, Sadowska-Krawczenko I, Serrano-Viñuales I, Krolak-Olejnik B, Ybarra MM, Morales-Betancourt C, Korček P, Teresa-Palacio M, Mosca F, Hergenhan A, Koksal N, Tsoni K, Kadri MM, Knöpfli C, Rafinska-Wazny E, Akin MS, Nordvik T, Peng Z, Kersin SG, Thewissen L, Alarcon A, Healy D, Urlesberger B, Baş M, Baumgartner J, Skylogianni E, Karadyova V, Valverde E, Bergon-Sendin E, Kucera J, Pisoni S, Wang L, Smits A, Sanchez-Salmador R, Rasmussen MI, Olsen MH, Jensen AK, Gluud C, Jakobsen JC, Greisen G. Cerebral oximetry monitoring in extremely preterm infants. N Engl J Med. 2023;388(16):1501–11.

20. Greisen G, Vannucci RC. Is periventricular leucomalacia a result of hypoxic-ischaemic injury? Hypocapnia and the preterm brain. Biol Neonate. 2001;79(3-4):194–200.

21. Liao SL, Lai SH, Chou YH, Kuo CY. Effect of hypocapnia in the first three days of life on the subsequent development of periventricular leukomalacia in premature infants. Acta Paediatr Taiwan. 2001;42(2):90–3.

22. Murase M, Ishida A. Early hypocarbia of preterm infants: its relationship to periventricular leukomalacia and cerebral palsy, and its perinatal risk factors. Acta Paediatr. 2005;94(1):85–91.

23. Shankaran S, Langer JC, Kazzi SN, Laptook AR, Walsh M. Cumulative index of exposure to hypocarbia and hyperoxia as risk factors for periventricular leukomalacia in low birth weight infants. Pediatrics. 2006;118(4):1654–9.

24. Dix LML, Weeke LC, de Vries LS, Groenendaal F, Baerts W, van Bel F, Lemmers PMA. Carbon dioxide fluctuations are associated with changes in cerebral oxygenation and electrical activity in infants born preterm. J Pediatr. 2017;187:66–72.e61

25. El-Dib M, Aly S, Govindan R, Mohamed M, du Plessis A, Aly H. Brain maturity and variation of oxygen extraction in premature infants. Am J Perinatol. 2016;33(8):814–20.

26. Van Hoften JCR, Verhagen EA, Keating P, Ter Horst HJ, Bos AF. Cerebral tissue oxygen saturation and extraction in preterm infants before and after blood transfusion. Arch Dis Child Fetal Neonatal Ed. 2010;95(5):F352–8.

27. Seidel D, Bläser A, Gebauer C, Pulzer F, Thome U, Knüpfer M. Changes in regional tissue oxygenation saturation and desaturations after red blood cell transfusion in preterm infants. J Perinatol. 2013;33(4):282–7.

28. O'Leary H, Gregas MC, Limperopoulos C, Zaretskaya I, Bassan H, Soul JS, Di Salvo DN, Du Plessis AJ. Elevated cerebral pressure passivity is associated with prematurity-related intracranial hemorrhage. Pediatrics. 2009;124(1):302–9.

29. Riera J, Cabañas F, Serrano JJ, Bravo MC, López-Ortego P, Sánchez L, Madero R, Pellicer A. New time-frequency method for cerebral autoregulation in newborns: predictive capacity for clinical outcomes. J Pediatr. 2014;165(5):897–902.e891

30. Soul JS, Hammer PE, Tsuji M, Saul JP, Bassan H, Limperopoulos C, Disalvo DN, Moore M, Akins P, Ringer S, Volpe JJ, Trachtenberg F, Du Plessis AJ. Fluctuating pressure-passivity is common in the cerebral circulation of sick premature infants. Pediatr Res. 2007;61(4):467–73.

31. Tsuji M, Saul JP, du Plessis A, Eichenwald E, Sobh J, Crocker R, Volpe JJ. Cerebral intravascular oxygenation correlates with mean arterial pressure in critically ill premature infants. Pediatrics. 2000;106(4):625–32.

32. Vesoulis ZA, Mathur AM. Cerebral autoregulation, brain injury, and the transitioning premature infant. Front Pediatr. 2017;5:7.

33. Alderliesten T, Lemmers PMA, Van Haastert IC, De Vries LS, Bonestroo HJC, Baerts W, Van Bel F. Hypotension in preterm neonates: low blood pressure alone does not affect neurodevelopmental outcome. J Pediatr. 2014;164(5):986–91.

34. Pellicer A, Greisen G, Benders M, Claris O, Dempsey E, Fumagalli M, Gluud C, Hagmann C, Hellström-Westas L, Hyttel-Sorensen S, Lemmers P, Naulaers G, Pichler G, Roll C, Van Bel F, Van Oeveren W, Skoog M, Wolf M, Austin T. The SafeBoosC phase II randomised clinical trial: a treatment guideline for targeted near-infrared-derived cerebral tissue oxygenation versus standard treatment in extremely preterm infants. Neonatology. 2013;104(3):171–8.

35. Evans N, Kluckow M. Early determinants of right and left ventricular output in ventilated preterm infants. Arch Dis Child Fetal Neonatal Ed. 1996;74(2):F88–94.

36. Skinner JR, Milligan DWA, Hunter S, Hey EN. Central venous pressure in the ventilated neonate. Arch Dis Child. 1992;67(4 SUPPL):374–7.
37. Noone MA, Sellwood M, Meek JH, Wyatt JS. Postnatal adaptation of cerebral blood flow using near infrared spectroscopy in extremely preterm infants undergoing high-frequency oscillatory ventilation. Acta Paediatr. 2003;92(9):1079–84.
38. Palmer KS, Spencer SA, Wickramasinghe Y, Wright T, Southall DP, Rolfe P. Effects of positive and negative-pressure ventilation on cerebral blood-volume of newborn-infants. Acta Paediatr. 1995;84(2):132–9.
39. Zaramella P, Freato F, Grazzina N, Saraceni E, Vianello A, Chiandetti L. Does helmet CPAP reduce cerebral blood flow and volume by comparison with infant flow driver CPAP in preterm neonates? Intensive Care Med. 2006;32(10):1613–9.
40. Lemmers PM, Toet MC, van Bel F. Impact of patent ductus arteriosus and subsequent therapy with indomethacin on cerebral oxygenation in preterm infants. Pediatrics. 2008;121(1):142–7.
41. Underwood MA, Milstein JM, Sherman MP. Near-infrared spectroscopy as a screening tool for patent ductus arteriosus in extremely low birth weight infants. Neonatology. 2007;91(2):134–9.
42. Bhatt M, Petrova A, Mehta R. Does treatment of patent ductus arteriosus with cyclooxygenase inhibitors affect neonatal regional tissue oxygenation? Pediatr Cardiol. 2012;33(8):1307–14.
43. Lemmers PMA, Molenschot MC, Evens J, Toet MC, Van Bel F. Is cerebral oxygen supply compromised in preterm infants undergoing surgical closure for patent ductus arteriosus? Arch Dis Child Fetal Neonatal Ed. 2010;95(6):F429–34.
44. Vanderhaegen J, De Smet D, Meyns B, Van De Velde M, Van Huffel S, Naulaers G. Surgical closure of the patent ductus arteriosus and its effect on the cerebral tissue oxygenation. Acta Paediatr. 2008;97(12):1640–4.
45. Pichler G, Urlesberger B, Müller W. Impact of bradycardia on cerebral oxygenation and cerebral blood volume during apnoea in preterm infants. Physiol Meas. 2003;24(3):671–80.
46. Alderliesten T, Lemmers PM, Smarius JJ, van de Vosse RE, Baerts W, van Bel F. Cerebral oxygenation, extraction, and autoregulation in very preterm infants who develop peri-intraventricular hemorrhage. J Pediatr. 2013;162(4):698–704 e692.
47. Cimatti AG, Martini S, Galletti S, Vitali F, Aceti A, Frabboni G, Faldella G, Corvaglia L. Cerebral Oxygenation and Autoregulation in Very Preterm Infants Developing IVH During the Transitional Period: A Pilot Study. Frontiers in pediatrics 2020;8:381.
48. Zhang Y, Chan GS, Tracy MB, Lee QY, Hinder M, Savkin AV, Lovell NH. Cerebral near-infrared spectroscopy analysis in preterm infants with intraventricular hemorrhage. Conf Proc IEEE Eng Med Biol Soc. 2011;2011:1937–40.
49. Noori S, McCoy M, Anderson MP, Ramji F, Seri I. Changes in cardiac function and cerebral blood flow in relation to peri/intraventricular hemorrhage in extremely preterm infants. J Pediatr. 2014;164(2):264–70. e261-263
50. Sorensen LC, Maroun LL, Borch K, Lou HC, Greisen G. Neonatal cerebral oxygenation is not linked to foetal vasculitis and predicts intraventricular haemorrhage in preterm infants. Acta Paediatr. 2008;97(11):1529–34.
51. Verhagen EA, Ter Horst HJ, Keating P, Martijn A, Van Braeckel KNJA, Bos AF. Cerebral oxygenation in preterm infants with germinal matrix-intraventricular hemorrhages. Stroke. 2010;41(12):2901–7.
52. Kochan M, McPadden J, Bass WT, Shah T, Brown WT, Tye GW, Vazifedan T. Changes in cerebral oxygenation in preterm infants with progressive posthemorrhagic ventricular dilatation. Pediatr Neurol. 2017;73:57–63.
53. Norooz F, Urlesberger B, Giordano V, Klebermasz-Schrehof K, Weninger M, Berger A, Olischar M. Decompressing posthaemorrhagic ventricular dilatation significantly improves regional cerebral oxygen saturation in preterm infants. Acta Paediatr. 2015;104(7):663–9.
54. Soul JS, Eichenwald E, Walter G, Volpe JJ, du Plessis AJ. CSF removal in infantile posthemorrhagic hydrocephalus results in significant improvement in cerebral hemodynamics. Pediatr Res. 2004;55(5):872–6.

55. Kaiser JR, Gauss CH, Pont MM, Williams DK. Hypercapnia during the first 3 days of life is associated with severe intraventricular hemorrhage in very low birth weight infants. J Perinatol. 2006;26(5):279–85.
56. Kaiser JR, Gauss CH, Williams DK. The effects of hypercapnia on cerebral autoregulation in ventilated very low birth weight infants. Pediatr Res. 2005;58(5):931–5.
57. Pryds O, Christensen NJ, Friis-Hansen B. Increased cerebral blood flow and plasma epinephrine in hypoglycemic, preterm neonates. Pediatrics. 1990;85(2):172–6.
58. Matterberger C, Baik-Schneditz N, Schwaberger B, Schmölzer GM, Mileder L, Pichler-Stachl E, Urlesberger B, Pichler G. Blood glucose and cerebral tissue oxygenation immediately after birth-an observational study. J Pediatr. 2018;200:19–23.
59. Mattersberger C, Schmölzer GM, Urlesberger B, Pichler G. Blood glucose and lactate levels and cerebral oxygenation in preterm and term neonates-a systematic qualitative review of the literature. Front Pediatr. 2020;8:361.
60. Wong J, Shah PS, Yoon EW, Yee W, Lee S, Dow K. Inotrope use among extremely preterm infants in Canadian neonatal intensive care units: variation and outcomes. Am J Perinatol. 2015;32(1):9–14.
61. Munro MJ, Walker AM, Barfield CP. Hypotensive extremely low birth weight infants have reduced cerebral blood flow. Pediatrics. 2004;114(6):1591–6.
62. Lemmers PMA, Zwanenburg RJ, Benders MJNL, De Vries LS, Groenendaal F, Van Bel F, Toet MC. Cerebral oxygenation and brain activity after perinatal asphyxia: does hypothermia change their prognostic value? Pediatr Res. 2013;74(2):180–5.
63. Peng S, Boudes E, Tan X, Saint-Martin C, Shevell M, Wintermark P. Does near-infrared spectroscopy identify asphyxiated newborns at risk of developing brain injury during hypothermia treatment? Am J Perinatol. 2015;32(6):555–64.
64. Thoresen M. Cooling the newborn after asphyxia—physiological and experimental background and its clinical use. Semin Neonatol. 2000;5(1):61–73.
65. Szakmar E, Smith J, Yang E, Volpe JJ, Inder T, El-Dib M. Association between cerebral oxygen saturation and brain injury in neonates receiving therapeutic hypothermia for neonatal encephalopathy. J Perinatol. 2021:1–9.
66. Goeral K, Urlesberger B, Giordano V, Kasprian G, Wagner M, Schmidt L, Berger A, Klebermass-Schrehof K, Olischar M. Prediction of outcome in neonates with hypoxic-ischemic encephalopathy II: role of amplitude-integrated electroencephalography and cerebral oxygen saturation measured by near-infrared spectroscopy. Neonatology. 2017;112(3):193–202.
67. Niezen CK, Bos AF, Sival DA, Meiners LC, Ter Horst HJ. Amplitude-integrated EEG and cerebral near-infrared spectroscopy in cooled, asphyxiated infants. Am J Perinatol. 2018;35(9):904–10.
68. Massaro AN, El-Dib M, Glass P, Aly H. Factors associated with adverse neurodevelopmental outcomes in infants with congenital heart disease. Brain and Development. 2008;30(7):437–46.
69. Hirsch JC, Charpie JR, Ohye RG, Gurney JG. Near-infrared spectroscopy: what we know and what we need to know-a systematic review of the congenital heart disease literature. J Thorac Cardiovasc Surg. 2009;137(1):154–9.e112
70. Neshat Vahid S, Panisello JM. The state of affairs of neurologic monitoring by near-infrared spectroscopy in pediatric cardiac critical care. Curr Opin Pediatr. 2014;26(3):299–303.
71. Andropoulos DB, Stayer SA, Diaz LK, Ramamoorthy C. Neurological monitoring for congenital heart surgery. Anesth Analg. 2004;99(5):1365–75.
72. Lee JK, Easley RB, Brady KM. Neurocognitive monitoring and care during pediatric cardiopulmonary bypass—current and future directions. Curr Cardiol Rev. 2008;4(2):123–39.
73. Toet MC, Flinterman A, Laar I, Vries JW, Bennink GB, Uiterwaal CS, Bel F. Cerebral oxygen saturation and electrical brain activity before, during, and up to 36 hours after arterial switch procedure in neonates without pre-existing brain damage: its relationship to neurodevelopmental outcome. Exp Brain Res. 2005;165(3):343–50.
74. Aly SA, Zurakowski D, Glass P, Skurow-Todd K, Jonas RA, Donofrio MT. Cerebral tissue oxygenation index and lactate at 24 hours postoperative predict survival and neurodevelopmental outcome after neonatal cardiac surgery. Congenit Heart Dis. 2017;12(2):188–95.

75. Stolwijk LJ, Lemmers PMA, Harmsen M, Groenendaal F, de Vries LS, van der Zee DC, Benders MJN, van Herwaarden-Lindeboom MYA. Neurodevelopmental outcomes after neonatal surgery for major noncardiac anomalies. Pediatrics. 2016;137:2.
76. Conforti A, Giliberti P, Mondi V, Valfré L, Sgro S, Picardo S, Bagolan P, Dotta A. Near infrared spectroscopy: experience on esophageal atresia infants. J Pediatr Surg. 2014;49(7):1064–8.
77. Cruz SM, Lau PE, Rusin CG, Style CC, Cass DL, Fernandes CJ, Lee TC, Rhee CJ, Keswani S, Ruano R, Welty SE, Olutoye OO. A novel multimodal computational system using near-infrared spectroscopy predicts the need for ECMO initiation in neonates with congenital diaphragmatic hernia. J Pediatr Surg. 2018;53(1):152–8.
78. Muñoz A, Tan J, Hopper A, Vannix R, Carter H, Woodfin M, Blood A, Baerg J. Cerebral and renal oxygenation in infants undergoing laparoscopic gastrostomy tube placement. J Surg Res. 2020;256:83–9.
79. Stienstra RM, McHoney M. Near-infrared spectroscopy (NIRS) measured tissue oxygenation in neonates with gastroschisis: a pilot study. J Matern Fetal Neonatal Med. 2022;35(25):5099–107.
80. Levy PT, Pellicer A, Schwarz CE, Neunhoeffer F, Schuhmann MU, Breindahl M, Fumagelli M, Mintzer J, de Boode W, Alarcon A, Alderliesten T, Austin T, Bruckner M, de Boode WP, Dempsey G, Ergenekon E, Fumagalli M, Greisen G, Gucuyener K, Hahn GH, Kalish BT, Kooi E, Lee-Summers J, Lemmers P, Levy PT, Liem KD, Hansen ML, Martini S, Naulaers G, Pichler G, Rhee C, Roehr CC, Roll C, Schwarz CE, da Costa CS, Szczapa T, Urlesberger B, Wolf M, Wong F, on behalf of the ESIGNIS. Near-infrared spectroscopy for perioperative assessment and neonatal interventions. Pediatr Res. 2021. [Epub ahead of print].
81. Franzini S, Brebion M, Crowe AM, Querciagrossa S, Ren M, Leva E, Orliaguet G. Use of combined cerebral and somatic renal near infrared spectroscopy during noncardiac surgery in children: a proposed algorithm. Paediatr Anaesth. 2022;32(12):1278–84.
82. Weber F, Scoones GP. A practical approach to cerebral near-infrared spectroscopy (NIRS) directed hemodynamic management in noncardiac pediatric anesthesia. Paediatr Anaesth. 2019;29(10):993–1001.

Part VI

Miscellaneous

Sub-Ependymal Pseudocysts and Lenticulostriate Vasculopathy

Frances M. Cowan and Lara M. Leijser

Abbreviations

cUS	Cranial ultrasound
CTN	Caudothalamic notch
GLC	Germinal layer cyst
GMC	Germinal matrix cyst
LSV	Lenticulostriate vasculopathy
SEC	Sub-ependymal cyst
SEP	Sub-ependymal pseudocyst

F. M. Cowan (✉)
Department of Paediatrics, Imperial College London, London, UK
e-mail: f.cowan@imperial.ac.uk

L. M. Leijser
Section of Newborn Critical Care, Department of Pediatrics, Cumming School of Medicine, University of Calgary, Calgary, AB, Canada
e-mail: lara.leijser@ucalgary.ca

© The Author(s) 2024
G. Meijler, K. Mohammad (eds.), *Neonatal Brain Injury*,
https://doi.org/10.1007/978-3-031-55972-3_18

18.1 For Parents

When cranial ultrasound scans are performed on your baby to check for changes in the brain, small cysts and thin linear bright white areas in the brain tissue may be seen. Cysts that are seen on the first routine ultrasound scan are mostly not of concern and rarely cause any problems if they are small, rounded (looking like beads of a necklace), few in number, and located near the front of the lateral ventricles (the normal fluid-filled spaces) in the brain. They are often called "sub-ependymal pseudocysts." They will not get much bigger and will not influence the later development of your child. However, if the cysts are seen in combination with other changes in the brain, if your baby is sicker than expected (e.g., for their prematurity), or if there was an infection during the pregnancy, extra investigations may be suggested by the medical team. The extra investigations are done to make sure there is no underlying reason for the cysts that may need treatment or could influence your child's development.

Small bright white areas may be seen on ultrasound scans in the central parts of the brain (called deep gray matter). They are often linear in shape, located in the walls of small blood vessels, and known as lenticulostriate vasculopathy (LSV). Small amounts of LSV are frequently seen in newborn babies. Like sub-ependymal pseudocysts, LSV is mostly not of concern and will not influence the development of your child. However, if LSV is seen in combination with other changes in the brain, if the bright areas are more widespread, non-linear, and located in other areas than the deep gray matter, or if your baby is sicker than expected, extra investigations may be needed, for the same reasons as for the cysts.

18.2 For Professionals

18.2.1 Sub-Ependymal Pseudocysts and Lenticulostriate Vasculopathy

Small cystic lesions located around the lateral ventricles (sub-ependymal pseudo-cysts [SEPs]), especially the frontal horns, and in the caudothalamic notch (CTN cysts) (Fig. 18.1) and linear echodensities along the trajectory of small central arteries, known as lenticulostriate vasculopathy (LSV) (Fig. 18.2), are common findings on cranial ultrasound (cUS) scans in newborn infants. SEPs and LSV are reported

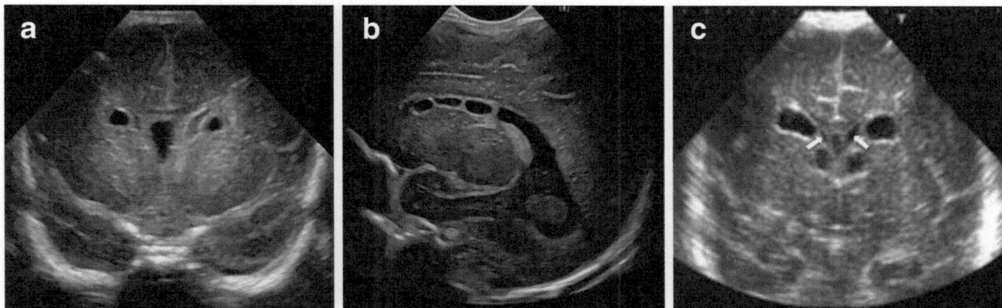

Fig. 18.1 Coronal and parasagittal cUS scans showing bilateral smooth-walled and rounded sub-ependymal cysts (SEPs) (**a**, **b**) and cysts in the caudo-thalamic notches (CTNs) (**c**). (**a**) Typical bilateral SEPs most commonly appear to be in the wall of the ventricle and can sometimes be difficult to differentiate from strands running across the anterior horns of the ventricles; (**b**) multiple small SEPs seen along the ventricular margin, often referred to as a "string of pearls"; (**c**) larger SEPs adjacent to very small lateral ventricles (arrows) in addition to cysts in both CTNs

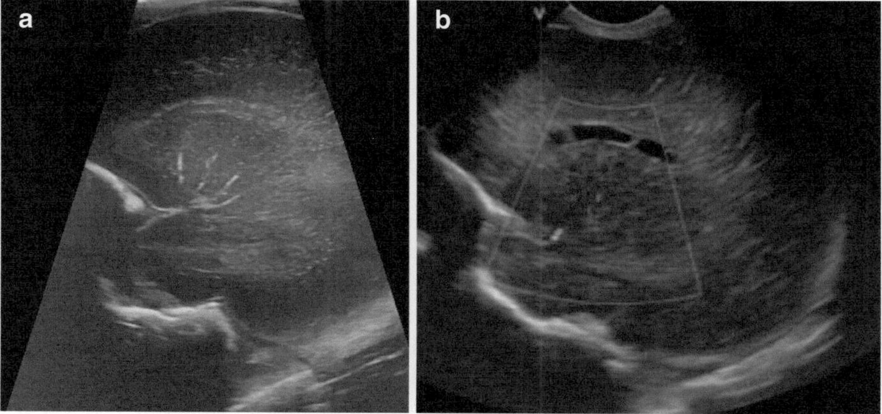

Fig. 18.2 Parasagittal cUS scans showing (**a**) mild lenticulostriate vasculopathy (LSV) in a well preterm twin; (**b**) LSV confirmed using Doppler ultrasound showing blood flow velocities within the echogenic lines in an infant with additional SEPs who had surgery for Ladd's bands

in 5–9% of newborns, being more common in preterm as compared to term-born infants [1–7].

SEPs, CTN cysts, and LSV can raise considerable concern, and it is important to assess their clinical significance. The lesions rarely cause a problem in themselves and reassurance to parents should be given about this. In particular when the cysts are small and single (though often bilateral) or the LSV is fairly faint and found on routine screening cUS in neurologically asymptomatic preterm infants, they are generally unrelated to any pathology or adverse long-term outcome. These findings are also more common in twins and triplets for reasons that are not clear, and in this context they seem benign. However, when cysts are multiple and LSV is marked and associated with more extensive echodensities in the deep gray and/or white matter that are also highly suggestive of calcifications, they can be markers of ante-natally acquired infection, such as cytomegalovirus (CMV; see below) or Rubella [8–13]. SEPs, CTN cysts, and LSV are also commonly seen in infants with genetic, developmental, or metabolic disorders [14–22]. Hence, the clinical context in which the lesions are seen and the timing of their appearance are very important in determining their clinical significance.

18.2.2 Sub-Ependymal Pseudocysts

Multiple and confusing terminologies for the small cysts located around or along the lateral ventricles are used. They can be called SEPs, sub-ependymal cysts (SECs), germinolytic cysts, germinal matrix or germinal layer cysts (GMCs and GLCs, respectively), or paraventricular cysts. If present at birth, the term connatal cysts can be used as an encompassing term. Similar looking cysts in the caudotha-lamic notches (CTN) are generally referred to by their location as CTN cysts (Fig. 18.1). There is no absolute distinction between the terminologies, and they are used alternatingly. Small cysts are generally better seen on cUS than on magnetic resonance imaging (MRI) [16].

18.2.2.1 Where Are the Cysts Located?

In general, SEPs are located inferior to a line drawn horizontally across the roof of the lateral ventricles, whereas cysts in the adjacent white matter due to injury, such as cystic periventricular leukomalacia/white matter injury and periventricular hem-orrhagic infarction, are located above that line (Fig. 18.3). SEPs are mostly bilateral, but if unilateral, they are more commonly located in the left than right hemisphere. In general they decrease in size over time [1]. Injurious white matter cysts on the other hand are usually located more laterally, often have more irregular margins, and/or are mostly larger than SEPs (Figs. 3.3 and 3.8 in Chap. 3). When referring to the SEPs, it is best to avoid the term "periventricular" as this may be taken to mean cystic periventricular leukomalacia/white matter injury, a condition that carries quite different etiologies and prognostic consequences. Small SEPs are not primar-ily in the white matter and have been mistakenly referred to as cystic periventricular leukomalacia/white matter injury in several publications (Chap. 5, "Preterm White Matter Injury") [4, 23, 24].

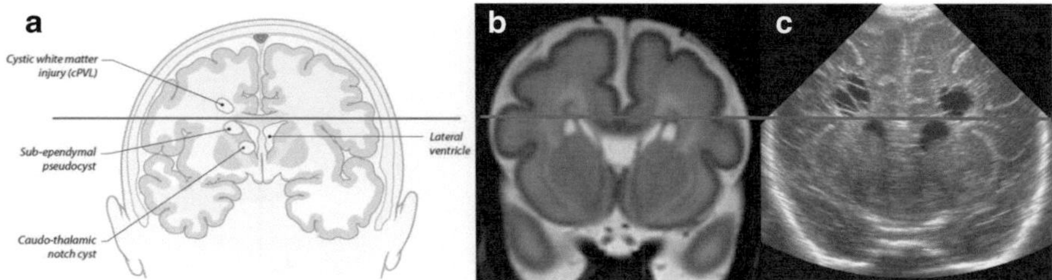

Fig. 18.3 (**a**) Schematic drawing showing SEPs, generally located below the level of the uppermost border of the lateral ventricle (represented by the green line), whereas cysts in cystic white matter injury are usually located above the green line and more laterally in the white matter. The location of CTN cysts is also shown; (**b**) coronal T2-weighted MR image of a preterm infant showing typical SEPs located below the green line. Although well seen on MRI in this example, SEPs and CTN cysts are often better seen on cUS; (**c**) coronal cUS scan showing cysts located in the white matter above the green line, typical of cystic white matter injury. (© Amanda Gautier-Ronopawiro)

18.2.2.2 Why Are Sub-Ependymal Cysts Often Called Pseudocysts?

The term "pseudocyst" is used because the sub-ependymal cysts are not lined with ependyma but develop in the germinal layer and have a wall consisting of germinal cells and glial tissue. The germinal layer lines the ventricles and gives rise to cells that migrate outwards in the second trimester to the cortex (Chap. 1, "Introduction on Development, Maturation and Vulnerability of the Neonatal Brain"). After the process of cell migration is complete, the germinal layer starts to involute, and SEPs may develop [25–27].

18.2.2.3 What Other Cysts Are Commonly Detected on cUS?

CTN cysts, having a similar appearance to SEPs, though often multilocular, are located between the head of the caudate nucleus and the thalamus. CTN cysts are best seen on a parasagittal view on cUS, just off the midline (Fig. 18.4). They are common in infants with CMV (congenital and acquired; Fig. 18.5) but may also develop in preterm infants a few weeks after birth, especially in infants with chronic lung disease. Most CTN cysts initially present as bilateral areas (but can be unilateral or asymmetric) of increased echogenicity, often mistaken for a late-onset germinal matrix hemorrhage. The echogenic areas progress to cysts that may persist for several weeks. In most cases, no clear cause is found for CTN cysts, and the cysts remain without developmental consequence. However, it is important to test for postnatally acquired CMV [28, 29]. Also, germinal matrix or germinal layer cysts (GMC/GLCs) that can develop following a germinal matrix-intraventricular hemorrhage (Fig. 18.6) are often located in the CTN. Brain MRI, in particular susceptibility-weighted imaging, can be helpful in differentiating CTN cysts from GMC/GLCs as in the case of CTN cysts, mostly no evidence of a germinal matrix-intraventricular hemorrhage is detected [30, 31].

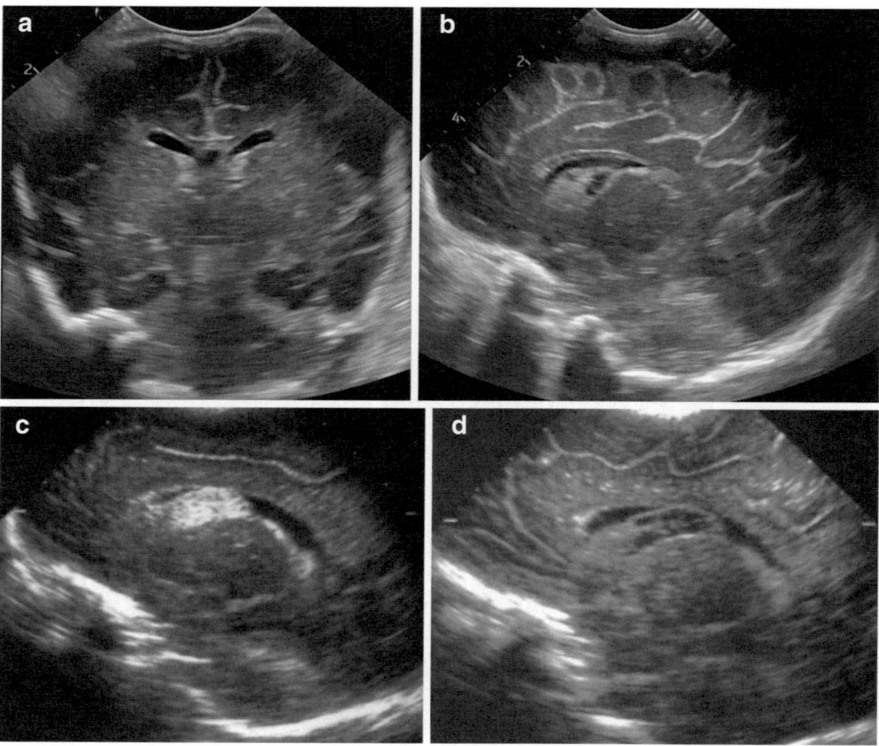

Fig. 18.4 Cranial ultrasound scans showing (**a**) bilateral echogenicity in the CTNs with some cystic development on coronal view at 6 weeks after birth in a preterm infant with chronic lung disease. These findings could be mistaken for a germinal matrix hemorrhage (GMH), but GMH generally occurs much earlier, and the appearance is not typical; (**b**) evolution of cysts in the CTN in the same infant on later parasagittal cUS scan; (**c**) large echogenic area with suggestion of some cystic change in the CTN in parasagittal view in the first postnatal week in a preterm infant (33 weeks' gestation). This could also be a large GMH but is atypically large; (**d**) parasagittal view in the same infant with overtly cystic evolution of the persisting echogenicity in the CTN over the course of several weeks. This infant was one of twins who both had similar findings on cUS, and were both positive for cytomegalovirus

Other types of cysts that are occasionally seen, in particular in preterm infants, are temporal horn cysts (Fig. 18.7) and choroid plexus cysts (Fig. 18.8) [27, 32–35].

Temporal horn cysts are not so common. They can be unilateral or bilateral and mostly resolve over time (Fig. 18.7). Their cause is often unclear, but they are reported in congenital CMV and Rubella for which testing is strongly recommended. There are also rare associations with leukoencephalopathies and Aicardi-Goutières syndrome [36], though seldom reported neonatally.

Choroid plexus cysts are nowadays mostly already seen on antenatal ultrasound scans and may persist and be seen on postnatal cUS (Fig. 18.8). In the vast majority of cases, choroid plexus cysts are benign and resolve or disappear spontaneously

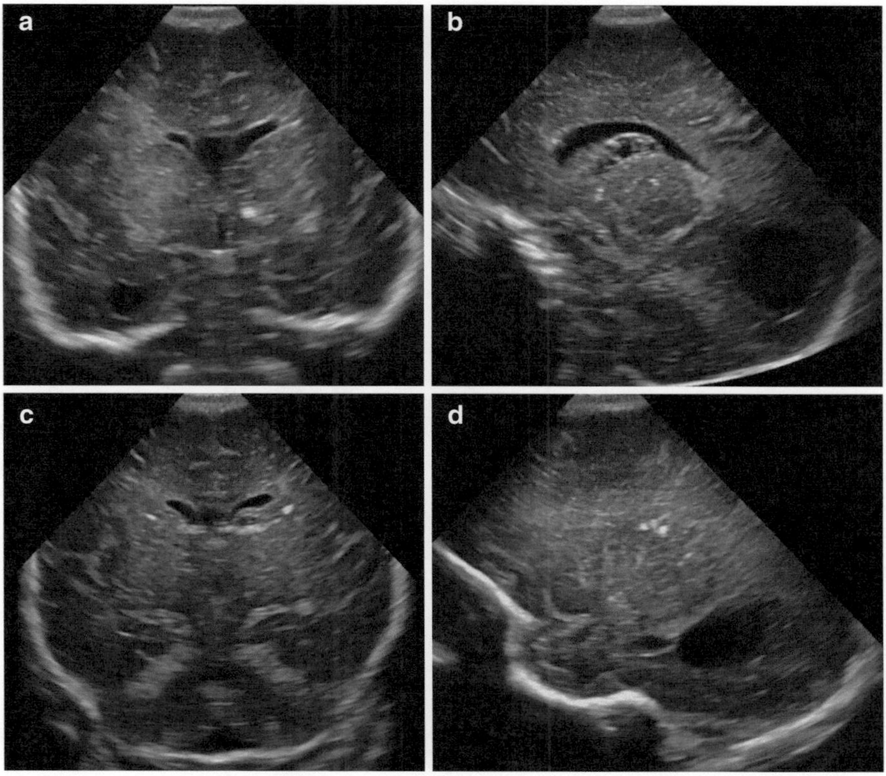

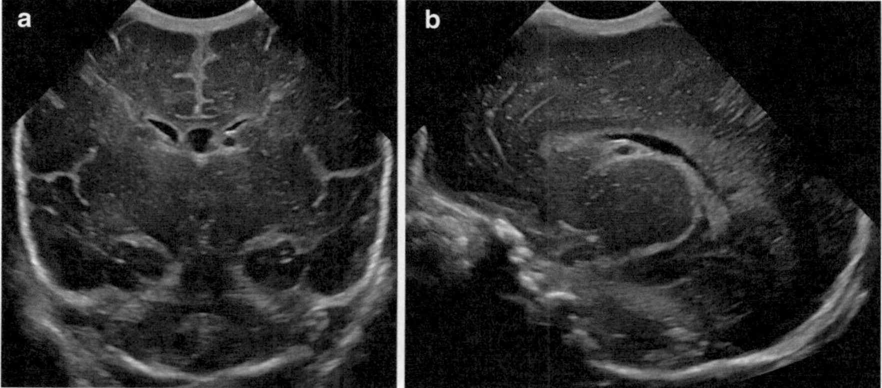

Fig. 18.5 Coronal (**a**, **c**) and left-sided parasagittal (**b**, **d**) cUS scans on day 2 in a term-born infant (39 + 4 weeks' gestation) with congenital CMV showing punctate/rounded echodensities, highly suggestive of calcifications, in the periventricular white matter and thalami, CTN cysts, subtle LSV, and dilation of the posterior and temporal ventricular horns

Fig. 18.6 (**a**) Coronal and (**b**) parasagittal cUS scans showing a small cyst that developed 2 weeks following a left-sided small germinal matrix hemorrhage in a preterm infant

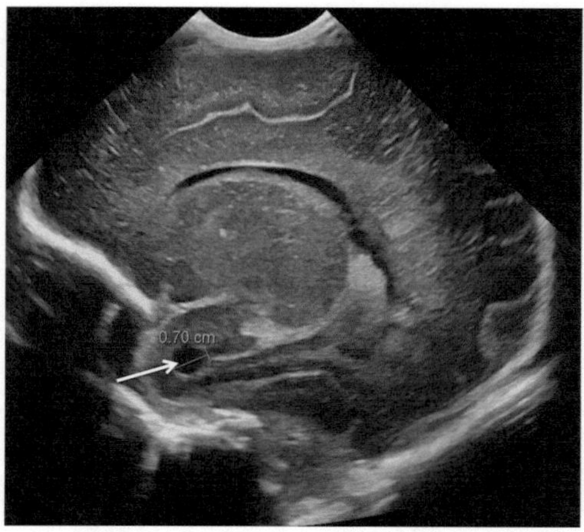

Fig. 18.7 Parasagittal cUS scan showing a cystic lesion adjacent to the temporal horn (arrow) in a well preterm infant (32 + 3 weeks gestation)

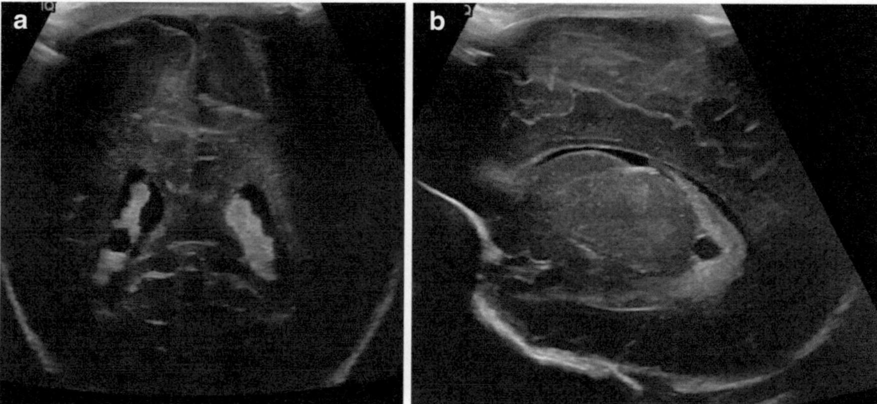

Fig. 18.8 (a) Coronal and (b) parasagittal cUS views showing a choroid plexus cyst on the right in a preterm infant (32 + 0 weeks' gestation) scanned on day 3. The choroid plexus on the left is somewhat irregular, but there was no evidence of a hemorrhage or later abnormality

without long-term consequences [37, 38]. However, in a small number of cases, in particular when there are multiple, large (>1 cm) cysts in the choroid plexus, the cysts can be an indicator of a chromosomal disorder (such as trisomy 18 or 21, Aicardi syndrome) or a metabolic disorder. In these cases, the underlying cause will determine the long-term consequences [27, 32, 39].

18.2.2.4 Neurodevelopmental Outcomes

SEPs and CTN cysts are mostly associated with normal neurodevelopmental outcomes, in particular when cysts are isolated, single (although bilateral), small, located in frontal brain areas, and without known etiology [7, 40, 41]. A recent study has shown that white matter microstructure is not different between infants with and without SEPs [42]. However, it is still strongly recommended to consider testing for CMV and other conditions in infants with SEPs and CTN cysts, in particular when cysts are large, multiple, extensive, and/or asymmetrical. While neurodevelopmental outcome may be normal in the case of multiple, large cysts, more extensive and asymmetrical cysts are more often associated with abnormal outcomes, being related to the underlying cause rather than to the cysts themselves. It is important not to miss a diagnosis with significant implications for treatment (in case of congenital CMV) and neurodevelopmental and behavioral outcomes [6, 43, 44] or that may lead to a genetic diagnosis with the possibility of recurrence in the family. An overview of more and less common conditions or lesions that can be associated with cystic lesions and calcifications and warrant further investigation in the appropriate clinical context is provided below.

18.2.3 Associations with Sub-Ependymal Pseudocysts

1. Germinal matrix hemorrhage may evolve into small cysts appearing within 1–2 weeks of the hemorrhage (Fig. 18.6). These cysts are relatively short-lived and are not associated with more adverse outcomes than might be anticipated for the gestational age of the infant, presence of intraventricular hemorrhage, illness severity, and any other brain abnormalities. Occasionally, if larger, they may obstruct the foramen of Monro and cause unilateral ventriculomegaly.
2. CTN cysts in preterm infants that appear around or after 1 month of birth and are unrelated to germinal matrix hemorrhage may be due to postnatally acquired CMV. However, in most cases no clear cause or definite adverse sequelae are identified (Fig. 18.4a, b).
3. Viral infections, in particular congenital CMV and Rubella [8–13]. These cysts are usually present at birth and most often located in the CTN. Initially the CTN can be echogenic and may gradually become multi-cystic over days to weeks; the resulting cysts can persist for many weeks (Fig. 18.5). Testing for CMV is strongly recommended when any small cysts in the CTN area are seen that are not clearly related to a prior germinal matrix hemorrhage (as seen evolve over serial cUS scans); see above. Even if antenatal testing for CMV was negative, late gestation or postnatal infection can occur, and re-testing should be done. Cysts, LSV, and other echogenicities suggestive of calcifications may appear in the same regions in both congenital and postnatally acquired CMV.
4. SEPs are more common in both mono- and dizygous twins, with the highest prevalence in the case of twin-to-twin transfusion syndrome [4, 45]. The cause of the association is unknown but seems benign.
5. In sick, symptomatic pre-term or term-born infants, particularly those who are encephalopathic, SEPS and CTN cysts can be markers of metabolic disorders such as Zellweger syndrome or mitochondrial disease [14–22]. In these cases, the cysts often co-occur with LSV and calcifications (Figs. 18.9 and 18.10).

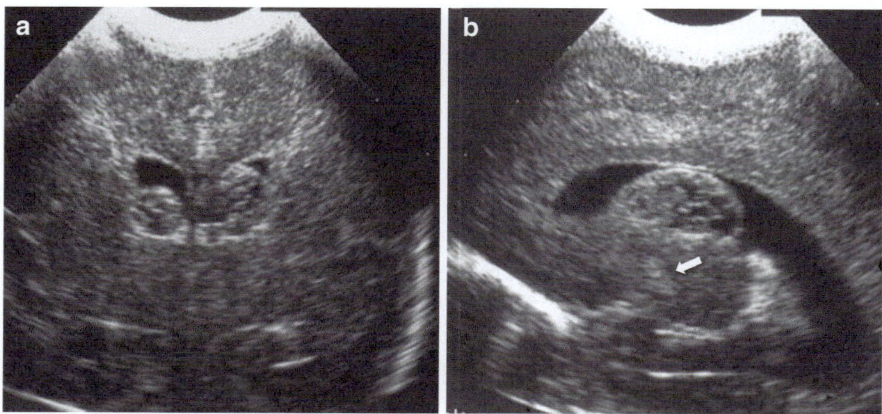

Fig. 18.9 (**a**) Coronal and (**b**) parasagittal cUS scans of a preterm infant (31 weeks' gestation) later diagnosed with a mitochondrial disorder (complex 1), showing bilateral large GLCs not preceded by intraventricular hemorrhage. There is additionally a small area of calcification in the basal ganglia seen on the parasagittal view (**b**; arrow) also commonly found with this disorder

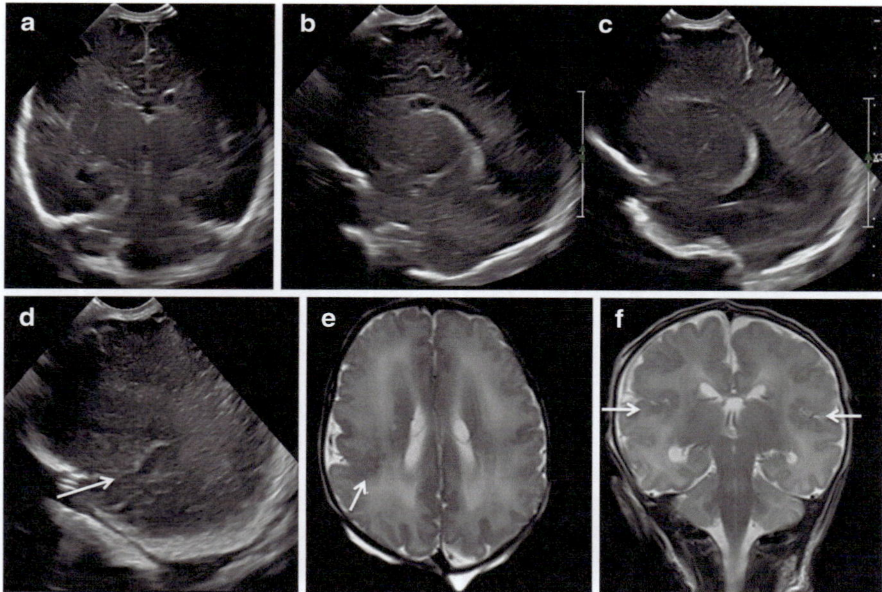

Fig. 18.10 Coronal and parasagittal cUS scans (**a–d**) and axial and coronal MR images (**e, f**) of a term infant born by uncomplicated planned C-section who presented with respiratory distress, persistent generalized hypotonia with hypermobile joints, as well as a broad nasal bridge, small chin, nuchal skin folds, and cryptorchidism; clinical seizures were confirmed electrographically. cUS on day 2 showed SEPs, CTN cysts, and subtle LSV (**a–c**) in combination with immature folding of the Sylvian fissures (**d**, arrow), suggestive of cortical dysplasia. The cysts were also seen on MRI (**e**) on day 3 together with extensive polymicrogyria (**e, f**; arrows). The cUS findings alone were highly suggestive of Zellweger syndrome which was later confirmed

18.2.4 Further, More Rare Associations with Cysts, in Particular SEPs and CTN Cysts

(Note: the table provides examples but is not all inclusive)

Disorder	Suggested investigations
Various chromosome disorders/syndromes, e.g. trisomy 18/21, 5p-, Schinzel-Giedion, Hirschhorn-Wolf	Karyotype and CGH array and whole exome sequencing (WES)
Mitochondrial spectrum disorders (Fig. 18.9), e.g. complex 1, or IV deficiency, pyruvate dehydrogenase deficiency (Fig. 18.11), pyruvate kinase deficiency-often have cysts, central gray matter calcifications, strands across the ventricles and abnormal cerebellar development	Lactate (repeated), muscle biopsy, brain proton magnetic resonance spectroscopy (MRS) for lactate. Mitochondrial gene panel
Organic acidemias, e.g. D-2-hydroxyglutaric aciduria, glutaric aciduria type 1, methylmalonic acidemia	Urine organic acids Carnitine
Peroxisomal disorders including Zellweger syndrome-often have cysts with LSV and abnormal appearance to the Sylvian fissures due to polymicrogyria (Fig. 18.10)	Very long chain fatty acids (VLCFAs)
Sulphite oxidase deficiency	**Fresh** urine for sulphite (false pos/neg occur). Low plasma homocysteine. Skin fibroblasts for lack of sulphite oxidase. Brain magnetic resonance imaging (MRI) extensive changes (HIE mimic)
Holocarboxylase synthetase deficiency	Urine organic acids, ammonia, acidosis HLCS gene (21q22.1)
Multiple acyl CoA dehydrogenase deficiency (glutaric aciduria type II)-mainly arachnoid cysts anterior to the temporal horns)	Urine organic acids; acyl carnitine profile
Carbohydrate glycosylation defects	Transferrin isoforms
Canavan's disease	High N-acetyl aspartate (NAA) on proton MRS
Alexander disease	No NAA on proton MRS
Phacomatoses, e.g. tuberous sclerosis, Gorlin basal naevus syndrome, Jadassohn's linear naevus syndrome	History and physical exam with a thorough assessment of the skin. Brain MRI, cardiac rhabdomyoma
Sotos syndrome	Large NSD1 gene
Proteus syndrome—more arachnoid than sub-ependymal cysts	Physical appearance; brain MRI
Neonatal lupus erythematosus	Maternal systemic lupus, Ro/SSA antibodies, heart block
Fetal cocaine exposure	History, neonatal behavior
Various brain malformations	Brain MRI
Pyridoxine-dependent seizures	Pyridoxine levels

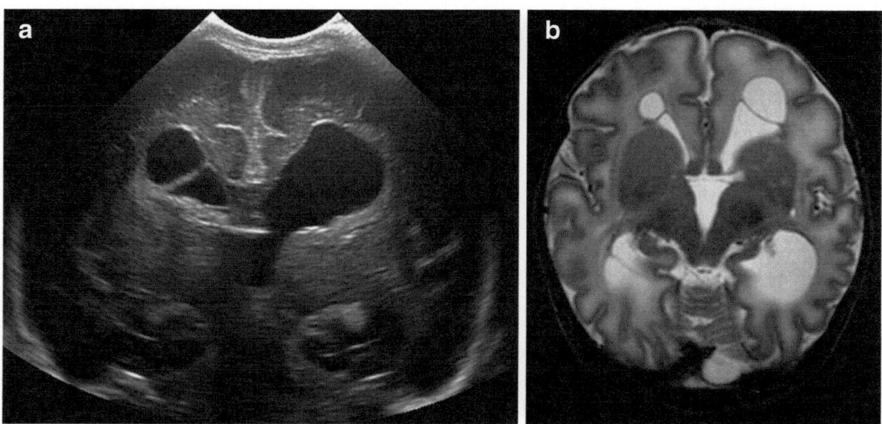

Fig. 18.11 Coronal cUS (**a**) and axial MR image (**b**) of an infant born at 42 weeks' gestation by normal vaginal delivery with good Apgar scores. The infant was admitted in the first week with cyanotic spells needing ventilation. The infant was microcephalic, had possible seizures and raised lactate levels of 4–6 mmol/L. Admission cUS (**a**) showed enlarged lateral and third ventricles with a strand across the right ventricle forming a loculated cyst. The MRI (**b**) confirmed this finding and also showed a similar strand forming a large cyst on the left as well as a strand across the right posterior horn. In this clinical context, such brain imaging findings are highly suggestive of pyruvate dehydrogenase deficiency, which was confirmed in this infant

18.2.5 Lenticulostriate Vasculopathy and Calcifications

Lenticulostriate vasculopathy (LSV) is seen on neonatal cUS scans as echogenic lines in a vertical or semi-vertical orientation within the basal ganglia. The lines follow the trajectory of the walls of medium-sized lenticulostriate vessels, which are early branches of the middle cerebral artery. One can often visualize blood flow through the vessels using Doppler ultrasound (Fig. 18.2). The hyperechoic appearance of LSV is probably due to intramural and perivascular deposits of amorphous basophilic material in the lenticulostriate vessels. The walls of the vessels are usually thickened and hypercellular but without fibrosis or hyalinization [46–51]. Mineralizing necrosis is described in some reports, but not all, and calcification may not be the only explanation for the echogenicity seen in LSV.

The occurrence of LSV seems to be increasing, with incidences of 1–5% described in older studies versus up to over 30% more recently. This is probably related to the improved quality of ultrasound scanners, enabling depiction of even normal vascular structures, higher incidence of more extreme prematurity, increased awareness, and better documentation [5, 6, 52, 53].

LSV, regardless of extent, is generally considered a benign finding in itself and can be seen on cUS scans of preterm infants as well as healthy term-born infants. A classification system for LSV was suggested by Sisman et al. in 2018 [54]. However, in their relatively small study of 40 preterm infants, the classification system was not associated with differences in outcomes at 18–36 months corrected age.

LSV that becomes apparent in preterm infants a few weeks after birth, especially when associated with SEPs, should lead to testing for postnatally acquired CMV. In addition to congenital infectious etiologies, there is some evidence for other non-infectious etiologies. LSV is seen more often in very preterm infants with a complicated neonatal course (related to bronchopulmonary dysplasia and necrotizing enterocolitis), being related to a marginally increased risk for adverse outcomes [54, 55]. Importantly, however, LSV, like small SEPs, is more common in a variety of disorders, most notably genetic syndromes, congenital viral infections, and metabolic diseases [56]. Thus detection of LSV on cUS may be helpful diagnostically in symptomatic infants.

Scattered small areas of echogenicity that are thought to be due to calcification, but not related to a vascular distribution or confined to the basal ganglia region, may be seen in the distribution of cells migrating to the cortex or demarcating abnormal cortical folding in infants with cortical dysplasia. Scattered calcifications can also be found in metabolic and genetic disorders and viral and other infections (examples in Figs. 18.5, 18.11, 18.12, and 18.13) [50, 51].

In summary, the clinical context in which LSV and/or echogenicity suggestive of calcification is observed and the timing of their appearance are very important in determining the clinical significance and appropriateness of further investigations. Of note, these abnormalities in the neonatal brain are better seen on cUS than on MRI. While MRI is not of added benefit for visualizing LSV and calcifications, it

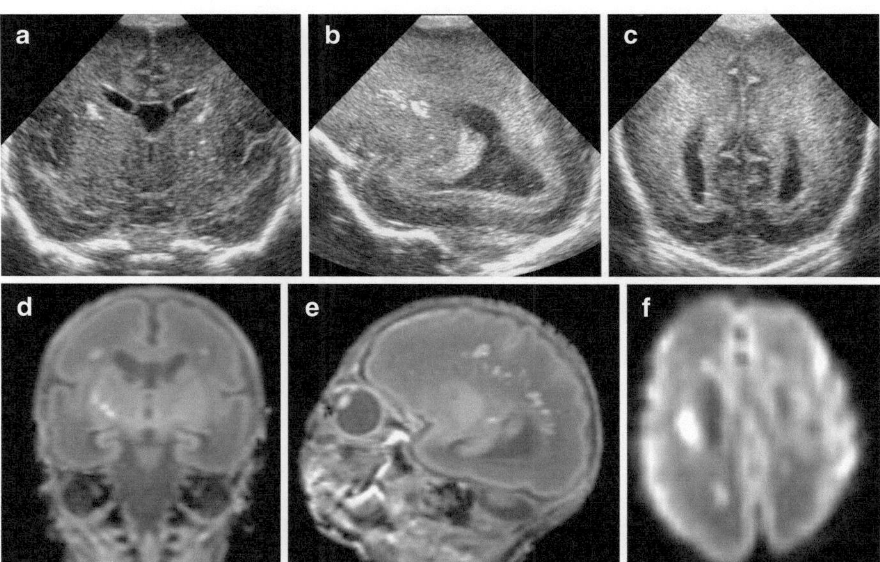

Fig. 18.12 cUS scan on the day of admission and MR images on day 11 in a severely growth restricted preterm infant (31 + 0 weeks' gestation) diagnosed with Aicardi-Goutières syndrome. (**a–c**) Coronal and parasagittal cUS scans showing extensive small irregularly shaped echogenicities in the basal ganglia and periventricular white matter; (**d**) coronal, and (**e**) sagittal T1-weighted MR image showing T1 shortening in corresponding areas; (**f**) axial diffusion-weighted image showing areas of diffusion restriction in the periventricular white matter

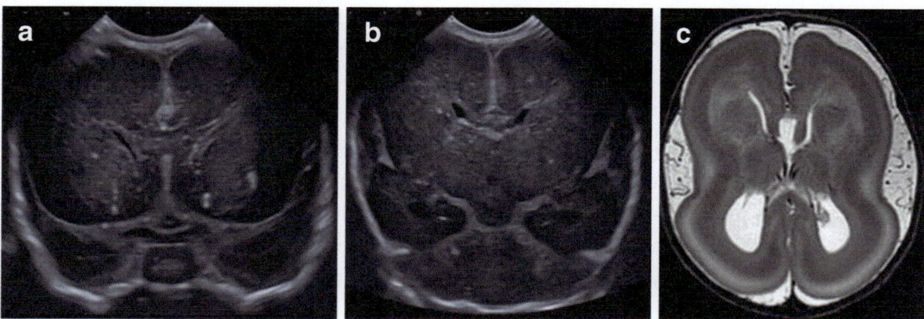

Fig. 18.13 Coronal cUS scans in a term-born infant showing linear echogenicities in the deep gray matter (**a**) and more scattered punctate echogenicities, suggestive of calcifications, in the deep gray matter, periventricular white matter, and cerebellum. There is limited cortical folding for a term-born infant and an abnormal appearance to the Sylvian fissures (**b**). (**c**) Axial MR image in the same infant showing lissencephaly

will contribute to assessing the presence and extent of associated lesions. Although computed tomography (CT) can show calcification, it is not required in addition to cUS and should be avoided in newborn infants due to the radiation exposure.

18.2.6 Associations with LSV and Echogenicities Suggestive of Calcifications Seen on cUS

(Note: the table provides examples but is not all inclusive)

Infections	Common:
	Cytomegalovirus (congenital and acquired)
	Rubella
	HIV
	Zikavirus
	Toxoplasma
	Bacterial meningitis
Metabolic disorders	Peroxisomal disorders
	Mitochondrial disorders
	Organic acidemias
	Carbohydrate glycosylation defects
	Hypoglycemia
Pregnancy related	Multiple births
	Twin-to-twin transfusion
	Non-immune fetal hydrops
Other conditions	Pre-natal drug and alcohol exposure
	Congenital cardiac disease
	Hypoxia-ischemia—late after injury in damaged tissue
	Neonatal lupus syndrome
	Diabetic fetopathy
	Chronic lung disease (bronchopulmonary dysplasia)
	Trisomy 21 and other chromosomal disorders
	Aicardi-Goutières syndrome (Fig. 18.12)
	Lissencephalies, e.g. miller-Dieker syndrome
	Tuberous sclerosis

References

1. Larcos G, Gruenewald SM, Lui K. Neonatal subependymal cysts detected by sonography: prevalence, sonographic findings, and clinical significance. AJR Am J Roentgenol. 1994;162(4):953–6.
2. Chang C-L, Chiu N-C, Ho C-S, Li S-T. Frontal horn cysts in normal neonates. Brain and Development. 2006;28:426–30.
3. Fernandez Alvarez JR, Amess PN, Gandhi RS, Rabe H. Diagnostic value of subependymal and choroid plexus cysts on neonatal cerebral ultrasound: a meta-analysis. Arch Dis Child Fetal Neonatal Ed. 2009;94(6):F443–6.
4. Cevey-Macherel M, Forcada Guex M, Bickle Graz M, Truttmann AC. Neurodevelopment outcome of newborns with cerebral subependymal pseudocysts at 18 and 46 months: a prospective study. Arch Dis Child. 2013;98(7):497–502.
5. Ballardini E, Tarocco A, Rosignoli C, Baldan A, Borgna-Pignatti C, Garani G. Universal head ultrasound screening in full-term neonates: a retrospective analysis of 6771 infants. Pediatr Neurol. 2017;71:14–7.
6. Lin YJ, Chiu NC, Chen HJ, Huang JY, Ho CS. Cranial ultrasonographic screening findings among healthy neonates and their association with neurodevelopmental outcomes. Pediatr Neonatol. 2021;62(2):158–64.
7. Carney O, Hughes E, Tusor N, Dimitrova R, Arulkumaran S, Baruteau KP, Collado AE, Cordero-Grande L, Chew A, Falconer S, Allsop JM, Rueckert D, Hajnal J, Edwards AD, Rutherford M. Incidental findings on brain MR imaging of asymptomatic term neonates in the developing human connectome project. EClinicalMedicine. 2021;38:100984.
8. Beltinger C, Saule H. Sonography of subependymal cysts in congenital rubella syndrome. Eur J Pediatr. 1988;148(3):206–7.
9. Tomà P, Magnano GM, Mezzano P, Lazzini F, Bonacci W, Serra G. Cerebral ultrasound images in prenatal cytomegalovirus infection. Neuroradiology. 1989;31:278–9.
10. Yamashita Y, Matsuishi T, Murakami Y, Shoji H, Hashimoto T, Utsunomiya H, Araki H. Neuroimaging findings (ultrasonography, CT, MRI) in 3 infants with congenital rubella syndrome. Pediatr Radiol. 1991;21:547–9.
11. de Vries LS, Gunardi H, Barth PG, Bok LA, Verboon-Maciolek MA, Groenendaal F. The spectrum of cranial ultrasound and magnetic resonance imaging abnormalities in congenital cytomegalovirus infection. Neuropediatrics. 2004;35(2):113–9.
12. Oosterom N, Nijman J, Gunkel J, Wolfs TF, Groenendaal F, Verboon-Maciolek MA, de Vries LS. Neuro-imaging findings in infants with congenital cytomegalovirus infection: relation to trimester of infection. Neonatology. 2015;107(4):289–96.
13. de Vries LS. Viral infections and the neonatal brain. Semin Pediatr Neurol. 2019;32:100769.
14. Russel IM, van Sonderen L, van Straaten HL, Barth PG. Subependymal germinolytic cysts in Zellweger syndrome. Pediatr Radiol. 1995;25(4):254–5.
15. Barkovich AJ, Peck WW. MR of Zellweger syndrome. AJNR Am J Neuroradiol. 1997;18(6):1163–70.
16. Leijser LM, de Vries LS, Rutherford MA, Manzur AY, Groenendaal F, de Koning TJ, van der Heide-Jalving M, Cowan FM. Cranial ultrasound in metabolic disorders presenting in the neonatal period: characteristic features and comparison with MR imaging. AJNR Am J Neuroradiol. 2007;28:1223–31.
17. Rohrbach M, Chitayat D, Maegawa G, Shanske S, Davidzon G, Chong K, Clarke JTR, Toi A, Tarnopolsky M, Robinson B, Blaser S. Intracerebral periventricular pseudocysts in a fetus with mitochondrial depletion syndrome: an association or coincidence. Fetal Diagn Ther. 2009;25:177–82.
18. Leshinsky-Silver E, Lev D, Malinger G, Shapira D, Cohen S, Lerman-Sagie T, Saada A. Leigh disease presenting in utero due to a novel missense mutation in the mitochondrial DNA–ND3. Mol Genet Metab. 2010;100(1):65–70.

19. Rossler L, Ludwig-Seibold C, Thiels CH, Schaper J. Aicardi-Goutières syndrome with emphasis on sonographic features in infancy. Pediatr Radiol. 2012;42:932–40.
20. Jain-Ghai S, Mishra N, Hahn C, Blaser S, Mercimek-Mahmutoglu S. Fetal onset ventriculomegaly and subependymal cysts in a pyridoxine dependent epilepsy patient. Pediatrics. 2014;133(4):e1092–6.
21. Brun N, Robitaille Y, Grignon A, Robinson BH, Mitchell GA, Lambert M. Pyruvate carboxylase deficiency: prenatal onset of ischemia-like brain lesions in two sibs with the acute neonatal form. Am J Med Genet. 1999;84(2):94–101.
22. Soares-Fernandes JP, Teixeira-Gomes R, Cruz R, Ribiero M, Magalhães, Rocha JF, Leijser LM. Neonatal pyruvate dehydrogenase deficiency due to a R302H mutation in the PDHA1 gene: MRI findings. Pediatr Radiol. 2008;38:559–62.
23. Al Rifai MT, Al Tawil KI. The neurological outcome of isolated PVL and severe IVH in preterm infants: is it fair to compare? Pediatr Neurol. 2015;53(5):427–33.
24. Riedesel EL. Neonatal cranial ultrasound: advanced techniques and image interpretation. J Pediatr Neurol. 2018;16:106–24.
25. Larroche JC. Sub-ependymal pseudo-cysts in the newborn. Biol Neonate. 1972;21(3):170–83.
26. Makhoul IR, Zmora O, Tamir A, Shahar E, Sujov P. Congenital subependymal pseudocysts: own data and meta-analysis of the literature. Isr Med Assoc J. 2001;3(3):178–83.
27. Epelman M, Daneman A, Blaser SI, Ortiz-Neira C, Konen O, Jarrín J, Navarro OM. Differential diagnosis of intracranial cystic lesions at head US: correlation with CT and MR imaging. Radiographics. 2006;26:173–96.
28. de Vries LS, Verboon-Maciolek MA, Cowan FM, Groenendaal F. The role of cranial ultrasound and magnetic resonance imaging in the diagnosis of infections of the central nervous system. Early Hum Dev. 2006;82(12):819–25.
29. Nijman J, de Vries LS, Koopman-Esseboom C, Uiterwaal CS, van Loon AM, Verboon-Maciolek MA. Postnatally acquired cytomegalovirus infection in preterm infants: a prospective study on risk factors and cranial ultrasound findings. Arch Dis Child Fetal Neonatal Ed. 2012;97(4):F259–63.
30. van Baalen A, Rohr A. From fossil to fetus: nonhemorrhagic germinal matrix echodensity caused by mineralizing vasculitis—hypothesis of fossilizing germinolysis and gliosis. J Child Neurol. 2009;24(1):36–44.
31. Dogan MS, Koc G, Doganay S, Dogan S, Özdemir A, Korkmaz L, Coskun A. Evaluation of symmetrical increased echogenicity of bilateral caudothalamic grooves detected on cranial ultrasonography by comparing with susceptibility-weighted imaging. Radiol Med. 2018;123:434–40.
32. Riebel T, Nasir R, Weber K. Choroid plexus cysts: a normal finding on ultrasound. Pediatr Radiol. 1992;22:410–2.
33. Cooper S, Bar-Yosef O, Berkenstadt M, Hoffmann C, Achiron R, Katorza E. Prenatal evaluation, imaging features, and neurodevelopmental outcome of prenatally diagnosed periventricular pseudocysts. Am J Neuroradiol. 2016;37(12):2382–8.
34. Scelsi CL, Rahim TA, Morris JA, Kramer GJ, Gilbert BC, Forseen SE. The lateral ventricles: a detailed review of anatomy, development, and anatomic variations. Am J Neuroradiol. 2020;41(4):566–72.
35. Mohammad K, Scott JN, Leijser LM, Zein H, Afifi J, Piedboeuf B, de Vries LS, van Wezel-Meijler G, Lee SK, Shah PS. Consensus approach for standardizing the screening and classification of preterm brain injury diagnosed with cranial ultrasound: a Canadian perspective. Front Pediatr. 2021;9:618236.
36. Nunes RH, Pacheco FT, da Rocha AJ. Magnetic resonance imaging of anterior temporal lobe cysts in children: discriminating special imaging features in a particular group of diseases. Neuroradiology. 2014;56:569–77.
37. Digiovanni LM, Quinlan MP, Verp MS. Choroid plexus cysts: infant and early childhood developmental outcome. Obstet Gynecol. 1997;90(2):191–4.
38. Yhoshu E, Mahajan JK, Singh UB. Choroid plexus cysts-antenatal course and postnatal outcome in a tertiary hospital in North India. Childs Nerv Syst. 2018;34(12):2449–53.

39. Naeini RM, Yoo JH, Hunter JV. Spectrum of choroid plexus lesions in children. AJR Am J Roentgenol. 2009;192(1):32–40.
40. van der Weiden S, Steggerda SJ, Te Pas AB, Vossen AC, Walther FJ, Lopriore E. Routine TORCH screening is not warranted in neonates with subependymal cysts. Early Hum Dev. 2010;86(4):203–7.
41. Unger S, Salem S, Wylie L, Shah V. Newborn frontal horn cysts: cause for concern? J Perinatol. 2011;31:98–103.
42. Wang M, Liu C, Li X, Liu H, Jin C, Tao X, Wang X, Zhao H, Cheng Y, Wu F, Zhang Y, Yang J. Isolated periventricular pseudocysts do not affect white matter microstructure development in neonatal stage: a retrospective case-control diffusion tensor imaging study. Eur J Radiol. 2019;116:152–9.
43. Chang H, Tsai CM, Hou CY, Tseng SH, Lee JC, Tsai ML. Multiple subependymal pseudocysts in neonates play a role in later attention deficit hyperactivity and autistic spectrum disorder. J Formos Med Assoc. 2019;118(3):692–9.
44. Sun C, Zhang X, Chen X, Wei X, Chen Y, Yang A, Zhu J, Wang G. Evaluation of MRI features and neurodevelopmental outcomes for prenatally diagnosed periventricular pseudocysts. Front Pediatr. 2021;9:681999.
45. Chang YL, Chang SD, Chao AS, Lien R, Cheng PJ, Chueh HY. Low rate of cerebral injury in monochorionic twins with selective intrauterine growth restriction. Twin Res Hum Genet. 2010;13(1):109–14.
46. Teele RL, Hernanz-Schulman M, Sotrel A. Echogenic vasculature in the basal ganglia of neonates: a sonographic sign of vasculopathy. Radiology. 1988;169:423–7.
47. Cabañas F, Pellicer A, Morales C, García-Alix A, Stiris TA, Quero J. New pattern of hyperechogenicity in thalamus and basal ganglia studied by color Doppler flow imaging. Pediatr Neurol. 1994;10:109–16.
48. Coley BD, Rusin JA, Bcue DR. Importance of hypoxic/ischemic conditions in the development of cerebral lenticulostriate vasculopathy. Pediatr Radiol. 2000;30:846–55.
49. El Ayoubi M, de Bethmann O, Monset-Couchard M. Lenticulostriate echogenic vessels: clinical and sonographic study of 70 neonatal cases. Pediatr Radiol. 2003;33:697–703.
50. Gonçalves FG, Caschera L, Teixeira SR, Viaene AN, Pinelli L, Mankad K, Alves CAPF, Ortiz-Gonzalez XR, Andronikou S, Vossough A. Intracranial calcifications in childhood: part 1. Pediatr Radiol. 2020a;50(10):1424–47.
51. Gonçalves FG, Caschera L, Teixeira SR, Viaene AN, Pinelli L, Mankad K, Alves CAPF, Ortiz-Gonzalez XR, Andronikou S, Vossough A. Intracranial calcifications in childhood: part 2. Pediatr Radiol. 2020b;50(10):1448–75.
52. Leijser LM, Steggerda SJ, de Bruïne FT, van Zuijlen A, van Steenis A, Walther FJ, van Wezel-Meijler G. Lenticulostriate vasculopathy in very preterm infants. Arch Dis Child Fetal Neonatal Ed. 2010;95(1):F42–6.
53. Hung YL, Shen CM, Hung KL, Hsieh WS. Lenticulostriate vasculopathy in very-low-birth-weight preterm infants: a longitudinal cohort study. Children. 2021;8(12):1166.
54. Sisman J, Chalak L, Heyne R, Pritchard M, Weakley D, Brown LS, Rosenfeld CR. Lenticulostriate vasculopathy in preterm infants: a new classification, clinical associations and neurodevelopmental outcome. J Perinatol. 2018;38:1370–8.
55. Sisman J, Leon RL, Payton BW, Brown LS, Mir IN. Placental pathology associated with lenticulostriate vasculopathy (LSV) in preterm infants. J Perinatol. 2023;43(5):568–72.
56. Cantey JB, Sisman J. Best practice guidelines: the etiology of lenticulostriate vasculopathy and the role of congenital infection. Early Hum Dev. 2015;91:427–30.